Rural Health

Edited by Umar Bacha

Published in London, United Kingdom

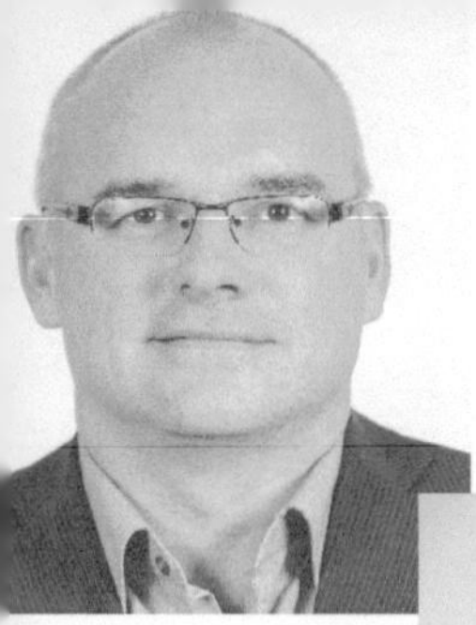
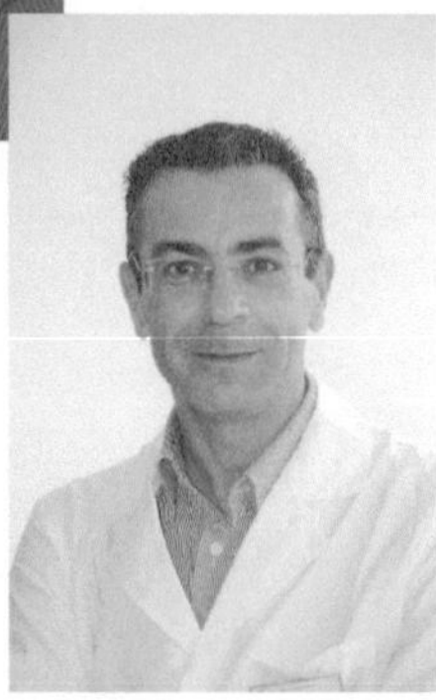
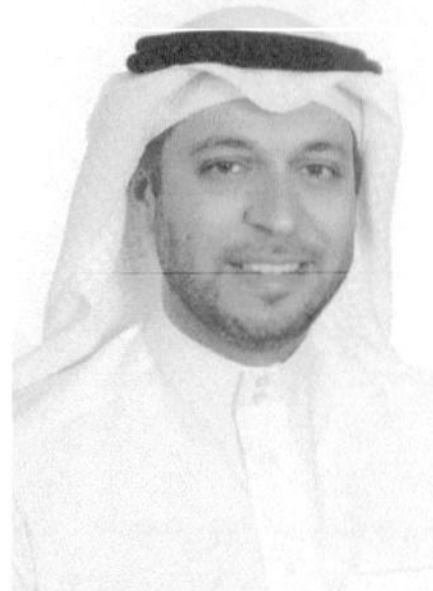
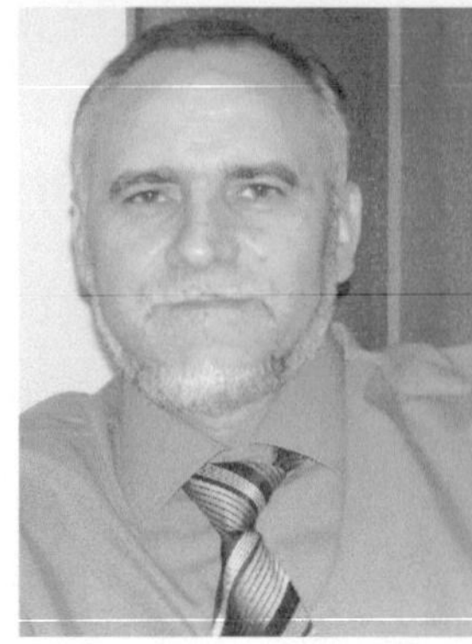
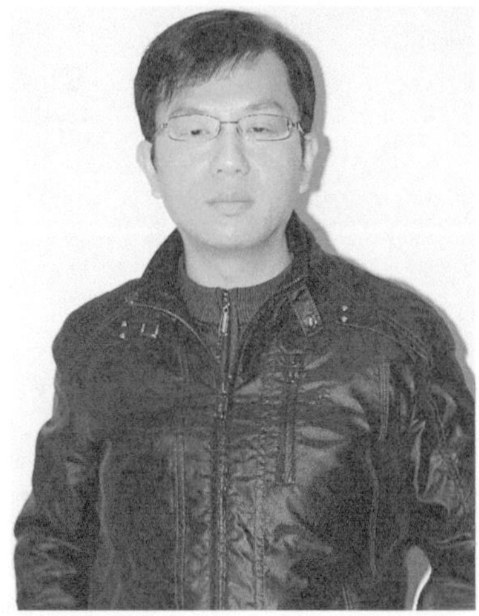
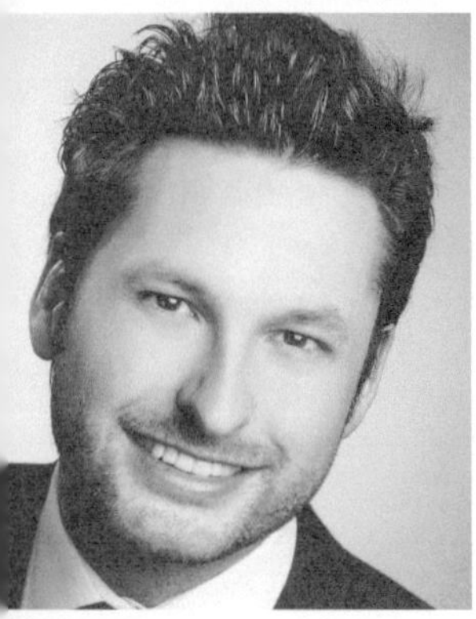
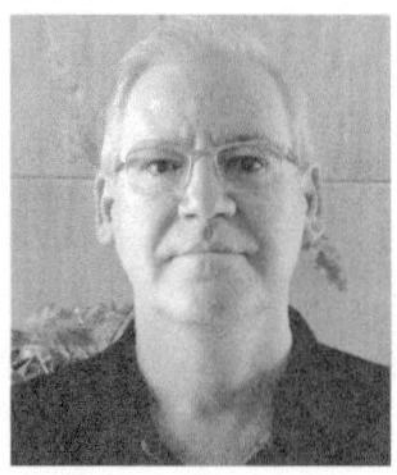

IntechOpen

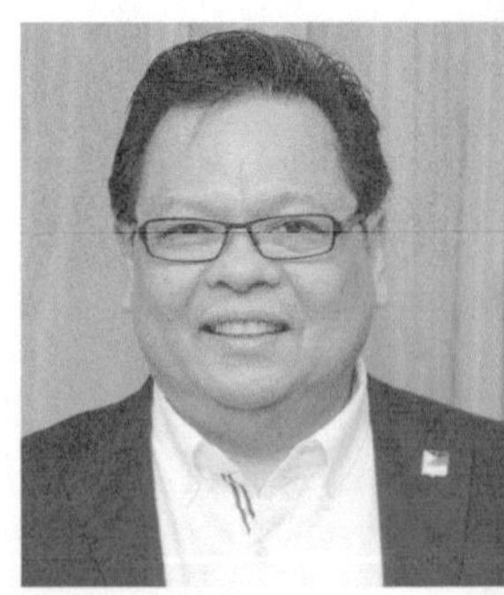
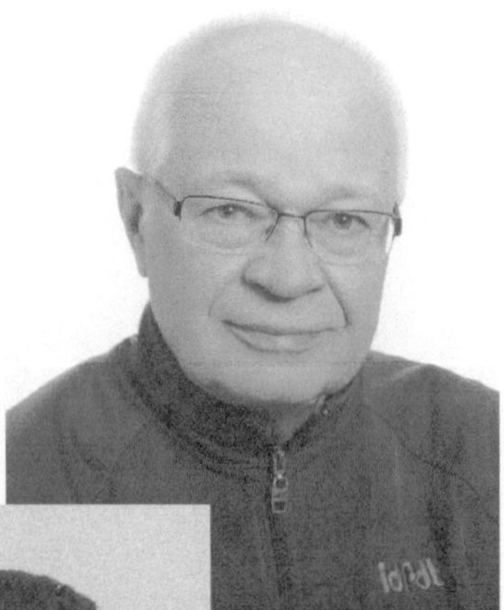
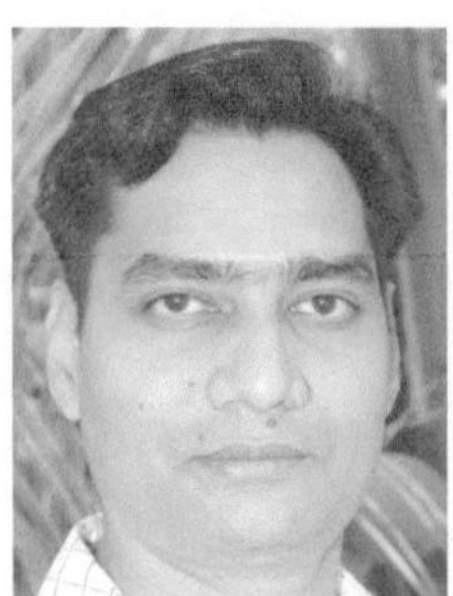
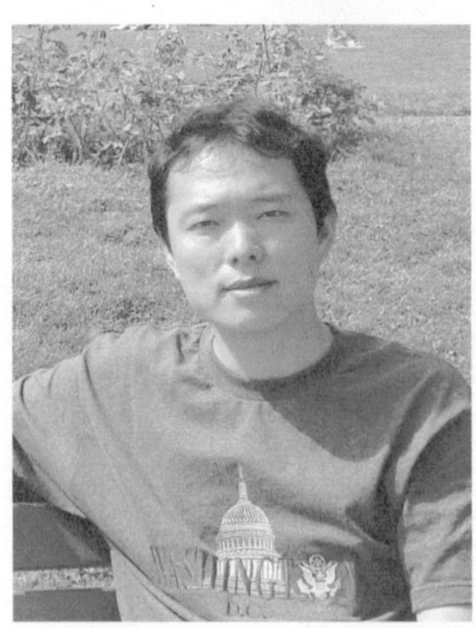
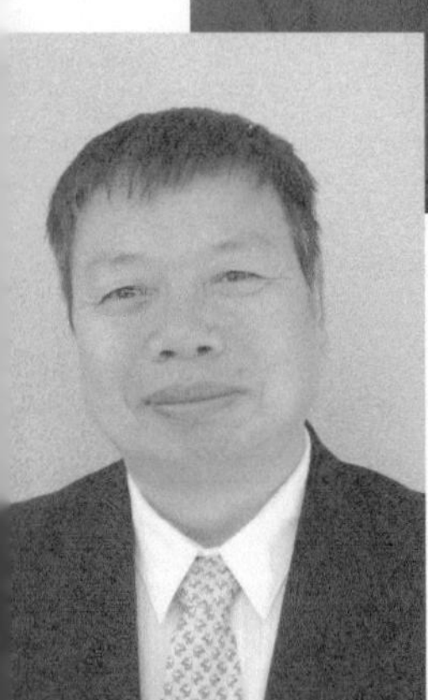
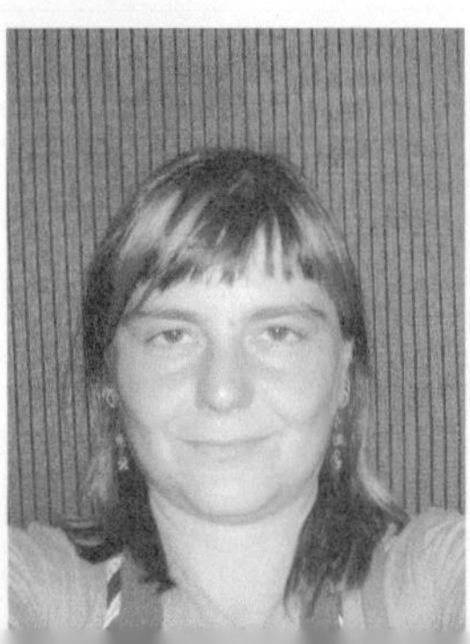

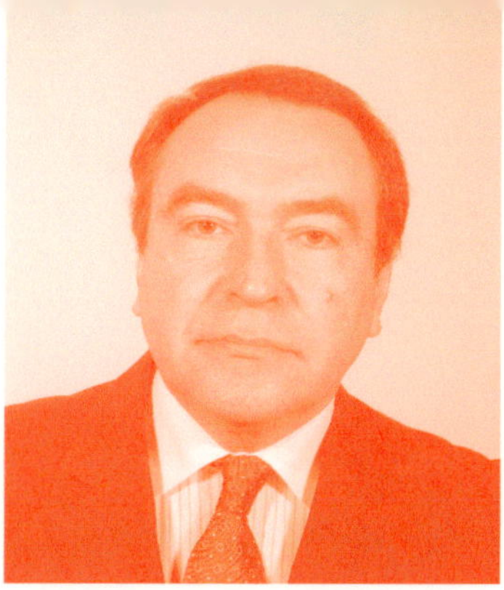
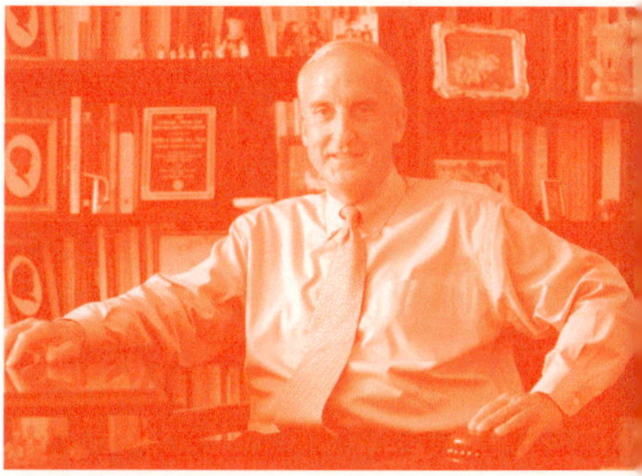
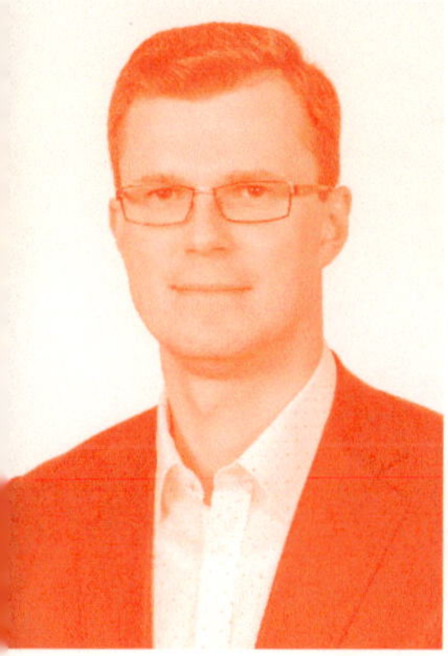
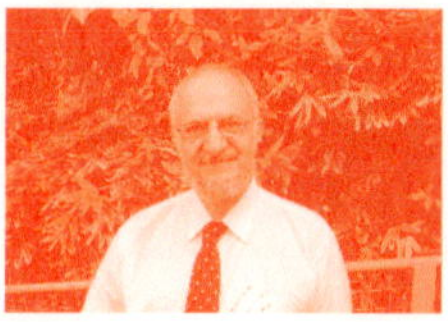
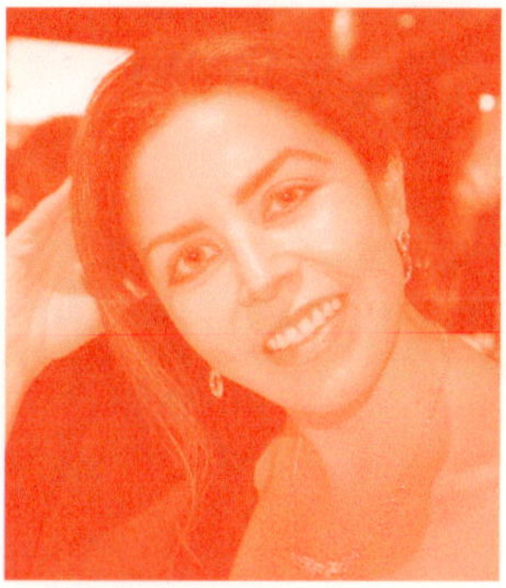

Supporting open minds since 2005

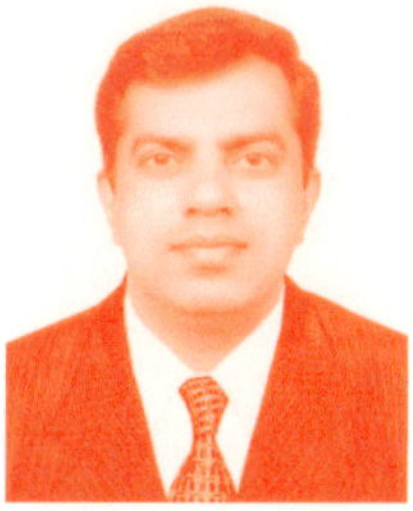
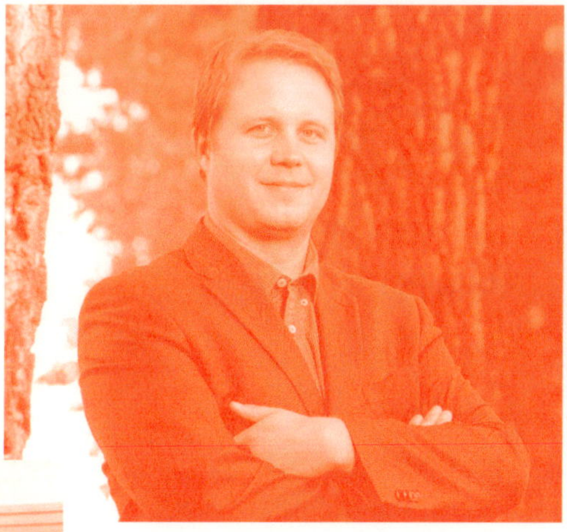
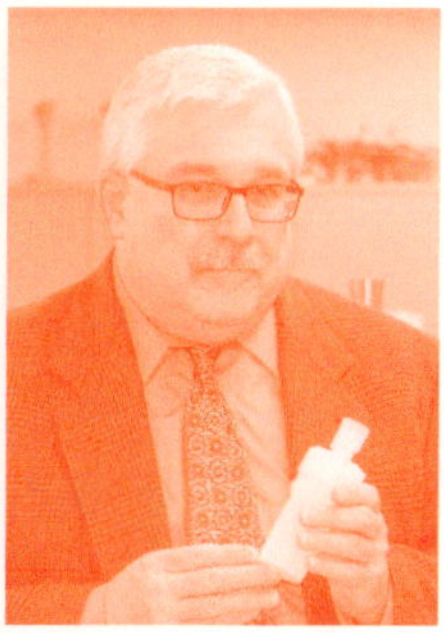
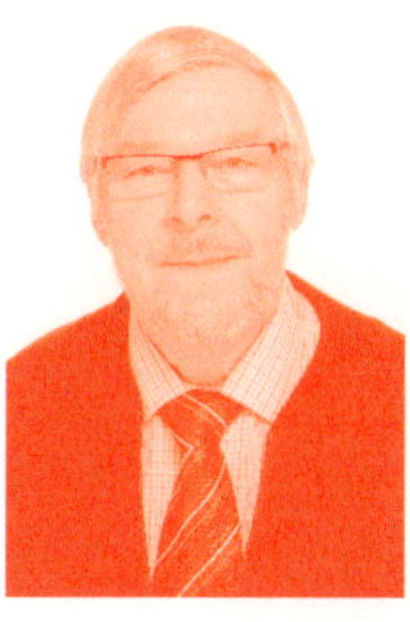
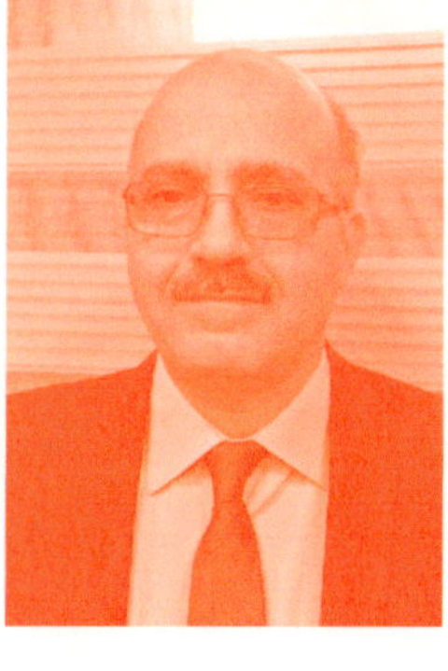
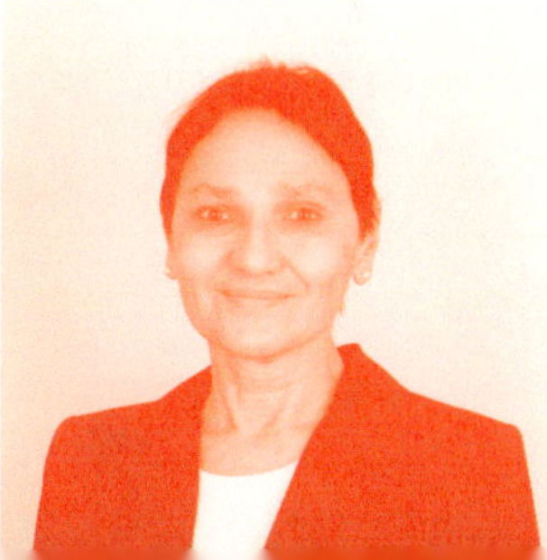
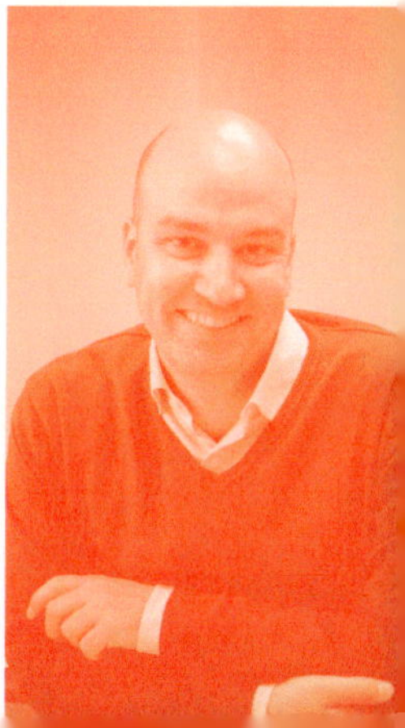

Rural Health
http://dx.doi.org/10.5772/intechopen.87618
Edited by Umar Bacha

Contributors
Tolulope Ebenezer Atalabi, Omotosho Taiye Lawal, Anastasia V. Simakova, Natalia V. Poltoraskaya, Irina B. Babkina, Tatyana N. Poltoratskaya, Alexander V. Shikhin, Tatyana M. Pankina, Juliet Waterkeyn, Nguyen Huy Nga, Victor K. Nyamandi, Ankeeta Menona Jacob, Khalid Sawalha, Nicholas Beresic, Shoaib Khan, Gilbert-Roy Kamoga, Awolu Adam, Adam Fusheini, Daniel Dramani Kipo-Sunyehzi, Paulo Henrique das Neves Martins Pires, Isaac Oluwafemi Dipeolu, Adetoro A. Adegoke, Godwin Y. Afenyadu, Fatima L. Adamu, Sally Findley, Chineme Michael Anyaeze, Knut Holtedahl, Muhammad Hanif, Siddra Khalid, Akhtar Rasul, Khalid Mahmood, Pradyot Ranjan Jena, Rajesh Kalli, Purna Chandra Tanti, Anbarasu Kannan, P.P. Mubthasima, Kaumudi Pande, Rajalakshmi Prakash

First published in London, United Kingdom, 2022 by IntechOpen
IntechOpen is the global imprint of INTECHOPEN LIMITED, registered in England and Wales, registration number: 11086078, 5 Princes Gate Court, London, SW7 2QJ, United Kingdom
Printed in Croatia

British Library Cataloguing-in-Publication Data
A catalogue record for this book is available from the British Library

Additional hard and PDF copies can be obtained from orders@intechopen.com

Rural Health
Edited by Umar Bacha
p. cm.
Print ISBN 978-1-83969-370-0
Online ISBN 978-1-83969-371-7
eBook (PDF) ISBN 978-1-83969-372-4

For EU product safety concerns:
IN TECH d.o.o., Prolaz Marije Krucifikse Kozulić 3, 51000 Rijeka, Croatia, info@intechopen.com or visit our website at intechopen.com.

Meet the editor

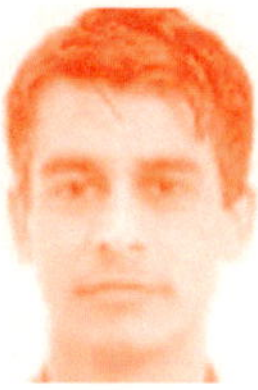

Umar Bacha is an associate professor at the School of Health Sciences, University of Management and Technology, Lahore, Pakistan. He obtained a BSc (Hons) in Biochemistry and an MPhil and Ph.D. in Nutrition. He has published several research papers and authored and co-authored several books. His fields of interest are nutrient and drug interactions with an emphasis on the effect of drugs on nutrient bioavailability and public health nutrition. Dr. Bacha has several national and international awards to his credit.

Contents

Preface

Rural health is the study of healthcare systems in rural settings. This book discusses rural healthcare systems, all-cause mortality rates in low- and middle-income countries, and the latest improvements in the field of rural health care using case studies, research, and comprehensive reviews. The book includes ten chapters that cover such topics as human resources, maternal mortality in developing countries, safety of healthcare workers, zoonotic and veterinary diseases, diagnosis and treatment of diseases like cancer, and many other subjects related to rural health care. The editor wishes to thank all contributing authors who dedicated their time and effort to make this book possible.

Dr. Umar Bacha
School of Health Sciences (SHS),
University of Management and Technology,
Lahore, Pakistan

Section 1

Health Structure and Facilities in the Rural Community

Chapter 1

Reducing Disease Burden in Rural Populations: Case Studies in Europe and Africa

Paulo Henrique das Neves Martins Pires

Abstract

In 1984, Portugal was a middle-income country, developing the primary health care system, based on family doctors, health centres and health posts, reaching almost all population, with infectious diseases as one of the main health problems. In 2006, Mozambique was a low-income country, with a national health service attaining 60% of the population (40% in rural areas), with a double burden of disease (infectious and non-communicable diseases). Working in primary health care in Europe and Africa, we compare several experiences of family medicine practice in rural populations, different in context, time, and methods: Portugal 1984–2006 and Mozambique 2007–2020, all with a strong component of community health education. Our descriptive case studies, summarise strategies, interventions, and results, reviewing reports and articles. Population' health indicators, and quality of life have improved, in different contexts with culturally tailored approaches. Participative societal diagnosis and multidisciplinary interventions are necessary to improve rural population health. Different rural populations and cultures are ready to learn and to participate in health promotion; empowering rural populations on health issues is an affordable strategy to better health indicators and services. Family Medicine is effective to extend primary health care to all rural populations, aiming universal health cover.

Keywords: empowerment, family medicine, health education, Mozambique, multidisciplinary, participative, Portugal, primary health care, rural medicine

1. Introduction

Since 1978, with the Declaration of Alma-Ata issued at the International Conference on Primary Health Care (PHC), the World Health Organisation (WHO) urgently recommended to the Ministries of Health (MH) in all countries, to organise their national health systems (NHSs) into two levels to protect and promote the health of all people of the world. First universal PHC services covering all populations in all territories, and then a secondary level of health care for more specialised interventions.

PHC was then defined as "essential health care based on practical, scientifically sound and socially acceptable methods and technology, made universally accessible to individuals and families in the community, through their full participation and at a cost that the community and country can afford to maintain at every stage of their development in the spirit of self-reliance and self-determination".

To attain the human right "health for all", WHO's member nations committed their governments to accept PHC as national policy [1].

In 2018, in commemoration of the 40th anniversary of Alma Ata, the Global Conference on Primary Health Care formulated the Astana Declaration on PHC, emphasising that "Strengthening PHC is the most inclusive, effective, and efficient approach to enhance people's physical and mental health, as well as social well-being, and that PHC is a cornerstone of a sustainable health system for universal health coverage (UHC) and the health-related Sustainable Development Goals (SDGs)" [2]. In 2019 WHO recommended that member countries' governments harness new funds to achieve these goals [3].

As a medical doctor, our professional, politic, and philosophic perspective, since university, has been to work with low-income populations in rural areas, those with less access to health care services. This has been our foundation throughout 36 years of practice, in many different contexts in Europe, Asia, and Africa. Our practice included a strong component of individual and community health education using a holistic approach to improve population health and reduce health disparities [4].

This chapter summarises different interventions attempting to reduce disease burden in rural populations, comparing methods and health results from distinct cases.

2. Portugal, 1984–2006

2.1 Background

In 1984, 10 years after the revolution (24 April 1974), the recently created NHS was expanding to cover all provinces and populations, even in isolated rural areas, developing the PHC system, based on family doctors, health centres and health posts. There were around 28000 medical doctors for 10 million inhabitants (average 1/357), but the majority was working in cities, many in private clinics, and family doctors were a small minority.

Portugal was a middle-income country, where infectious, contagious, and parasite diseases were the main problems. Coming out of 40 years of dictatorship, the rural population had no access to public health services, was poorly educated, and had little information regarding hygiene and nutrition. Since the creation of the NHS, the country has made impressive progress in health indicators, such as reducing infant mortality and increasing life expectancy by four years to 81.3 years (longer than the European Union average).

Montalegre administrative division (806 Km^2), in the northern Portuguese region of Barroso, Trás-os-Montes province, on the frontier with Galicia (Spain), was a markedly isolated area, in the mountains, with one health centre (built in 1985) and nine decentralised health posts, covering around 30.000 people living in 35 villages. Ambient temperature ranges from negative 10 °C in winter to 38 °C in the summer. There were no industries, and the main activities were subsistence agriculture, cattle breeding, and forestry. Family houses had no running water, no indoor toilet or bathrooms, no sanitation and electricity had arrived only one year before in 1983. There was no public transportation, few roads and low accessibility to products and services.

We started working in Montalegre as a private General Practice physician and received family medicine (FM) speciality in the NHS from the Portuguese MH Institute of General Practice after four years. We worked at Montalegre' s Health Centre (MHC), and at two other health posts, assisting an average of 577 families (1927 persons), in Cabril and Salto villages; emergency room coverage and wards rounds were done weekly, assisting a population around 14.000 persons at MHC.

2.2 Methods

During the last two years of our medical training at Louvain Catholic University, in Brussels, Belgium, with the help of professors in the disciplines of Tropical Medicine and Public Health, we developed a base line study about health issues in the Cabril administrative division, a mountain area in the Penêda-Gerês National Park (PGNP). The survey identified the main population health problems, high maternal mortality (with 92% of home deliveries) and child mortality (89 deaths per 1000 births), alcohol abuse (86% consumers with 31% abuse), and high prevalence of arthrosis (25%) in the older population. We then developed an implementation research project, aimed at improving these health indicators. The project included activities in health education and support, adolescent, and youth cultural and sport activities, and agricultural diversification to improve family income.

2.2.1 Health education and support

- Daily practice: preventive medicine, diagnosis, treatment, rehabilitation, health education and promotion of healthy behaviours.

- Implementation research: clinical and community health research, evaluation, and program interventions and adaptations.

- Community health education programmes: interventions with local authorities to furnish running water; promote sanitation and organize a rubbish collection and treatment system; interventions with school boards to organize health fairs and student health extension activities in the villages; weekly radio broadcast on local health issues.

- Alcohol abuse prevention programme: systematic screening and behavioural counselling; [5] focus group discussions with the families in the villages, with adolescents, pregnant women, and men, and in schools (primary and secondary) with pupils and teachers, male, and female.

2.2.2 Adolescent and youth cultural and sport activities

- A Cabril Youth Cultural and Sportive Association was established. This new institution edited and distributed a monthly newspaper in 17 villages, organized a small library and history museum, and produced a one-hour film about the history of the region.

- Local screening of films along with debates, photography expositions, football championships, and swimming competitions, were implemented in the villages.

- Theatre groups were trained and performed in primary and secondary schools.

2.2.3 Family agricultural diversification

- Honey production was a traditional activity in most families (2 kg/year/beehive). With the PGNP support, we trained farmers on modern beekeeping. Within the cooperative equipment was acquired and distributed. One year after, farmers were collecting 25 kg/year/hive).

- All families bread some cattle (average 2 cows, 3 pigs, 8 goats, 10 chicken). The local typical horse known as "*Garrano do Gerês*" had almost disappeared. We looked farther afield to find some female and male horses of this type and brought them to Cabril. We began breeding them to spend half of the year in the village (Autumn and Winter), and the other six months free in the mountain of Gerês, with weekly surveillance. Interaction with veterinary authorities led to the classification of the horses as a species threatened with extinction, and so the Ministry of Agriculture paid a yearly subsidy per animal to farmers. This increased the number of local breeders and produced a new source of family income.

- The magnificent landscape of PGNP (the only national park in Portugal), was perfect for developing tourism. The unpolluted environment boasts vast lakes of quiet clear water, a wide ecological diversity including eagles, wolfs, snakes, fish, medicinal plants, and alpine vegetation. There are several large dams providing hydroelectric power. The rich cultural heritage of the area was on display. There are ruins from the middle-ages, sacred religious monuments, and scattered granite sculptures. Story tellers, popular games, traditional theatre, and local wool and linen producers abound. Given all this it was decided to develop an eco-tourism cooperative. *TG – Trote Gerês, cooperativa de ocupação de tempos livres, crl*, built a camping-site, an hippic centre, and organised different tours, with small groups, either by foot, horse and occasionally with the support of a van. Later other lodging and restaurant services were begun employing 50 workers of local families.

2.3 Results

- Endemic outbreaks of tuberculosis, brucellosis, and rickettsia were stopped.

- Family planning and contraception was used by 90% of women between 15–50 years of age.

- By building a trusting and ongoing relationship with families, we saw all pregnant women went attending ante-natal visits and delivering at the maternity unit. All children were followed through family medicine visits, and the child mortality rate was zero in 2001 (**Table 1**). Maternal mortality (3.3 deaths/1000 livebirths) approached zero in 2006 [6].

- Alcohol abuse behaviours diminished, notably in pregnant women.

- Arthrosis was prevented with health education on weight carrying and viral infections prevention and treated with local medicinal plants.

- The emphasis on the region's typical culture and environmental quality increased population' self-esteem and attracted many visitors.

- Diversification of economic activities resulted in increased family income, along with better nutrition, housing and child and adolescent education.

Child mortality rates Year	1981	1996	2001
Deaths of children <1 year/1.000 live births	18.1	10.5	0

Table 1.
Child mortality rate in Montalegre, Portugal, 1981–2001.

2.4 Conclusion

This was our contribution to improve health indicators in the rural communities of Cabril and Salto, Montalegre. We saved lives of mothers and children. At only a small increase in health costs we significantly raised the population's quality of life.

But we observed a quick penetration of the modern consumer society model into the area. In came roads, money, television, and returning emigrants. The new NHS was tailored to the treatment of the infectious diseases burden and the hierarchy was resistant to adaptations or innovations. With this change in lifestyle, non-communicable diseases such as hypertension, obesity, diabetes, became prominent in this population, and there was not an efficient response from the NHS.

Between 2000 and 2017, the country reduced public health expenditure, thus preventing modernization of services. Private medical care was increased contributing to a loses of the public medical workforce. The NHS no longer meets the needs of a substantial part of the population [7].

3. Mozambique, 2007–2020

3.1 Background

Mozambique is a low-income country (gross domestic product - GDP per Capita 458 USD), [8] with a NHS reaching only 60% of the population (40% in rural areas), with a double burden of disease (infectious-contagious and non-communicable diseases, NCDs). In 2007, Mozambique had a high birth and fertility rate (42 births / 1000 inhabitants and 5.7 pregnancies /women, respectively), high maternal mortality rate (500 deaths / 100000 live births) and high child mortality rate (94 deaths/1000 live births), with an average life expectancy of only 51 years. The population was growing at 2.5% /year. To face these critical situations, the MH has been developing a country wide information and education campaign in health promotion [9]. They are targeting malaria prevention, maternal and child health, tuberculosis, and human immunodeficiency virus (HIV) infection.

The country has several ethnic groups, with over 10 languages and 30 dialects, though the population speaking the official language (Portuguese) is only around 30%; 50% have no school education. Most of the population live in rural areas (70%), with low access to media (10% with television, 50% with radio, 2% with internet). Running water reaches 34% of family homes, sanitation 46% and electricity 10%. Population density is low (25.3 inhabitants/Km^2), and 47% has less than 14 years of age; 56% are Christian and 18% Islamic.

In 2020 there were only around 4000 physicians for 30 million inhabitants (average 1/7500), but half of them practice in the capital (Maputo) and in the country' biggest city near-by (Matola). Many districts with more than 100000 inhabitants have only one doctor, and the PHC system depends almost exclusively on medical technicians and nurses with just three years of training.

3.2 Methods

PHC Mozambican interventions followed three phases.

The first (2006–2007), in a rural area of Matola district, in the South, was implemented as a health promotion campaign. Most of these families had little formal education, no regular employment income, and were living from subsistence agriculture and informal small business. During 2006–2007, in association with a local non-governmental association (NGO), ADEL Maputo, a local economic development association, funded by the Galician Government (Spain), we used a participatory action approach with the community to get an idea of what health issues were present. We then built, equipped, and furnished the consumables for the first Health Promotion Centre in Mozambique. It had a water reservoir, meeting room, two offices, and WC.

Then we trained a group of 50 adolescent and youth boys and girls, in basic health research. This included design and application of questionnaires, along with management of health promotion and disease prevention activities. The activities included hygiene, nutrition, food security, fruit trees culture, and sexual transmitted infections (STIs). This group implemented an information and screening campaign on the street. It included malaria, HIV, malnutrition, obesity, hypertension, diabetes, and STIs. They visited families delivering health promotion key messages and gave five fruit trees (three rich in calories, two rich in vitamins and minerals) to each of 1075 families, in the rural area of *Zona Verde* (Green Zone). At the same time a media campaign was developed and broadcast online (global), on radio, on TV, and in newspapers (regional and national). Locally they distributed banners and leaflets. Key messages were adapted to different target populations such as children, adolescents, youth, adult men and women, seniors, and elders. Local public authorities and companies (private and cooperative) were project partners. They cooperated in health key messages diffusion. The MH started a health post at the Health Promotion Centre.

The second phase from 2007–2010 was in the 16 rural districts of Zambézia province, in central Mozambique. It aimed to reduce HIV incidence through expansion of antiretroviral treatment (HAART). This intervention was an initiative of the Vanderbilt University Institute for Global Health (Nashville, USA) funded by the President's Emergency Plan for Acquired Immunodeficiency syndrome (AIDS) Relief (PEPFAR). Working initially as a family doctor consultant, later as a clinical site coordinator and district clinic advisor, and ultimately as a clinical program manager, we contributed to the design of a base line study, which surveyed the health facilities, the health professionals (HPs), and reviewed some of NHS data. Subsequently, an implementation plan was designed. It targeted primary HIV prevention, testing, patient's treatment (expanding HAART) and follow-up. It also included up-grading health facilities and laboratory support, training of HPs and research. Team building for project's field implementation was multicultural and interdisciplinary. Activities were varied:

- AIDS and HIV literature review, cultural research, summary of national official and social impact and response to HIV.
- Research and discussion on methods and strategies for health systems and program development.
- Establishing partnerships and coordinating with the MH, local administration, and international NGO's.
- Health infrastructure and laboratory planning, development, implementation, and evaluation.
- Design of teaching tools for health workers in PHC and health promotion.
- Constitution of a new local NGO (FGH, Friends in Global Health, LLC), modelling appropriate team management, evaluation tools, social interventions, partnerships, communication, information systems, and community mobilization.

- Planning, coordination, implementation and evaluation of the participatory action derived community information and operational research done in community health. We stressed use of evidence-based medicine, family epidemiology, and various types of sampling methods.

- Planning, coordination and evaluation of health and health promotion education programs, including resources preparation, identification of sources, institutional partnerships, economic management, action plans and reports, risk assessment.

- Planning and execution of training activities for HPs on HIV/AIDS/HAART/opportunistic infections (OI), principles of FM, prevention of mother to child transmission (PMTCT), volunteer counselling and testing (VCT), tuberculosis (TB) and STIs, including counselling and therapeutic adherence.

- Counselling in health care systems management and development and HAART expansion techniques was given to AIDS care in six rural Zambezian under resourced districts. This was done in partnership with MH, local administration as well as local, national, and international NGO's. The initial target population was 1250000 patients, later in 12 districts with a target population of 2350000 and most recently in 18 health centres.

The third phase (2011–2020), was in Lúrio University (UniLúrio), Nampula province in northern Mozambique. It was aimed at implementing a FM residency training program and improving health extension in peri-urban and rural populations. The Faculty of Health Sciences (FHS) is the oldest (14 years) and bigger faculty in this public university, and the board recognised the need to broadly implement the PHC system with family doctors, to change the country health paradigm towards UHC. As assistant lecturer at UniLúrio we developed several activities:

- Preparation and proposal approved for the specialisation of Mozambique general practitioners in Family and Community Medicine by Mozambican Medical College and the MH.

- Development of proposals for curriculum in Community Health and Scientific Research Methodology.

- Development of the One Student One Family Program (1-EF) for all the FHS courses (Medicine, Dentistry, Pharmacy, Nutrition, Nursing, Optometry), and organising a medical records database system. This program links every new student entering the FHS (200/year), to a family living in rural Natikiri (around the Campus). The student will visit periodically during a full term, and every term right from the first year, for health education extension and occasional referrals of acute or chronic cases to the NHS.

- Training of FHS lecturers and students in operational and implementation research methods, and bioethics.

- Health emergencies strategies (human and natural catastrophes) design and training for private initiative, students, and lecturers.

- Faculty board counselling, pedagogic assessment and development, quality assessment and development, member of evaluation boards (candidate lecturers, Nutrition, Optometry and Pharmacy degrees).

- Lecturing on Family and Community Medicine concepts to the 2nd, 4th and 5th year of Medicine students and overseeing rural medical internships (6th year). (Note that students enter the Medical degree program directly from high school).

- Planning and execution of operational and implementation research (Maternal and child health, Hansen disease, tuberculosis, cholera, HIV, mental health).

- FHS Scientific Committee work which included development and implementation of a research policy, reviewing lecturers' and students' research protocols and manuscripts.

3.3 Results

Health promotion and education of rural populations was achieved on the three phases, but at different locations and times, using different methods, producing several outputs. Below is a summary of the main results.

3.3.1 Phase 1

- 10000 persons were interviewed, screened, and given the health promotion key messages: 24% were positive for malaria, 16% had dermatologic diseases, 13% were positive for HIV, 10% had cholera, 8% TB, 8% hypertension, 7% diarrhoea, 4% STI and 4% arthrosis. Those with these issues were informed about specific prevention activities, about treatment methods, and referred to the NHS services.

- Using the local language, 2121 participants in community health extension activities, were reached in 37 interventions (27 local communities, 6 primary schools, 3 markets, 1 pre-school nursery).

- 1075 rural families received, planted, and farmed 5375 fruit trees in their courtyards, serving around 6000 people.

- The first Health Promotion Centre in Mozambique was built, equipped, and staffed with a trained team and in cooperation with MH, a new health post for disease screening and reference to NHS was launched.

3.3.2 Phase 2

Health infrastructure evaluation and development in 36 health centres and hospitals in 16 rural districts of Zambézia, providing water, power, installation of prefabricated health units and laboratory equipment [10].

The working team in the 16 districts reached 263 people, supporting their families (1315 persons), and innovating with three new positions in the NHS: social assistant, case manager, data manager.

HPs trainings on HIV, counselling, TB, PMTCT, OI reached 350 NHS workers and 210 HP students.

Patient followed with a positive HIV result increased from 9000 to 46000, and those on HAART increased from 3000 to 8000 (**Table 2**).

Testing pregnant women for HIV to prevent mother to child transmission (PMTCT) increased from 2000 to 60000 thousand, and their HIV prevalence reduced 8% (**Table 3**).

HIV	Year		Progress
Indicator	2006 (n)	2008 (n)	%
HIV+	9310	46202	496
Initiating HAART	400	2702	676
Total in HAART	2979	7722	259

n – number of participants; % - percentage.

Table 2.
High Activity Antiretroviral Treatment services expansion, in rural districts of Zambézia province, Mozambique.

PMTCT	Year		Progress
Indicator	2006 (n)	2009 (n)	%
Pregnant women tested for HIV	1995	60697	3042
Pregnant women HIV+	338	5655	1673
HIV prevalence	16.9	9.3	55

n – number of participants; % - percentage.

Table 3.
Prevention of Mother to Child Transmission of HIV services expansion, in rural districts of Zambézia province, Mozambique.

Local traditional healers were trained and engaged in research, preventive health activities, and health promotion.

Social local organizations entrepreneurship training was delivered to 75 male and female rural youth in the 16 rural districts.

3.3.3 Phase 3

Quality of students' research protocols and manuscripts improved.

Number of students completing health studies increased.

Number of student presentations of health research studies increased.

FHS scientific publications rose by 300%.

Health education teaching by students with rural families increased in number, and targeted major local health problems [11].

The implementation research on maternal and child health, Alert Community to a Prepared Hospital (ACPH) project (an international collaboration with a team from Canada), improved several indicators in Natikiri rural population (**Table 4**) [12].

The culturally adjusted and focused data collection methods used in this implementation research project, demonstrated that the ACPH project was an efficient extension tool in population health education, and in continuing education of HPs with vocational training [13].

Pregnant women attending ante-natal visits reported care improvements at the local NHS facilities (**Table 5**).

Local health facility indicators in maternal care showed a significant increase in access and quality (**Table 6**).

Family and Community Medicine training at UniLúrio in Nampula, a four-year residency program for accrediting Mozambican General Practitioners just implemented in 2021, is set to change the country' health paradigm, from hospital care in cities to PHC reaching populations all over the country.

	Adolescents			Adults		
	Oct 2017 (n = 30)	Jun 2018 (n = 140)	*p-value*	Oct 2017 (n = 61)	Jun 2018 (n = 221)	*p-value*
Knowledge (%)						
Sexual & Reproductive Health	41	56	0.135	63	76	0.0425
ACPH key messages	11	47	<0.001	50	90	≤0.001
Attitude (%)						
Contraceptives access	56	75	0.0361	63	83	<0.001

Oct – October; Jun – June; n – number of participants.

Table 4.
Adult and adolescent sexual and reproductive health and family planning knowledge, and attitude, before and after the interventions.

		2017 (n = 100)	2018 (n = 78)	2019 (n = 131)		
Question	**Response (%)**	**Baseline**	**Post 4 trainings**	**Post 8 trainings**	**Evolution (%)**	***p***
How do you evaluate your experience at ANV?	Great	5.0	39.7	42.5	+750	<0.001
	Good	69.0	56.4	48.0	−30	
	Not very satisfied	26.0	3.8	8.7	−66	
	Not satisfied	0.0	0.0	0.8	(−)	

n – number of participants; % - percentage.

Table 5.
Users' opinions about their ante-natal visits (ANVs) experience.

Indicator	2016	2019	Indicator	Number ANVs (standard deviation)	95% CI	*p*
1rst ANV	1882	2393	1rst ANV (2016–2019)	2.028 (253.7)	1624.3–2431.8	0.001
4 ANVs	405	1155	4 ANVs (2016–2019)	780 (325.7)	261.7–1298.3	0.017

ANV – Ante-natal visits; CI – Confidence interval.

Table 6.
Statistically significative improvement of antenatal visits indicators in Marrere Health Centre.

3.4 Conclusion

A variety of new PHC approaches have been implemented with good results. They need to be replicated and reinforced at all health facilities and in all communities, and in all the university health care programs.

With a population over 30 million (2019), a poorly resourced health system (low funding, few health professionals), and a double burden of diseases, [14] Mozambique, urgently needs to develop new approaches. This situation, though, has been aggravated by wars (north and centre), climate crises, and the SARS-CoV-2 pandemic. Though the country had an exceptionally low number of Covid-19 cases and deaths, access to public health services significantly decreased due to lockdowns.

Access to water and sanitation contribute to child and maternal mortality outcomes, and if the country is to seriously address the SDG of reducing child and maternal mortality, then improved water and sanitation accesses are key strategies [15].

Family planning (FP) is an efficient primary preventive intervention to reduce maternal mortality in developing countries, and this practice must be reinforced from its current low levels [16].

The MH must consolidate PHC by placing family doctors all over the country, supporting, motivating, and stabilising them and their HPs teams in rural areas [17]. A stronger commitment to PHC and FM is needed to change the actual unfavourable health paradig [18].

4. Discussion

Rural populations are the most affected by health system and other inequalities. They suffer the greatest disease burden and have the least access to health services, in both low and middle-income countries (LMIC). Following the continuing importance of PHC strategies it is necessary to strengthen the commitment to PHC and its associated services to achieve a more efficient, effective, and equitable health care system [19].

All the interventions mentioned above benefited from a community based participatory action assessment and implementation method, especially including the target populations, from needs assessment, to intervention design, implementation method, and evaluation [20].

Forms of communication, adapted to local cultural contexts and language, through media campaigns, were strong and beneficial tools in all interventions.

HP training must be a recurrent and continuous exercise of update and spur innovation, motivating them to practice continuous professional development and higher levels of workplace and career satisfaction.

In LMIC, community health workers (including traditional healers), [21] are essential and are effective groups to reach rural populations and improve their health and social stability [22, 23].

FM in PHC has shown to be an efficient strategy to improve rural population health and their quality of life [24].

The burden of NCDs is growing, and must be approached with robust research, to provide locally relevant evidence, to organise preventative activities and deliver care [25]. The new orientations for PHC set out in the 2005 Declaration of Montevideo, are a response to the challenge of burgeoning communicable and chronic NCDs, with health services that remain generally underfunded [26].

The introduction of electronic clinical files by NHSs in PHC, will better health services and patient care [27, 28].

Research is an indispensable tool to monitor epidemiologic transitions, to tailor patient centred care, and to adapt health promotion interventions [29].

Governments must integrate their health policies with broader plans for poverty reduction, economic and sustainable development, [30] as well as increase NHS funding, [31] to achieve resiliency and greater efficiency and effectiveness [32].

5. Conclusions

Improved health services are possible with well-conceived and designed programs. Community based participatory assessment of health issues is essential to attain good implementation results to improve population health.

Multidisciplinary, simple, and complex interventions are necessary to improve rural population health. Widely varied types of rural populations and cultures are all ready to learn and to participate in health promotion and management, in cooperation with their NHSs.

Empowering rural populations on health issues and with decision making is an affordable strategy to better health indicators and services.

NHSs must innovate to respond to fast changing local and global contexts, like climate emergency, migration, and pandemics. Located, stable and well-trained HP teams are important to assure efficient PHC, and all-in collaboration with local health service education organizations, community-based groups, an NGOs.

FM is an excellent tool to extend effective PHC to all rural populations, aiming at UHC.

Reducing poverty and a strong investment in infrastructures (water, sanitation, health facilities, roads, and communications) is necessary to attain UHC.

A healthy population demands a continuous investment in information and education.

Acknowledgements

We acknowledge the contributions of David Zakus and Ronald Siemens, from Canada, reviewing English editing.

This manuscript had no external funding.

Conflict of interest

The authors declare no conflict of interest.

List of abbreviations

ACPH	Alert Community to a Prepared Hospital
AIDS	Acquired immunodeficiency syndrome
FM	Family medicine
GDP	Gross domestic product
HAART	High activity antiretroviral therapy
HIV	Human immunodeficiency virus
HP	Health professional
HT	Hypertension
LMIC	Low- and middle-income countries
MH	Ministry of Health
MHC	Montalegre health centre
NCD	Non communicable disease
NGO	Non-governmental organization
NHS	National health system
OI	Opportunistic infection
PGNP	Penêda-Gerês National Park.

PHC	Primary health care
PMTCT	Prevention of mother to child HIV transmission
SDG	Sustainable development goals
STI	Sexually transmitted infection
TB	Tuberculosis
UHC	Universal health cover
UniLúrio	Lúrio University
USD	United States of America dollar.
VCT	Volunteer counselling and HIV testing
WHO	World Health Organization

Author details

Paulo Henrique das Neves Martins Pires
Faculty of Health Sciences, Lúrio University, Nampula, Mozambique

*Address all correspondence to: druidatom@gmail.com

References

[1] Rifkin SB. Alma Ata after 40 years: Primary Health Care and Health for All—from consensus to complexity. BMJ Glob Health 2018;3:e001188. doi:10.1136/bmjgh-2018-001188.

[2] Flinkenflogel M, Kiguli-Malwadde E, De Maeseneer J. From Alma Ata to Astana: Family Medicine is at the centre of the progress that has been made in developing primary health care in sub-Saharan Africa. Africa Health, January 2019. p11-14.

[3] Carter M, Emmet A. The Global Community Has Pledged to Achieve Universal Health Coverage: What's It Going To Take? Global Health Policy. September 23, 2019. DOI: 10.1377/hblog20190920.827005.

[4] Wallerstein N (2006). What is the evidence on effectiveness of empowerment to improve health? Copenhagen, WHO Regional Office for Europe (Health Evidence Network report). http://www.euro.who.int/Document/E88086.pdf.

[5] U.S. Preventive Services Task Force. Screening and Behavioral Counseling Interventions to Reduce Unhealthy Alcohol Use in Adolescents and Adults: Recommendation Statement. American Family Physician June 15, 2019. Volume 99, Number 12. www.aafp.org/afp.

[6] https://www.pordata.pt/DB/Municipios/Ambiente+de+Consulta/Tabela. Accessed 13.01.2021.

[7] The Lancet. National health care in Portugal: a new opportunity. www.thelancet.com. Vol 394 October 12, 2019.

[8] INE. Resultados definitivos do Censo 2017 IV Recenseamento Geral da População e Habitação. Instituto Nacional de Estatística. República de Moçambique. Maputo. 2019. www.ine.gov.mz.

[9] Abdula N. Estratégia Nacional de Promoção de Saúde 2015-2019 [2024]. Direcção Nacional de Saúde Pública. Ministério de Saúde. República de Moçambique. Maputo. 2015.

[10] Moon T, Burlison J, Pires P, et al. Lessons learned in the implementation of an HIV/AIDS follow-up and treatment program in rural Mozambique. Retrovirology: Research and Treatment 2010, 3: 1-14.

[11] Pires P, Duran S, Siemens R. Community-Based Health Sciences Learning: A Curriculum Assessment and the Development of Family and Community Health Program. Basic Research Journal of Medicine and Clinical Sciences. ISSN 2315-6864 Vol 4 (5) pp 140-145. May 2015. http://www.basicresearchjournals.org.

[12] Pires P, Siemens R, Mupueleque M. Improving sexual and reproductive health and practice in Mozambican families with media campaign and volunteer Family Health Champions. Fam Med Com Health. 2019; 7:e000089. Doi: 10.1136/fmch-2018-000089.

[13] Pires P. Implementation research methods: an extension tool in health education and information. International Journal of Family & Community Medicine, Volume 4 Issue 2. MedCrave. 2020. https://medcraveonline.com/IJFCM/IJFCM-04-00183.pdf.

[14] Ciccaci F, Orlando S, Majid N, et al. Epidemiological transition and double burden of diseases in low-income countries: the case of Mozambique. Pan African Medical Journal. 2020;37(49). 10.11604/pamj.2020.37.49.23310. Available on-line at: https://www.panafrican-med-journal.com//content/article/37/49/full

[15] Cheng J, Schuster-Wallace C, Watt S, et al. An ecological quantification of the

relationships between water, sanitation and infant, child, and maternal mortality. Environmental Health 2012, 11:4 doi:10.1186/1476-069X-11-4.

[16] Ahmed S, Li Q, Liu L, et al. Maternal deaths averted by contraceptive use: an analysis of 172 countries. The Lancet. 2012;380;111-125.

[17] WHO. Increasing access to health workers in remote and rural areas through improved retention: global policy recommendations. World Health Organization 2010. ISBN 978 92 4 156401 4 (NLM classification: WA 390).

[18] WHO. The world health report 2008: primary health care now more than ever. World Health Organization. 2008. ISBN 978 92 4 156373 4 (NLM classification: W 84.6), ISSN 1020-3311.

[19] OECD (2020), Realising the Potential of Primary Health Care, OECD Health Policy Studies, OECD Publishing, Paris, https://doi.org/10.1787/a92adee4-en.

[20] WHO. Universal health coverage, Primary health care towards universal health coverage. Executive Board, 144th Session, 13 December 2018. Provisional agenda item 5.5. World Health Organization.

[21] Zhang K, Sharan A, Espinosa S, et al. The Path Toward Integration of Traditional and Complementary Medicine into Health Systems Globally: The World Health Organization Report on the Implementation of the 2014-2023 Strategy. The Journal of Alternative and Complementary Medicine Volume 25, Number 9, 2019, pp. 869-871. DOI: 10.1089/acm.2019.29077.jjw.

[22] Mash B, Ray S, Essuman A, et al. Community-orientated primary care: a scoping review of different models, and their effectiveness and feasibility in sub-Saharan Africa. BMJ Global Health 2019;4:e001489. doi:10.1136/bmjgh-2019-001489.

[23] McPake B, Edoka I, Witter S, et al. Cost–effectiveness of community-based practitioner programmes in Ethiopia, Indonesia and Kenya. Bull World Health Organ 2015; 93:631-639A. DOI: http://dx.doi.org/10.2471/BLT.14.144899.

[24] Mash R, Pressentin K. Strengthening the district Health system through Family physicians. SAHR. 2018.

[25] Cowan E, D'Ambruoso L, Merwe M, et al. Understanding non-communicable Diseases: combining Health surveillance with local knowledge to improve rural primary health care in South Africa. Global Health Action. 2021 Vol 14, 1852781. https://doi.org/10.1080/16549716.2020.1852781.

[26] Martin C. Chronic disease and illness care. Canadian Family Physician. Le Médecin de famille canadien. Vol 53: December, décembre 2007.

[27] Processo clínico eletrónico melhora cuidados de saúde. Journal of General Internal Medicine. 2012-10-15.

[28] American Board of Family Medicine. ABFM to simplify MOC for family physicians and make it more meaningful: a family medicine registry. Ann Fam Med 2015; 13:288-290. DOI: 10.1370/afm.1793.

[29] Hickner J, Kuzel A, Weidner A. Building research capacity in Departments of family medicine: Pearls from NAPCRG 2013. Association of Departments of Family Medicine. Annals of Family Medicine vol. 13, no. 2, March/April 2015. www.annfammed.org.

[30] Binagwaho A, Ghebreyesus T. Primary healthcare is cornerstone of universal Health coverage. BMJ 2019; 365:l2391. DOI: 10.1136/bmj.l2391.

[31] WHO. Primary Health care: transforming vision into action. Operational framework, Draft for consultation. Technical series on primary Health care. World Health Organisation. UNICEF. 2019.

[32] Loewenson R, Accoe K, Bajpai N, et al. Reclaiming comprehensive public Health. BMJ Global Health 2020; 5:e003886. DOI:10.1136/bmjgh-2020-003886.

Section 2

Rural Health Care System

Chapter 2

Healthcare Delivery Systems in Rural Areas

Ankeeta Menona Jacob

Abstract

Health care is a fundamental right of every human being. About half of the world's population (An estimated 3.4 billion of the world's 7.6 billion in 2018) lived in rural areas. Individuals in rural areas often have poor access to healthcare because of poor accessibility and availability of standard healthcare systems and socio-cultural factors affecting their perception of health compared to the urban population. Though there is a projected decrease in the absolute percentage of the world's population dwelling in rural areas by 2050, there is also a projected increase projected increase needing of prioritizing rural health. This chapter shall discusses the critical factors that disadvantage the rural population. It also considers the methods used to work out rural healthcare delivery strategies to decrease this disparity in rural areas' health care facilities.

Keywords: Rural Health services, Telemedicine, Health services accessibility, Telemedicine, Health Policy

1. Introduction

Healthcare is a fundamental right of every human being and everyone's responsibility [1]. When healthcare is viewed as a right and a responsibility, the state's active role in maintaining its people's health becomes even more pro-active more pro-active. This remedies the often-neglected individual's responsibility toward his/her health. There has always been an inverse distribution of healthcare services in rural when compared to the urban population, which is often referred to as the inverse care law or Pareto's Law. Pareto's law of distribution applied to healthcare (according to the British General practitioner Julian Hart in 1971) hypothesized that those in the greatest need of medical services in healthcare get the lowest quality possible healthcare and at the very end [2].

The term rural population also differs from country to country and is defined by the country's statistical office. In 2019, the world bank estimated that about 3,397,467,990 individuals were residing in rural areas globally. However, the global increase in rural population has been less than 1% per annum [3]. Even though these population growth rates in rural areas are minuscule there is also a projected increase in population. The existing deficiencies in the healthcare delivery system rural areas will only compound the problems with further urbanization and the healthcare policies favoring healthcare privatization [4]. There is also a growing need to create rural communities which are healthy and at par with healthcare facilities in urban areas [5]. Therefore, prioritizing rural health is imperative and will be a dire necessity for the future.

2. Definitions in rural healthcare

Rural healthcare delivery systems are often deficient in human resource, infrastructure structure, equipment, and financial support. These are essential to provide quality clinical and community healthcare services to the population they cater to. Some countries define healthcare services provision in areas (or communities) that are at a distance of more than 80 km or more than one hour by road from a designated healthcare facility (providing round the clock anesthesia, surgical and obstetrical facilities) [5]. This phenomenon, however, is relative to urban healthcare delivery systems and not an absolute absence of healthcare facilities. The services providers in rural areas are mainly the state or the government. The rest of the health care providers in rural regions are primarily indigenous systems of medicine with or without formal training in healthcare provision.

Remote healthcare is a term often used interchangeably with rural healthcare. Remote healthcare refers to hard to reach areas geographically. This happens mainly in the rural areas where access via roads are challenging [5, 6]. These areas may benefit from a remote health monitoring system, especially for health conditions and diseases that need long-term healthcare. These regions, however, would be significantly helped by the use of Telemedicine, given information and communication technology widely available. Whenever access to healthcare for an emergency or serious condition is required, these remote areas would need referral-service access to a secondary or a tertiary healthcare facility.

Rural Healthcare access is the ability of rural communities (or individuals residing in such communities) who can be promptly approached for health promotive, preventive, curative, and rehabilitative services. This works on the tenets of availability, utility, acceptability, feasibility, and equitability [7].

Barriers to healthcare access are systematic hindrances that may interfere with access to healthcare systems. In rural health systems, they could be broadly classified as structural (Infrastructure, human resources and time-related inadequacies), financial (leading to catastrophic expenditures, unaffordability of medical aid, or lack of completeness in treatment due to inability of money) or personal or socio-cultural (Physical and/or physiological hindrances, socio-cultural inappropriateness) [8].

Social Acceptability of rural health services may be defined as the individual's subjective-attitudinal perception of health care service provision and providers [9]. Acceptability may also refer to the pertinent interaction and client satisfaction accompanying service provision in the socio-cultural context of the rural areas [10].

3. History of rural healthcare delivery systems

China: An excellent example of a rural healthcare delivery system was the "Barefoot doctors" of China. In 1965 Urban doctors trained young farmers in Shanghai's Chiang Chen Province in primary medical care. These later formed the backbone of China's medical aid services [11, 12]. After a training period of three to six months and regular skill up-gradation with in-service and apprenticeship programs, these part-time healthcare providers. The healthcare provision in these areas enjoyed the local Chinese population's support [12]. They were trained in preventive, promotive, and rehabilitative healthcare provision in traditional Chinese and Modern (or Western) Medicine, alongside providing medical care. These part-time healthcare providers, also developed a robust system for referral for complex medical and surgical cases to a secondary or tertiary healthcare facility [4]. The financial support for such healthcare providers was both from a collective and mutual aid basis. However, in 1978 major health reforms in China heralded a new breed of barefoot doctors to medically more qualified "Village health Doctors" and medically lesser qualified "rural health workers" (through an annual assessment) that led to the downfall of this system [13].

The financial moratorium also changed from a collective and mutual aid basis (through a rural cooperative medical system) to a paid service model. The new system in China rolled back many positive health reforms. These reforms included reduced mortality, improved life expectancy for almost three decades and most importantly widening the already existing urban and rural health disparity [14].

India: The concept of Community Health Worker (C.H.W.) was introduced under the "National Village Health Guide Scheme" much before the idea of primary Healthcare (through the Alma Ata declaration at Kazakhstan in 1978) was proposed [15]. However, lack of affiliation to a formal health system, poorly defined job responsibilities, and poor financial remuneration plagued the Village Health Guide scheme's success.

In India, maternal and child health, especially midwifery and childbirth assistance, was mainly through the "Traditional Dai" system. However, lack of formal training in midwifery and safe delivery practices led to significant mortality and morbidity among mothers and infants. Training of these traditional birth attendants in 2006 under the National Rural Health Mission (NRHM) was an essential step toward providing trained birth assistance and improving mothers and newborn health in rural areas.

The paradigm shift in India's healthcare provision was through the National Rural Health Mission effort in health activism through ASHA (Accredited Social Health Activist). Through local community participation, an ASHA worker proficient in various aspects of preventive, promotive, rehabilitative services largely concentrated in maternal and child health through local community participation. The ASHA worker also collaborates with local rural bodies to improve health, sanitation, and nutrition in India's rural communities, a bottom-up approach [16].

The healthcare system in India had stressed the need for primary healthcare right from the pre-independence era (The Joseph Bhore Committee report in 1946) [17]. The Health Survey and Development Committee report (or the Bhore Committee Report) laid down the blueprint for a three-tier system to deliver healthcare at centers in India before the first national health policy, in the year 1983. The unique nature of the Indian healthcare sector is the blend of traditional(commonly called the AYUSH system- made up of Ayurveda, Yoga, Unani, Siddha and Homeopathy medicine) and allopathic medicine that is made available through a myriad of public and private healthcare providers. However, these healthcare services are also negatively skewed toward the rural areas where more than 60% of the population resides.

The three-tier healthcare system is divided into the primary or first point of contact of healthcare through the sub-centers that cater to a population of 3000 to 5000 [17]. The sub-centers are then linked to the Primary Health Centers (P.H.Cs.) established in the rural and urban areas for a population of 30,000 in plains and 20,000 in hilly and tribal areas. The first point of referral for the Primary health centers in the Community Health Centers (C.H.C.) is set up for every 1,20,000 population in plain areas. Every 80,000 people in hilly, tribal areas form the second tier of the public health system in India. The third tier of healthcare providing tertiary healthcare is the First Referral Units (F.R.U.)s that are set up at district or sub-district levels with round- the-clock services for healthcare. These public healthcare centers were plagued with human resource and infrastructural deficiencies. They suffered a vital mechanism for referral of patients and follow-up from higher level healthcare centers, with less than 11.5% seeking healthcare at these centers [18]. However, the private healthcare sector and the non-governmental healthcare agencies also contribute to addressing the population's healthcare needs. Because of financial and other infrastructural strengths, these healthcare facilities are often beyond the reach of many, especially in rural areas [18]. Under the country's National Health Mission (N.H.M.), through the National Health Policy of 2017, recommended the establishment of "Health and Wellness Centers (H.W.C.)" for delivery of Comprehensive Primary Healthcare (CPHC) by up-gradation of sub-centers and Primary Health Centers as shown in **Figure 1**. The deficiencies seen in the implementation of rural healthcare seen earlier would now be overcome by improved spending to up to 70% of the budgetary allocation, institutional and governmental mechanisms under the flagship of National Health Mission (N.H.M.) for Primary Health care for Universal Health Coverage (UHC) in India and the Pradhan Mantri Jan Arogya Yojana (PMJAY).

Australia: The Australian Whitlam Labour government in 1972 pioneered setting up policies for the rural and remote regions of Australia, especially those residing in Australia's suburban areas. The Hawke Labour government of 1982 renewed its commitment to healthcare services' access and equity in Australia's remote and rural areas. The national conference at Toowoomba to design and set up a policy of initiatives for rural health in the late 1980's paved the way for the National Rural Health Strategy of 1994 that the Australian Health Ministers Council promulgated.

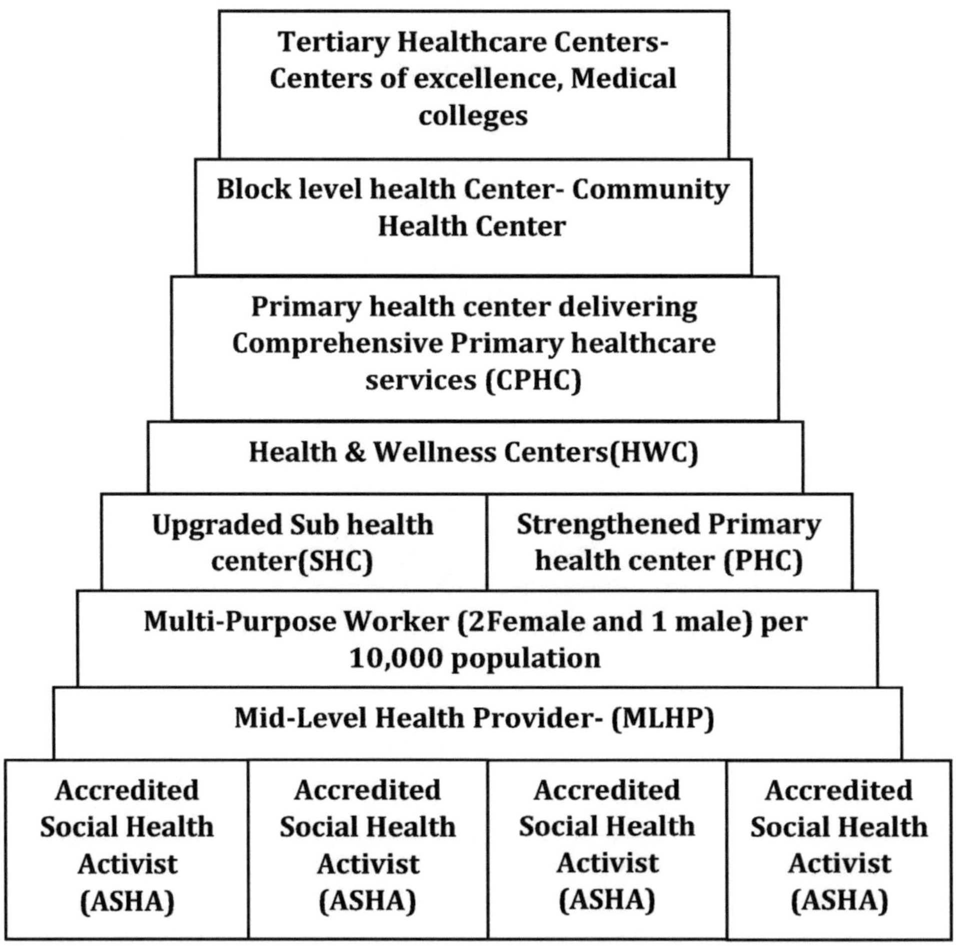

Figure 1.
Re-organization of public healthcare facilities for Rural India under the Ayushman Bharath scheme in India [18].

The National Rural Health Strategy through the RHSET programme, the Rural Incentives Program and the collective efforts of the doctors, nurses, Allied health professionals' associations worked toward healthcare service delivery in the remote and rural areas of Australia along with a Non-governmental rural health body called the National Rural Health Alliance. Although these efforts were primarily focused on incentivizing doctors and other paramedical staff of rural and remote Australia, it was ineffective in satisfying the rural health concept. This was because of issues of financial, infrastructural resource allocation to this programme, as indicated by the performance indicators measuring the remote and rural Australians' health.

The Australian rural and remote health program underwent a radical change through a dedicated policy framework improvement keeping in mind the provision of health services in these areas by 2008 and Healthy Horizons. This programme currently supports the implementation of local programs that are culturally sensitive, practical forging partnerships in the community and the health care providers by equipping the physical and social capabilities of rural and remote health care service centers in Australia [5].

United States of America -through rural public health began to rise in the early 1700s, the focus was more on improving and maintaining water supplies and sanitary conditions. However, in the late 1800s, with the spread of diseases from urban to rural communities, the focus shifted to improving rural health facilities from 1908 to the end of World War II. The Hill-Burton Act of 1945 promoted healthcare delivery access in rural areas via rural community hospitals [19].

Mexico: The social service year reform of 1930 was sponsored by President Lazaro Cardenas, where medical students had to compulsorily put in 5 months of rural healthcare service as part of their graduation. This helped bridge the health-related gaps in rural areas. Though there was a significant improvement in rural health, a lack of cultural impressionability caused setbacks in the desired outcome as anticipated by the medical graduates. Influenced by the Alma Ata declaration of 1978, the Coplamar system, a Social Protection of Marginal Groups program, was launched, wherein community-based health practitioners were trained in maternal and child health by ensuring community participation in rural communities. However, within years of introduction, the scheme suffered significant losses in funding and the scheme lost its popularity. The Coplamar system was later re-christened as the Opportunities program, a conditional cash-based transfer system that continues to function in rural Mexico [20].

4. Definition of rural health and its impact on health-seeking behavior

The World Health Organization (WHO) defines health as "The state of complete physical, mental and social wellbeing and not merely the absence of disease or infirmity". Perception of health was considered "working hard, staying busy, exercising, drinking water and eating well". Being healthy often referred to a more subjective consciousness of self-dependence to carry out their daily living activities in rural areas. A relative inability to carry out Daily activities to maintain a household or to perform farm-related chores was considered ill health. This perception of subjective health and wellbeing is particularly true in rural elderly. Physical, mental, social, and spiritual wellbeing are knitted into a mosaic of the everyday life fabric of rural elderly [21]. There is a distrust, especially in seeking professional help for mental health-related issues. The presence of indigenous systems of healthcare usually handles the burden of preventive and promotive health services. However, they are generally not trained or qualified in managing emergency medical conditions and have an inadequate system for referral for these conditions.

The intuitive feeling of health compounded with a low level of trust in the medical healthcare system, decreased demand for services for the "non-urgent" health issues" by healthcare providers, long waiting periods at hospitals for health-related issues. These factors often translate to neglect and apathy toward health-seeking at in the health care institutes in rural areas [21]. This perception of health and disease in rural residents goes a long way in planning healthcare service provision in rural areas [21].

5. Situational analysis of rural healthcare delivery system

Disparities exist among urban and rural healthcare delivery systems, but within the healthcare systems, there exist socio-cultural and ethnic differences in the accessibility and utilization of healthcare facilities [22]. The situational analysis will focus on aspects of any healthcare system, i.e., accessibility, utilization, acceptability, feasibility, and equity.

5.1 Differences in urban and rural healthcare service delivery systems

5.1.1 Accessibility

Healthcare services in rural areas are less accessible than the urban areas, which could be attributed to the topographical differences [5, 23]. Studies from the Indian subcontinent show that the bed population ratio, percentage of trained medical practitioners, and healthcare provision infrastructure are substantially lesser in rural areas compared to urban areas [4]. Even with a sharp increase in the need for emergency services for rural residents when compared to the incremental rise among urban residents in need of emergency services [24], more trained emergency physicians were present in urban areas than rural areas [25]. The number of healthcare professionals and availability of medical services in remote areas is sparse [5]. The problems with transport facilities and communication technologies further compound the problem of poor healthcare accessibility [23].

5.1.2 Utilization

The factors that enabled healthcare service utilization in Africa's urban areas were motivational benefits, the individuals' current health status, and services availability. However, in rural areas, geographical adjacency, free or low-cost healthcare availability, health insurance, ethnicity, and and family income, influence the rural residents' health services utilization [26]. In general, the individuals would preferred to be treated by healthcare personnel of the local areas, though often under-staffed or resource-constrained [23]. The underutilization has also been attributed to the lack of quality-assured healthcare services sensitive to people's health needs in rural areas [27].

5.1.3 Acceptability

The concept of acceptability has frequently been intermingled with availability and affordability of healthcare service provision and patient satisfaction [10]. The concept of trust in the healthcare provider, endorsement of the provider by leaders in the rural community in addition to early community interaction and home visits were found to improve the acceptability of maternal and child healthcare services in rural Uganda [28]. In rural northeast India, facilities for safe and sound quality healthcare services were linked to healthcare service acceptability [29].

5.1.4 Feasibility

The availability of healthcare-related services was substantially lesser in institutes providing rural healthcare vis a vis with their urban counterparts [30].

5.1.5 Equity

Equity in healthcare within rural areas also play an essential role in the rural healthcare delivery system. In the Republic of Suriname, a study conducted showed that equitable resource distribution for primary healthcare services was comparable in rural and urban areas. However, factors like perceived need, female gender, and socioeconomic status contributed to inequity for services related to chronic healthcare-related issues within the Republic of Suriname's rural areas [31].

Provision and upgrading healthcare-related insurance schemes and policies positively contributed to reducing the inequitable distribution of healthcare services [31]. The Development of tailor-made healthcare services addressing these principles to provide timely, socio-culturally appropriate, economically sustainable and equitable services in rural areas is necessary [5, 32].

6. Challenges in healthcare delivery in rural areas

The healthcare facilities in rural and remote areas are often deficient in core or essential health services, especially for support and local outpatient basis treatment [33]. The problem of shortages in trained global healthcare force and support, provision of geriatric and mental health services, infrastructure for timely healthcare services have affected rural healthcare services more than urban services [5]. The lack of healthcare insurance and the treatment costs incurred compounded with the insufficient healthcare expenditure of Gross National Product (G.N.P.) on health has worsened this situation [34]. The rural population of elderly, sick, uninsured and suffering from chronic diseases is significantly higher than its urban counterpart, which need to be addressed [33].

7. Ideal system of rural health service delivery

Planning rural healthcare services need an optimum mix of primary and secondary healthcare services at the community and individual levels. An ideal system delivering rural healthcare services should focus on "core healthcare services" or basic health-related amenities for maternal, child health, oral health. This must also include primary health care providers and emergency services for stabilizing patients needing urgent medical care with a timely referral system that provides a continuum of care [35]. The health systems should be locally sourced through community-based organizations, depending on the rural community's health care needs through a formal inquiry vide community- healthcare- needs assessment [35]. The aim of delivering healthcare in rural areas should not be limited only to improve the quantum of services provided but also the quality of healthcare services [35]. The Institutes of Medicine (I.O.M.) quality in healthcare can be approached through an integrated prioritized public health intervention at individual, family, community levels [29]. There should be provision for a support system for the healthcare service delivery personnel and the communities they serve through appropriate education, financial incentives, human resource, and infrastructural capacity. The feasibility and acceptability of Information and

Communication Technology (I.C.T.), especially for diagnostic emergencies like Acute abdomen, Myocardial infarction, Stroke etc., should be explored, especially in remote areas [34]. These systems of I.C.T., if feasible and planned correctly, can be used for monitoring of chronic that arise in Non-communicable and communicable diseases [34]. Leveraging the concept of a "healthy village" like the RURBAN initiative in India needs to be looked at while planning services in these areas [27].

A health care team providing these services, which are community-based with sustainable financial sourcing, can ensure healthcare facilities from seemingly simple medical issues to complex health conditions needing sophisticated tertiary care health system interventions, need to be planned too. The rural health care services need to be backed up by community participation with leaders and members of both health and non-health-based organizations in the rural community. The above system would also need to be socio-culturally sensitive and appropriate, catering to the rural community's health needs. This healthcare provision will depend on the healthcare funding through the nation's allocation of funds for health for rural and urban areas [28, 29].

8. Devising a rural healthcare delivery system

As emphasized by the Alma Ata declaration of 1978 in Kazakhstan, any healthcare system's precept should be based on primary healthcare [36]. Scarce resources are allocated in terms of human resources, infrastructure, and money for rural healthcare delivery, equitable healthcare provision can be made possible only by improving accessibility and acceptability of healthcare services among rural communities [18]. Sustainable healthcare delivery in rural areas can be possible only if the focus is shifted from providing healthcare service to providing a continuum of care in rural areas [6].

The Continuum healthcare delivery should be planned through a three-tier system of primary, secondary, and tertiary healthcare. This can be coordinated through collaboration and socially accountable healthcare institutes in these areas. In a consultation forum with Australia, Brazil, South Africa, Nepal, and India on A consultation forum with Australia, Brazil, South Africa, Nepal, and India on delivery of rural-primary healthcare, showed that geographically accessible, socio-culturally acceptable, family-centered healthcare needs to be developed. Integrating these concepts based on preventive, promotive, and curative, sensitive to the perceived requirements of the rural communities, need to be crafted. Creating a rural healthcare delivery system should begin with community healthcare needs and demands assessment that identifies potential strengths, weaknesses, threats, and opportunities in terms of human resource, infrastructure, and costs in building a sustainable rural healthcare delivery system sensitive to local healthcare needs. Once the healthcare-related needs are identified, prioritizing these needs based on either a nominal group technique or the Hanlon's basic priority rating system, or an intervention mapping can be employed. Implementing a healthcare system engaging community partners, a community-based organization ensuring the fullest community participation in making healthcare decisions through sustainable healthcare and financial incentivization schemes would be the next challenge to overcome.

When appropriate linkages being forged with referral systems, higher budgetary spending on healthcare by the states, healthcare insurance that improves affordability to build and empower healthcare teams providing rural healthcare [32]. With a shortage of trained rural healthcare professionals on health emergency and maternal and child health, individuals sourced from the local rural communities like the ASHA workers in India [16], Barefoot doctors in China [6, 12] could be looked at as potential bridges to the healthcare-related gap in rural areas. However, adequate and regular training and accreditation of rural healthcare providers who are sensitive to the family-centered practice of evidence-based medicine are paramount [32].

A concept of extended-community-care team sourced from trained staff of urban social and healthcare professionals who provide their skill and expertise prevalent in Scotland's remote and rural areas [6]. Research models for developing such extended healthcare teams in rural and remote with evidence through health impact assessment can ultimately translate to advocacy for policy-orientation prioritizing rural health.

Dissemination of information in rural healthcare delivery systems in research is also paramount for other rural communities to develop or adapt such models to achieve the best healthcare-related outcomes.

9. Role of telemedicine in rural healthcare delivery

Telemedicine has leveraged the benefits of advanced telecommunication and computer technologies, which can provide diagnostic and therapeutic support to patients residing in remote and rural areas [6, 37, 38]. Modern technology like Clinical Decision Systems (C.D.S.), Picture Archiving and Communication Systems (P.A.C.S) that capture, store, and disseminate health-related information from patients in rural and remote areas to healthcare providers on a real-time basis. These systems can help in making immediate and urgent healthcare decisions in these areas [37]. Information and Communication technologies improve accessibility to primary health care needs, maximizes service delivery, transfer and sharing of appropriate technology for instruction, training, continued education of healthcare service providers is also maximized in rural and remote areas [39, 40].

The characteristics of a programme that supports information and communication technology in remote and rural healthcare systems (which helps in return to improve health especially in developing countries are as follows:

1. Use of appropriate technology that is locally applicable to rural and remote health infrastructure

2. Leveraging and strengthening existing systems in the rural and remote communities

3. Demonstrating the benefit of using such health related information and communication technologies through showcasing of approaches in I.C.T delivery

4. Capacity building to innovate, develop and demonstrate the effectiveness of Information and Communication Technologies

5. Monitoring and evaluation through Participatory and Rapid Rural Appraisal

6. Designing better methods of communication strategies for delivery of healthcare in rural and remote areas

7. Continued research and information sharing regarding the strengths and challenges faced in setting up such technologies in rural and remote areas [40].

The three-pronged benefits that can be reaped by use of Information and Communication Technology (I.C.T.) would be in

1. **Improvement in functioning of health care systems**- of order/billing and electronic health record systems development

2. **Improvement of delivery of healthcare** through use of telemedicine and e-health that help in diagnostic, clinical decision making, quality assurance systems, disease surveillance

3. **Improving communication about health** in health-related research, health advocacy, patient information retrieval and dissemination [40].

The information and communication technology can also aid in lifelong learning, improvement and retraining in healthcare delivery system's accountability [38]. The establishment of electronic health records using barcoding and other such indexing systems for an individual also helps in maintaining the patients' continuity of care [37]. The WHO e-health strategy envisages, e- health-solutions exploration by identifying and addressing needs, innovative methods and research. This provides evidence, information, guidance, best practices and management of such solutions in rural and remote areas [40].

The challenges in implementation of Information and Communication technology like telemedicine, e-health include:

1. The lack of access to internet and mobile connectivity

2. The ack of credible and culturally sensitive information and communication technologies,

3. Insufficient political commitment toward establishment of a sustainable system for health information and communication

4. The need of extensive co-operation from stakeholders at the local, regional and national levels,

5. Paucity of foreign development investment for establishment of information and communication technologies.

10. Conclusions

Rural and remote healthcare delivery is essential to achieve a "Healthy Nation" through quality-assured core or basic healthcare centered on preventive, promotive, curative and rehabilitative service delivery. The healthcare- delivery system's focus on a constraint resource setting, lies in developing tailor-made models for the sustainable provision of healthcare facilities in rural and remote areas. Healthcare research into factors affecting accessibility, utilization, the feasibility of healthcare delivery models in rural areas should be encouraged to provide advanced insights into what works and what does not work in rural areas. The opportunities offered by information and communication technology, (including Telemedicine) bridge the gaps in rural and remote areas.

Conflict of interest

The authors declare no conflict of interest.

Author details

Ankeeta Menona Jacob
K S Hegde Medical Academy, a Constituent College of NITTE (Deemed to be) University, Deralakatte, Mangalore, Karnataka, India

*Address all correspondence to: nishankeeta@gmail.com

References

[1] Werner D, Thuman C, Maxwell J. Where there is no doctor: a village health care handbook. Rev. ed. Palo Alto, Calif., U.S.A: Hesperian Foundation; 1992. 512 p.

[2] Hart JT. The inverse care law. Lancet. 1971 Feb 27;1(7696):405-412.

[3] Rural population | Data [Internet]. [cited 2021 Mar 30]. Available from: https://data.worldbank.org/indicator/SP.RUR.TOTL

[4] Yadav K, Jarhyan P, Gupta V, Pandav CS. Revitalizing Rural Health Care Delivery: Can Rural Health Practitioners be the Answer? Indian J Community Med. 2009 Jan;34(1):3-5.

[5] Kilpatrick S, Liaw S-T. A textbook of Australian Rural Health. 1st ed. Canberra, A.C.T.: Australian Rural Health Education Network; 2008. 305 p.

[6] National Health Service in Scotland, Remote and Rural Steering Group, Scotland, Scottish Government. Delivering for remote and rural healthcare: the final report of the remote and rural workstream. 1st ed. Edinburgh: Scottish Government; 2008. 116 p.

[7] Chapman JL, Zechel A, Carter YH, Abbott S. Systematic review of recent innovations in service provision to improve access to primary care. Br J Gen Pract. 2004 May;54(502):374-381.

[8] Institute of Medicine (US) Committee on Monitoring Access to Personal Health Care Services. Access to Health Care in America [Internet]. Millman M, editor. Washington (DC): National Academies Press (US); 1993 [cited 2021 Apr 6]. Available from: http://www.ncbi.nlm.nih.gov/books/NBK235882/

[9] Dillip A, Alba S, Mshana C, Hetzel MW, Lengeler C, Mayumana I, et al. Acceptability – a neglected dimension of access to health care: findings from a study on childhood convulsions in rural Tanzania. BMC Health Serv Res. 2012 May 9;12:113.

[10] Goudge J, Gilson L, Russell S, Gumede T, Mills A. Affordability, availability and acceptability barriers to health care for the chronically ill: Longitudinal case studies from South Africa. BMC Health Services Research. 2009 May 9;9(1):75.

[11] Sidel VW. The Barefoot Doctors of the People's Republic of China. New England Journal of Medicine. 1972 Jun 15;286(24):1292-1300.

[12] Wen C. Barefoot doctors in China. Nurs Dig. 1975 Feb;3(1):26-28.

[13] Woodruff JE. China's 'barefoot' health care crumbles. Sun. 1986 May 27;299(8):1A,4A.

[14] Hu D, Zhu W, Fu Y, Zhang M, Zhao Y, Hanson K, et al. Development of village doctors in China: financial compensation and health system support. Int J Equity Health. 2017 Jul 1;16(1):9.

[15] Strodel RJ, Perry HB. The National Village Health Guide Scheme in India: lessons four decades later for community health worker programs today and tomorrow. Human Resources for Health. 2019 Oct 28;17(1):76.

[16] Sanjay V K. Strengthening Primary Health Care Through Asha Workers: A Novel Approach in India. Primary Health Care [Internet]. 2014 [cited 2021 Apr 1];04(01). Available from: http://www.omicsgroup.org/journals/strengthening-primary-health-care-through-asha-workers-a-novel-approach-in-india-2167-1079.1000149.php?aid=25013

[17] Chokshi M, Patil B, Khanna R, Neogi SB, Sharma J, Paul VK, et al. Health systems in India. J Perinatol. 2016 Dec;36(Suppl 3):S9-12.

[18] AYUSHMAN BHARAT-Comprehensive Primary Health Care through Health and Wellness Centers Operational Guidelines [Internet]. National Health Systems Resource Centre (NHSRC), New Delhi; [cited 2021 Apr 17]. Available from: http://nhsrcindia.org/sites/default/files/Operational%20Guidelines%20For%20Comprehensive%20Primary%20Health%20Care%20through%20Health%20and%20Wellness%20Centers.pdf

[19] Meit M, Knudson A. Why Is Rural Public Health Important? A Look to the Future. Journal of Public Health Management and Practice. 2009 Jun;15(3):185-190.

[20] Medcalf A, Bhattacharya S, Momen H, Saavedra M, Jones M. Health for all: the journey of universal health coverage [Internet]. 2015 [cited 2021 Apr 1]. 168 p. Available from: http://www.doabooks.org/doab?func=fulltext&rid=17456

[21] Gessert C, Waring S, Bailey-Davis L, Conway P, Roberts M, VanWormer J. Rural definition of health: a systematic literature review. BMC Public Health. 2015 Dec;15(1):1-14.

[22] James CV, Moonesinghe R, Wilson-Frederick SM, Hall JE, Penman-Aguilar A, Bouye K. Racial/Ethnic Health Disparities Among Rural Adults — United States, 2012-2015. MMWR Surveill Summ. 2017 Nov 17;66(23):1-9.

[23] Strasser R. Rural health around the world: challenges and solutions. Family Practice. :7.

[24] Greenwood-Ericksen MB, Kocher K. Trends in Emergency Department Use by Rural and Urban Populations in the United States. JAMA Netw Open. 2019 Apr 12;2(4):e191919.

[25] Hall MK, Burns K, Carius M, Erickson M, Hall J, Venkatesh A. State of the National Emergency Department Workforce: Who Provides Care Where? Ann Emerg Med. 2018 Sep;72(3):302-307.

[26] Oladipo JA. Utilization of health care services in rural and urban areas: a determinant factor in planning and managing health care delivery systems. Afr Health Sci. 2014 Jun;14(2):322-333.

[27] Panagariya A. The Challenges and innovative solutions to rural health dilemma. Ann Neurosci. 2014 Oct;21(4):125-127.

[28] Singh D, Cumming R, Negin J. Acceptability and trust of community health workers offering maternal and newborn health education in rural Uganda. Health Education Research. 2015 Dec 1;30(6):947-958.

[29] Saikia D, Das KK. Access to Public Health-Care in the Rural Northeast India. The NEHU journal. 2014 Dec;12(2):77-100.

[30] Croll Z, Gale J, Huggins C. Community Impact and Benefit Activities of Critical Access, Other Rural, and Urban Hospitals, 2018. 2018;5.

[31] Smits C, Toelsie J, Eersel M, Krishnadath I. Equity in health care: An urban and rural, and gender perspective; the Suriname Health Study. AIMS Public Health. 2018 Feb 27;5(1):1-12.

[32] Mohan P, Kumar R. Strengthening primary care in rural India: Lessons from Indian and global evidence and experience. J Family Med Prim Care. 2019;8(7):2169.

[33] Weisgrau S. Issues in Rural Health: Access, Hospitals, and Reform. Health Care Financ Rev. 1995;17(1):1-14.

[34] Omotosho A, Ayegba P, Emuoyibofarhe J, Meinel C. Current State of ICT in Healthcare Delivery in Developing Countries. Int J Onl Eng. 2019 May 14;15(08):91.

[35] Institute of Medicine (U.S.), editor. Quality through collaboration: the future of rural health. Washington, D.C: National Academies Press; 2005. 267 p.

[36] Rifkin SB. Alma Ata after 40 years: Primary Health Care and Health for All—from consensus to complexity. BMJ Glob Health [Internet]. 2018 Dec 20 [cited 2021 Apr 8];3(Suppl 3). Available from: https://www.ncbi.nlm.nih.gov/pmc/articles/PMC6307566/

[37] Burney AS, Mahmood N, Abbas. Information and Communication Technology in Healthcare Management Systems: Prospects for Developing Countries. IJCA. 2010 Jul;4(2):27-32.

[38] Chandrasekhar CP, Ghosh J. Information and communication technologies and health in low income countries: the potential and the constraints. Bulletin of the World Health Organization. 2001;6.

[39] Nyasulu C, Chawinga WD. The role of information and communication technologies in the delivery of health services in rural communities: Experiences from Malawi. S Afr j inf manag. 2018 Sep 18;20(1):1-10.

[40] Chetley A, Davies J, Trude B, McConnell H, Ramirez R, Shields T, et al. Improving Health, Connecting People: The Role of ICTs in the Health Sector of Developing Countries- A framework paper. 2006 p. 65. Report No.: Working paper No. 1.

Chapter 3

Common Genitourinary Fistulas in Rural Practice: Treatment and Management

Chineme Michael Anyaeze

Abstract

Acquired genitourinary fistulas are common in rural practice. They are pathological communications between the urinary and genital tracts, or between either of the tracts and gastrointestinal tract or skin. Vesicovaginal fistula is the commonest and most devastating. They may result from prolonged and obstructed labor, injuries during obstetric, gynecologic, pelvic and urologic procedures, circumcision, fall from heights, road traffic accidents and female genital mutilation. They present as urinary leakage with characteristic odor. Diagnoses are mainly clinical and confirmed by dye tests, contrast radiography and endoscopy. Treatment is individualized according anatomic sites and etiology. Timing of repair is of essence; delayed repair for obstetric and early for focal injuries. Multidisciplinary team approach and cooperation is encouraged in the management of some of these cases. The sustenance of the 2 – way referral system is emphasized in cases beyond the scope of rural practice. Repairs when undertaken by skilled compassionate fistula surgeons with attention to principles of fistula management and surgical treatment, success rate can approach 90%. Interposition of vascularized grafts have improved success rate. The burden of this condition will be reduced through integration of rural practitioners in the preventive strategies of health education of the public and girlchild; improvement of healthcare, education and transportation infrastructures.

Keywords: Common, Genitourinary, Fistula, Rural, Practice

1. Introduction

Genitourinary fistulas are abnormal tracts between the genital and urinary tracts. Abnormal tracts connecting the urinary system to any structure of the pelvic floor [1], gastrointestinal tract and the skin are also regarded as urinary fistulas [2]. Obstetric fistula is an abnormal hole connecting the vagina to the bladder (VVF), the rectum (RVF), the ureter (UVF) or a combination of these which leads to uncontrollable leakage of urine or feces or both through the vagina, and resulted usually as a complication of difficult labor. Urinary fistulas are severe physical, social and psychological debilitating conditions [3]. It presents as a surprise, taking the patient and caring physician unawares. The commonest type, vesicovaginal fistula (VVF) is still very common in the rural areas especially in Northern Nigeria, [4] and Ethiopia [5]. Thus, this condition is basically a rural disease. Rural area is characterized by meager earnings, low education and poor infrastructure [6]. In the developing countries the attending healthcare worker may be a Traditional Birth Attendant (TBA), traditional healer, quack, midwife, medical officer, obstetrician and gynecologist, surgeon or urologist. In the context of this work, the rural practitioner is a qualified medical doctor practising in the rural area, and is available and accessible to those who suffer from genitourinary fistulas.

The questions are, "will the integration of rural practitioners in the efforts towards elimination of obstetric fistulas reduce the prevalence and burden of the conditions?" What roles will the rural practitioner play in the treatment and management of genitourinary fistulas?

The true incidence of genitourinary fistulas in the developing countries is not known, [7] but some authors have put rates for VVF at 1–3 per 1000 deliveries [8], 3.5 per 1000 births [9] and 5–10 per 1000 deliveries [10]. In contrast VVF is no longer common in the developed countries as a result of improved obstetrics care; and results mainly as a complication of pelvic surgery, malignancy and radiotherapy [11].

This chapter will dwell on fistulas caused by trauma, including obstetric and iatrogenic, and its aim is to highlight the strategic position of rural practitioners in the prevention of genitourinary fistulas, the benefits that will be derived from their education and training on the subject matter, and to suggest a framework for their roles in the treatment and management of these conditions.

1.1 Objectives

The objectives of this work are to:

a. Rekindle attention to the burden of genitourinary fistulas in the rural areas.

b. Emphasize the importance of preventive strategies and stratify them for easy identification of roles and levels of participation by rural practitioners and specialized centers.

c. Empower the rural practitioner with information to identify and specify complex fistula varieties that require referral to specialized centers.

d. Prepare the rural practitioner to initiate informed early treatment and care for the genitourinary fistula patient.

e. Rekindle advocacy and solicit for regular fistula missions to reduce the prevalence and number in the waiting list.

f. Engage and train interested rural practitioners on effective preventive strategies and efficient fistula surgery, as they are more available and accessible to these rural fistula patients.

2. Etiology

2.1 Causes of genitourinary fistulas

Obstructed labor is the main cause of VVF in the rural areas accounting for between 56 and 97.88% in some series [4, 12–16].

Other causes of genitourinary fistulas in the developing world are well reported, [4, 5, 7, 9, 10, 12–17], and shown on **Table 1**.

SN	Etiology	Type(s)
1	**Obstetric** Obstructed labor. Injury to the bladder during cesarean section. Uterine rupture into the bladder. Perineal tear during childbirth. Forceps lacerations	Vesicovaginal fistula, Rectovaginal fistula, urethrovaginal fistula. VVF, vesicocervical fistula. Vesicouterine fistula. Rectovaginal fistula. VVF, RVF urethrovaginal fistula.
2.	Gynecologic surgery. Abdominal hysterectomy. Vaginal hysterectomy. Myomectomy. Surgery on the cervix	VVF, ureterovaginal fistula. VVF, ureterovaginal fistula. Vesicouterine Vesicocervical fistula.
3	Other pelvic surgery	VVF, ureterovaginal ureterocervical.
4	Harmful cultural practices. Gishiri cut, female circumcision	VVF, Urethrovaginal fistula
5	Miscellaneous Prolonged and neglected suprapubic catheter. Male circumcision Malignancy Infections Coital injury	Vesicocutaneous fistula Urethrocutaneous fistula. VVF, RVF VVF, VVF

Table 1.
Etiology of genitourinary fistulas in rural practice.

Table 2 summaries the etiology of genitourinary fistulas encountered by the author in rural practice from January 2000 to December 2020. Two of the VVF cases were associated with big vesical calculi; one of them had also vesicocutaneous fistula. Urethrovaginal fistulas are not common as noted in **Table 2**. They were complications of vaginal hysterectomy and consequences of vaginal procedures by quacks and homeopaths.

Rectovaginal Fistulas and other urinary fistulas are less common. RVF resulted from trauma mostly, and when it occurred during obstructed labor, it was associated with VVF. Urethrocutaneous fistulas in infants resulting from circumcision mishaps were not rare. These procedures were performed by traditional health attendants, hospital attendants, nurses, midwives and medical officers. The surgical residents at the Federal Medical Center Owerri, Nigeria perform circumcision under the supervision of team consultants since 2000. The less commonly occurring vesicouterine fistula (VUF) and vesicocervical fistula are complications of difficult cesarean sections (CS) [16], and uterine rupture. When urinary fistula occurs as a complication of treatment the effect is devastating to the trained care giver even though the propensity for medicolegal litigation is very low in the rural areas. The patient often stays isolated, withdrawn, miserable and depressed. The husbands and relatives of patients in my experience have been supportive and cooperative in contrast to other reports especially from northern Nigeria [3–10, 18].

2.1.1 Risk factors

The risk factors related to the development of urogenital fistulas in the rural areas that appear in the literature, [7, 12, 14, 16–23] are enumerated in **Table 3**. Other factors especially in the developed world include periurethral bulking, Burch Culpo suspension, urethral diverticulum repair, and loop excision of the cervix [24–28]. Endometriosis, gynecologic cancer, pelvic irradiation, schistosomiasis, intrauterine device and neglected pessary have also been reported [12, 14].

SN	Etiology	Type(s) of Fistulas(s)	No. of cases	Remarks
1. a b c d e	Obstetrics Obstructed labor Cesarean section Uterine rupture into the bladder Perineal tear Forceps injury	VVVF 30, RVF 2 VVF 9, UVF 7, VUF2 VUF 2, VCF 2 RVF 6 VVF 2, RVF 1	32 18 4 6 3	Referred by medical officers, obstetrician and gynecologists, midwives or directed by relatives or friends. There were attempted repairs in 19. The RVFs occurred in association with VVF.
2 a b c	Post gynecologic surgery Abdominal hysterectomy Vaginal hysterectomy Myomectomy	UVF 6, VVF 4 VCF 2 VVF4, Ur VF 3, EVF 1 VVF 4	12 8 4	Referred or invited by gynecologists Referral from gynecologists.
3 a b c 4 a b	Pelvic and inguinal surgeries General surgery Urology Inguinal herniorrhaphy Complications of procedures by unqualified personnel Homeopaths Quacks	VCuF 2 RUF 1, VCuF 8 VCuF 7 VVF 2 VVF 2, UrVF 1	2 9 7 2 3	The fistulas from urology procedures arose from the wounds of suprapubic cystostomies that failed to close spontaneously after removal of catheter. Injury to bladder sliding with hernial sac. Treating cystocele Treating Uterovaginal Prolapse
4	Circumcision	Ur C F 12	12	Infants.
5	Fall From height	VRF 2, RUF 2	4	Fell astride sharp pointed object. All males
6 a b	Violence Gunshot Stab injury	RUF4, UrCF3, VEF2, VCuF 1: from base of bladder to upper left thigh. RUF 2	10 2	One patient was shot with locally made hand shotgun forcefully inserted in his anus by armed robbers One patient was pinned in a bent over position at the waist and stabbed through the anus with a dagger.
7 a b c d	Miscellaneous Retained gauze After vaginal surgery Occupational hazard Infection Foreign body in the urethra Total	VVF 1 RVF 1 UrCF 1 UrVF 1 142	1 1 1 1	Lady farmer fell onto a cassava stem stump while harvesting cassava root by uprooting method.

Key: VVF = Vesicovaginal fistula, RVF = Rectovaginal fistula, VUF = Vesicouterine fistula, UVF = Ureterovaginal fistula, VCF = Vesicocervisal fistula, UrVF = Urethrovaginal fistula, RUF = Rectourethral fistula, VRF = Vesicorectal fistula, UrCF = Urethrocutaneous fistula, VCuF = Vesicocutaneous fistula, EVF = Enterovaginal fistula, VEF = Vesicoenteric fistula.

Table 2.
Genitourinary fistulas encountered by the author in rural practice.

Contributory factors to this burden are poor transport infrastructure, lack of skilled medical personnel and collapsed public healthcare delivery system [6]. Specialists in surgery and obstetrics and gynecology show little interest in fistula surgery, and rarely practice in rural areas. Bad roads prolong the time interval between onset of labor and arrival to hospital or make it impossible for the journey [7, 9].

SN	RISK FACTORS
1	**Sociocultural and general considerations**
	Young age [7–10].
	Early marriage [3–10, 18].
	Early pregnancy [3–10, 18, 20, 21].
	Pregnancy [14–18].
	Cephalopelvic disproportion [7].
	Female genital mutilation [3–7].
	Ignorance [18].
	Illiteracy [7–18, 21, 22].
	Poverty [18].
	Late presentation to hospital [14–18].
	Violence, youth restiveness, armed robbery banditry, armed conflicts.
	Cultural restrictions of women's movement [18].
2	**Obstetric**
	Prolonged labor [3–5, 9, 21, 23].
	Obstructed labor [3–5, 9, 12].
	Cesarean hysterectomy [12–15].
	Cesarean section [10–12].
	Repeat Cesarean Section.
	Operative vaginal delivery [12].
	Unskilled obstetrics care [14, 18].
	Inappropriate obstetrics care (labor at home, in the church).
3	**Gynecologic**
	Hysterectomy [4, 5, 9, 12, 15, 21, 23].
	Anterior colporrhaphy.
	Myomectomy.
	Induced abortion.
	Urinary bladder stone.
	Infections: Schistosomiasis, Tuberculosis, Lymphogranuloma venereum.
	Vaginal foreign body.
	Retain gauze after vaginal surgery.
	Urethral and bladder foreign body.

Table 3.
Risk factors related to the development of genitourinary fistulas in rural areas.

In southern Nigeria many roads are not passable during the peak of rainy season: July–September. Brain drains affect developing countries seriously as their trained healthcare professionals relocate or emigrate to Europe, America, Canada, Saudi Arabia for greener pastures [29, 30]. In this situation, these hapless young pregnant women turn to the familiar, available and accessible traditional healers, quacks, traditional birth attendants and poorly trained midwives whom they can afford their services for obstetrics care.

2.2 Classification and pathogenesis of genitourinary fistulas

The anatomic classification of urinary fistulas has been mentioned in **Table 2**. **Figure 1** shows them graphically.

The exact pathological mechanism in the formation of obstetric fistula is not clear. However, the compression of maternal soft tissues of bladder base, urethra, cervix vagina and rectum posteriorly, against the unyielding pubis and sacral spine during prolonged obstructed labor; with the resultant ischemia, epithelial necrosis and subsequent sloughing had been postulated as the pathophysiologic process in the formation of obstetric fistulas by many workers in the developing world [4–10, 14, 16, 20–22, 24].

Arrowsmith et al. described obstetric fistula formation within the spectrum of "obstructed labor injury complex" [20]. Urinary fistulas arising from surgical complications, wounding from accidents and stabbing are focal injuries [7]. Gunshots are more complex as they are associated with the phenomena of "tract cavitation and expansion" injuries [31]. Fistulas resulting from obstetric and high velocity gunshot injuries are larger. Ischemia, erosion and migration maybe responsible for the formation of fistulas by foreign bodies in the vagina, bladder, urethra or retained gauze during vaginal surgery.

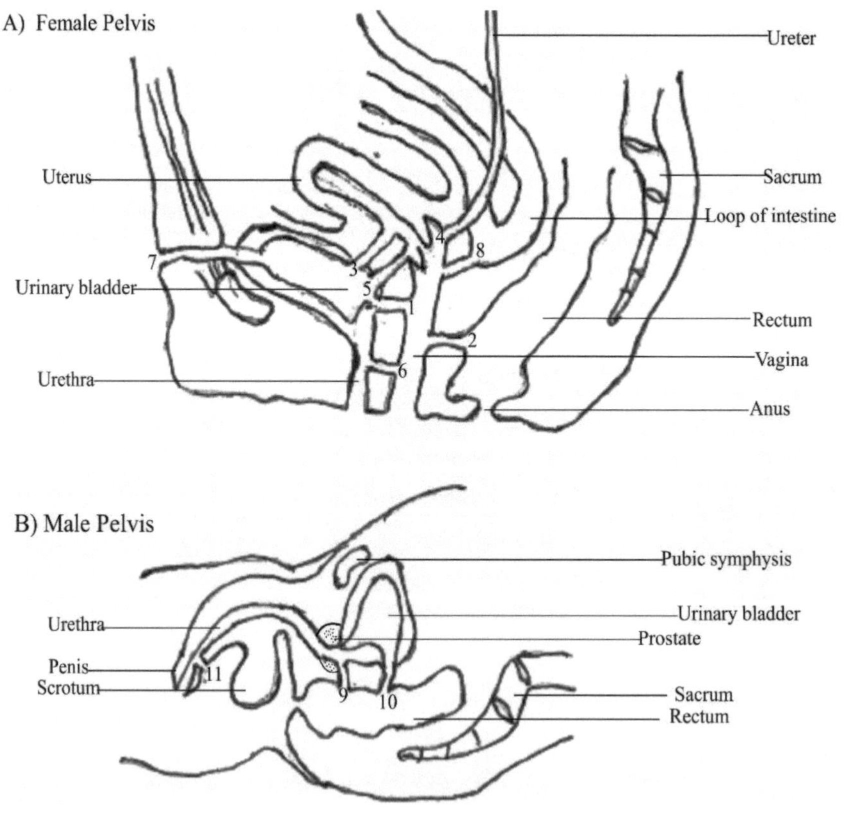

Figure 1.
(A and B): Anatomic sites of Urinary fistulas. 1-Vesicovaginal fistula, 2-Rectovaginal fistula, 3-Vesicouterine fistula, 4-Ureterovaginal fistula, 5-Vesicocervical fistula, 6- Urethrovaginal fistula, 7- Vesicorectal fistula, 8-Enterovaginal fistula, 9-Rectouethral fistula, 10-Vesicorectal fistula, 11-Urethrocutaneous fistula, Vesicoenteric fistula is not shown.

3. Clinical features

3.1 Clinical presentation

Leakage of urine is the usual complaint. Discharge of feces from the vagina indicates rectovaginal fistula, alone or in association with VVF. The genitourinary fistulas are associated with offensive urine odor. There may be leakage of urine from the vagina, anus or through a hole in the skin depending on the type and location of the fistula. The patient may give a history of prolonged or obstructed labor prior to the leakage by 3 to 10 days in the case of VVF. History of assisted vaginal delivery, before the leakage may indicate VVF [17]. Cesarean section, hysterectomies or any other pelvic surgery may precede the urinary leakage by 10-- 14 days. VVF, UVF, VCF, VUF, VCuF and RUF may result from these obstetric and pelvic surgeries. The differential diagnoses of VVF include stress, urge and over flow incontinence. Pain is not usually associated with VVF, and urinary leakage in VVF may commence immediately after catheter is removed.

VVF may present many weeks after pelvic surgery. A 65 years old lady presented to the author with offensive vaginal discharge and urinary retention 10 weeks after vaginal hysterectomy by a gynecologist. It turned out to be VVF resulting from eroding infected gauge that migrated into the bladder and pointing at the tip of the urethra. The gauze probably used to pack away the bladder must have been forgotten in the wound during the surgery. The patient may present with with a referral letter indicating the definitive or provisional diagnosis. In developing countries difficult urinary fistulas are referred to the urologist or fistula centers. Frequency, urgency, dysuria, vaginal discharge, bleeding or pain during coitus may be present. There may be irritation, rash or dermatitis and whitish crystal formation on the skin surrounding the fistula, **Figure 2**.

History of accidentally falling astride a sharp object, stab, or gunshot injury and sustaining a penetrating injury in the perineum or suprapubic region may be elicited; leakage of urine from the anus may suggest VRF or RUF.

3.2 History

History from clinical presentation as noted above will guide the clinician towards the likely fistula he/she is dealing with.

3.3 Physical examination

A general examination should be performed noting nutritional state of the patient and comorbidities. In rural practice nutritional anemia is common and they need to be addressed to enhance wound healing.

3.4 Pelvic examination

Inspection of the perineum for sinuses, fistulas or associated tears; followed by digital bimanual and bivalve speculum examination which assist in identifying the fistula; and provides the opportunity to note the location, size, number and whether simple or complex. An idea about inflammation, fibrosis and pliability of tissue surrounding the fistula and that of the introitus and vagina are ascertained during the examinations. Stenosis and fibrosis of the introitus and vagina sometimes complicate VVF [7, 32].

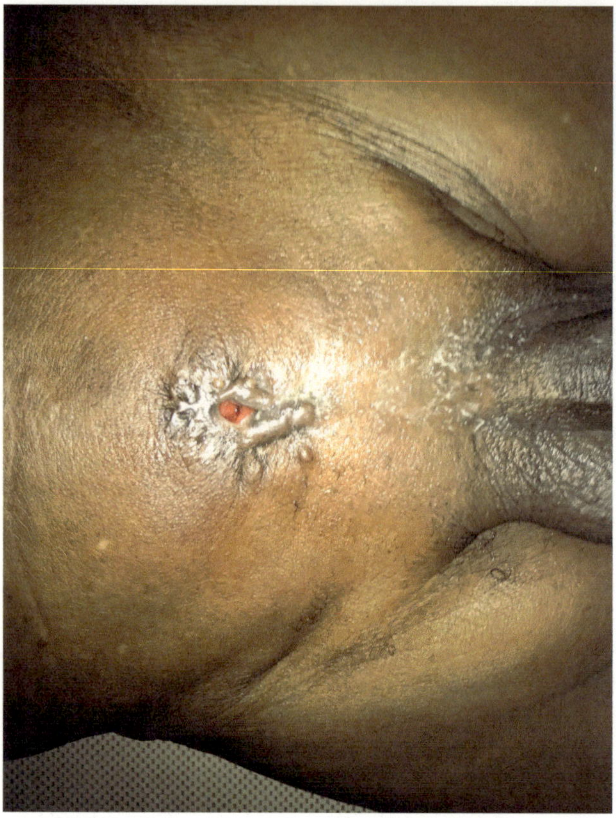

Figure 2.
Vesicocutaneous fistula showing whitish phosphate crystals.

Ongoing inflammation, infection and induration around the fistula are contra-indications for immediate repair.

4. Assessment and diagnoses of genitourinary fistulas

4.1 Dye test in VVF management

Indications

i. Confirmation or identification of small and hidden fistulas that cannot be verified by direct vision examination.

ii. To differentiate between VVF and UVF

iii. Differentiate between urogenital fistula and urinary incontinence

Method

It can be performed in the treatment room or theater. Methylene blue or indigo carmine is mixed with sterile water and instilled into the urinary bladder under gravity without spillage. A sterile gauze or cotton ball is placed at the vault, mid and distal vagina. Patient is asked to walk about and return for inspection after 30 minutes.

Interpretations

- If the gauze at the vault is wet and not stained, a ureterovaginal fistula is suspected.
- If the gauze at the vault is stained, a high VVF is suspected
- If the gauze at the mid vagina is stained a mid-vesicovaginal fistula is suspected
- Staining at the most distal part of the gauze in the distal vagina near the introitus suggests urinary incontinence.
- If the staining of the gauze at this distal vagina spares the most distal portion a urethrovaginal fistula is suspected.
- In the case where UVF is strongly suspected the vagina is carefully cleaned and test is performed again with fresh gauze in the vagina and intravenous indigo carmine given. Blue staining of the proximal end of the gauze confirms UVF. An intravenous urogram can also be used to confirm it where it is available.

4.2 Cystoscopy

Ideally cystoscopy should be performed for patients presenting with VVF. However, in the setting of rural practice in developing countries of Africa, such necessary services are not always available. The author uses a hand-held battery-operated portable cystoscope, **Figure 3**, to scope urinary fistula patients whenever necessary in the rural setting. It is very cheap to operate. Apart from visualizing the fistula, it helps in assessing the location, and size, whether simple or complex, and location of the ureteric orifices in relation to the fistulas. This is important in planning and choosing the approach for the repair [2, 32].

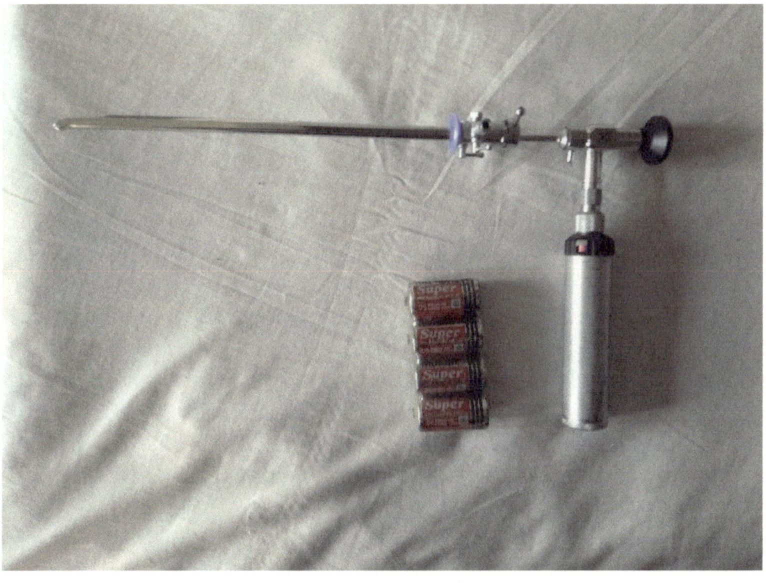

Figure 3.
Portable hand-held battery-operated cystoscope (TRICOMED Surgical Limited, England).

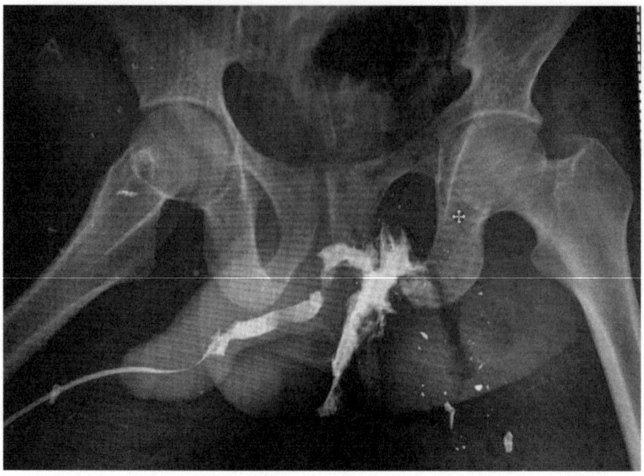

Figure 4.
Retrograde urethrogram showing a fistulous connection between bulbo-membranous urethra and rectum.

4.3 Imaging

Imaging may be needed, but most hospitals in rural practice lack imagine facilities. Patients who could afford contrast studies are referred to facilities that have them to access studies as intravenous urogram, with cystogram in UVF and VVF, retrograde urethrogram (RUG), **Figure 4** and micturating cystourethrogram (MCUG) in RUF, urethrovaginal, urethrocutaneous, and vesicocutaneous fistulas; barium enema, vaginography in RVF, and contrast CT scan. Many of our patients are poor and cannot afford these tests. In the rare situation where the fistulas could not be identified with office procedures despite a suggestive history, Rony A Adam [32] described a process where the patient is given phenazopyridine. (Pyridium) and wear a series of gauze at home over a long period. The gauze balls are placed separately in different plastic bags and brought for inspection later. Patients are instructed on proper conduct of the test in order not to contaminate the gauze during insertion.

5. Prevention

Urinary fistulas especially obstetric when they occur is associated with misery and isolation, expensive and difficult to treat. Healthcare financing is low in many developing countries [33] and may not be able to accommodate the management of genitourinary fistulas. Nigeria is perceived to bear the world's heaviest burden of obstetric fistulas, followed by Ethiopia, Uganda and Sudan [34]. In Nigeria, 12,000 fresh cases occur annually while 150,000 in the pool await repair [35]. Only 43% of births are attended to by skilled medical personnel in Nigeria [36]. Thus, some of these common genitourinary fistulas are avoidable. Hence some authors, National strategic Framework for Elimination of Obstetric Fistula in Nigeria, Fistula Foundation, and Professional groups recommended preventive strategies for genitourinary fistulas [34, 36]. The rural area is the veritable ground for it, and rural practice is one of the best channels to use.

Three perspectives can be recognized: primary, secondary and tertiary.

5.1 Primary prevention

The goal is to remove or stop the factors known to cause or contribute to urinary fistula formation. Health education and improvement on community health.

Involve community healthcare stakeholders as traditional rulers, village heads, women, youth and religious leaders, teachers and traditional birth attendants, traditional healers and heads of healthcare facilities in this program. Emphasis should be to discourage girlchild marriage, early pregnancy, delivery at home or in the church, conducting labor for a long time before referring to a superior facility, and female genital organ mutilation. Educate the community to embrace the attitude to have deliveries in suitable and efficient healthcare facilities. Encourage the girlchild to go to school and be able to comprehend the dangers in early marriage and pregnancy. Government to upscale health and transportation infrastructures to ensure timely comprehensive emergency obstetric care to all women as is obtainable in developed countries where the condition is eradicated. Effective training of midwives to conduct safe vaginal deliveries, and medical doctors to conduct safe vaginal deliveries, cesarean sections, gynecologic and pelvic surgeries. Regular workshops for public and private primary healthcare staff to monitor and recognize prolonged labor for quick referral. Multidisciplinary team approach for anticipated difficult cases. It can be rewarding to invite an experienced specialist or expert to the local center. The author has been invited by gynecologists and medical officers to join their surgeries in more than 35 instances. Part time or visiting appointments can be offered to such experts.

5.2 Secondary prevention

The goal is to recognize and repair injuries caused to urinary and genital tracts during surgeries; and to offer early attention and treatment to genitourinary injuries from other causes. The use of appropriate suture material and size in the surgery on urinary tract; and safe surgical conduct. Improved operating light is very important. Many theaters in rural practice use improvised theater lamp [6]. The author uses LED head light gear, **Figure 5** to augment whatever light that is available. It is pertinent for the pelvic surgeon to appreciate the applied anatomy of pelvic structures, and note that the trigone is situated at the anterior aspect of upper 1/3 of the vagina, and the cervical os is at the base of the trigone (inter ureteric ridge).

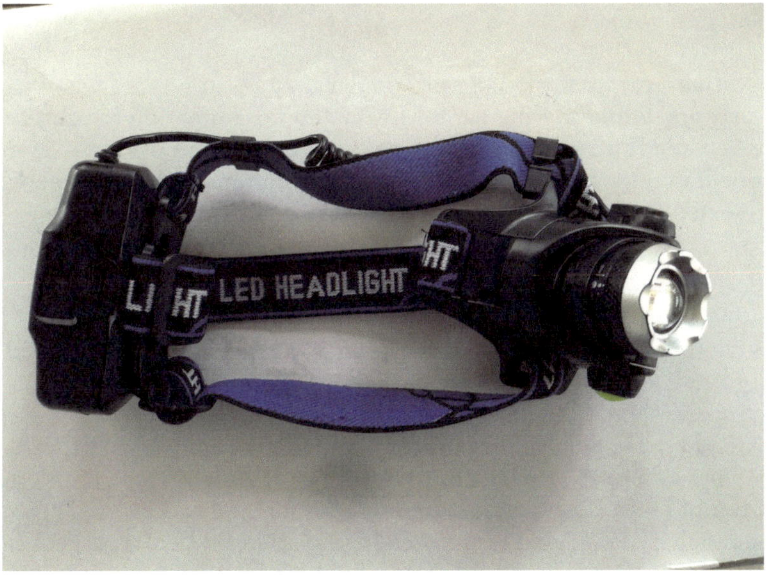

Figure 5.
Rechargeable LED operating headlight gear.

5.3 Tertiary prevention

Involves interventions geared towards prevention of complications from urinary fistulas. Treat infections, skin care, nutritional support, correction of nutritional deficiencies and anemia, social support and community reintegration to avert depression, abandonment and divorce. Advocacy for bilateral cooperation and collaboration to sponsor obstetric fistula repairs and training for more fistula surgeons. Repairs should be undertaken by skilled fistula surgeons. Nigeria|Fistula Foundation in her recent report stated that it has provided 9,464 fistula repair surgeries to Nigeria women since 2010 [36].

6. Treatment

6.1 Principles of fistula management

In addition to thorough evaluation of the genitourinary fistula patient, the following management principles are important. They should have adequate nutrition, successful treatment of infection, effective urinary drainage, removal or by pass of any distal obstruction and rule out any associated malignancy [2, 32, 37]. Adherence to the principles of surgical repair of urogenital fistulas is paramount to successful repair [2, 4, 5, 7–10, 14, 32, 37]. These include optimal operating light, adequate exposure of the fistula, excision of devitalized and ischemic tissues, removal of foreign bodies from the fistula, careful dissection, keeping to anatomical plane between organ cavities, use of small sized delayed absorbable sutures on small automatic needles, water tight closure, use of well vascularized flaps for repair and support, multilayer closure, non-overlapping tension free suture lines, stenting of urinary tract, adequate drainage after repair, prevention and treatment of infection, and adequate hemostasis.

6.2 Treatment of vesicovaginal fistula

6.2.1 Conservative method

Conservative treatment though not popular may be attempted when patient presents early and while waiting for infection and inflammation to subside. The author has recorded success on a few cases that ranged from 0.5 cm – 1.5 cm, **Table 4**. Small fistulas with oblique tracts have been reported to be amenable to conservative management [2].

6.2.2 Surgical repair of VVF

VVF is commonly classified as vesicocervical, juxtacervical, midvaginal suburethral, VVFs [8]. Other classification methods exist [38, 39].

Fistula repairs should be undertaken by "tutored and trained fistula surgeon" who has passion to ameliorate the suffering of patients. Some medical officers belong to this group [38]. The best opportunity to achieve a successful repair is at the first attempt [2–8]. There should be no room for trial and error. The trainee surgeon should be assisted and monitored by experienced fistula surgeons. In rural surgery for VVF, the best outcomes do not often come from trained specialists as obstetrician and gynecologists; general surgeons, urologists and plastic surgeons.

SN	Age	Sex	Etiology	Type	Time between onset of symptoms or injury and presentation (Days)	Intervention	Duration of treatment (weeks)
1	65	F	Erosion of retained vaginal wound gauze into the bladder.	VVF	8	Extraction of the gauze, urethral catheterization, appropriate antibiotic cover.	5
2	28	M	Stab injury through the anus	Rectourethral fistula	4	Urethral catheterization/stent	4
3	12	M	Fall from height with penetration of stick stump through the rectum into the bladder	Vesico-rectal fistula	3	Suprapubic cystostomy with continuous bladder drainage, defunctioning colostomy, appropriate antibiotics.	6
4	13	M	Accidental gunshot injury to the pelvis with exit wound at the perineum	Vesico-rectal fistula.	2	Defunctioning colostomy, Suprapubic cystostomy with continuous bladder drainage. appropriate antibiotics cover.	6

Table 4.
Cases of genitourinary fistulas treated with conservative method.

Timing of repair

In rural practice, obstetric fistula is commonest. Patients arrive late [18–10]. In the case of those who arrive early, we allow 8–12 weeks. If the fistula was iatrogenic or resulted from any other focal injury, we close the fistula as soon as infection is controlled. Controversies surround the timing of repair of VVF [4, 8, 14, 37, 38].

Approach

Whoever is undertaking VVF repair must be familiar with both vaginal and abdominal approaches, techniques and maneuvers. One approach may not be suitable for every case [40]. Most surgeons in the developing world use the vaginal approach [4–9, 12, 16, 37, 38].

6.2.2.1 Anesthesia

Anesthesia should be simple, safe and easy in rural practice. Heavy 0.5% Bupivacaine spinal and intravenous (iv) Ketamine anesthesia; conscious sedation with diazepam and pentazocine injections with local infiltration anesthesia of 1 or 2% lidocaine or lignocaine with or without adrenaline are commonly used. Sometimes iv Ketamine is used to supplement spinal anesthesia in lengthy surgical sessions. Ketamine is safe, 1–2 mg/kg for induction and 25–50 mg iv boluses in titrated doses [41]. Atropine 0.6 mg, diazepam 5 mg stat and given 30 minutes before the start of operation. Atropine prevents secretions and bradycardia, while diazepam prevents dysphoria and psychotomimetic effects during recovery. Bupivacaine spinal anesthesia may last up to 3 hours and is superior to 2% heavy lidocaine spinal anesthesia which may last for 90 minutes. Endotracheal intubation anesthesia is rarely used in rural practice [6].

6.2.2.2 Tools for VVF-repair

Tools for VVF repair is shown on **Table 5**. Two assistants are required in prone position. One will be holding up the posterior vaginal wall with a Sim's speculum [37].

6.2.2.3 Preoperative counseling

It is done in the language she will understand when conservative management has failed. Expectations are discussed, especially that the repair may fail, but hope will not be lost. The need for catheterization for 2–3 weeks, length of hospital stays; possible post-operative frequency, urgency, urgency incontinence for some time after removal of catheter. Patient is counseled thoroughly on informed consent and reminded that challenges may warrant change of plans intraoperatively.

SN	Item	Average quantity required
1	Operating table with stirrup accessories	1
2	Size 3, 12 cm, Bard parker handle	2
3	Sizes 10, 11 and curved 12 surgical blades	2 each
4	Medium and large sim's speculum	1 each
5	Short-blade Auvard (weighted) vaginal speculum	2
6	Long-blade Langenback retractors	2
7	Mosquito artery forceps: curved and straight	4 each
8	12 cm curved slender artery forceps with fine tips	4
9	Tissue forceps: Vulsellum, Allis	2 each
10	Curved 20 cm (McIndoe) light scissors	2
11	Straight stitch scissors	2
12	Standard needle holders	2
13	2- way foley catheters: sizes 16, 12, 10, 8	2 each
14	Methylene blue	1 bottle
15	Sterile water or normal saline	1, 000 mls
16	A small funnel for the catheter	1
17	Good suction machine with tubing	1
18	Sutures: 5/0 poliglecaprone (monocryl) or polyglyconate (Maxolon) or polydiaoxanone (PDS II); 4/0 polyglactin (vicryl) or polyglycolic acid (Dexon), 3/0 polyglactin .	6 each
19	Adrenaline 1: 1000	1 ampule
S20	2% lidocaine: plain and with Adrenaline	1 bottle each
21	Assistants	2
22	Scrub Nurse	1

Table 5.
Tools for VVF repair.

Choice of suture materials

Small size delayed absorbable sutures ranging from 5/0–4/0, monofilament and braided multifilament from 4/0 to 3/0 with 3/8 and 5/8 atraumatic needles are recommended, **Table 5**. This minimizes the amount of suture material in the wound and still provides adequate closure of wound edges [42].

6.2.2.4 Position for repair of VVF

This depends on the preference of the surgeon.

6.2.2.4.1 Prone position

Prone position is used in many fistula centers where skilled and experienced anesthetists will perform cuffed endotracheal intubation inhalation general anesthesia. The specifics of prone position are well illustrated in primary surgery volume one, edited by Maurice King et al. [37].

6.2.2.4.2 Lithotomy position

Exaggerated lithotomy position with slight head down position, buttocks just beyond the edge of the table.

6.2.2.5 Repairing technique of VVF

The principal steps are: dissecting out the fistula, mobilizing the vaginal skin from the bladder and precervical fascia, mobilization of precervical (pubovesical) fascia, if possible, attention to ureteric orifices, closure of bladder wall, doing a second layer with the precervical fascia over the first suture layer, placement of vascularized graft when indicated and closing the vaginal skin.

6.2.2.5.1 Steps in vaginal approach

i. After spinal anesthesia, antibiotic prophylaxis is given.

ii. Exaggerated lithotomy position.

iii. Skin preparation and draping.

iv. Pass size 16, 2- way Foley catheter, inflate the balloon and connect to a urine bag.

v. Infiltrate the layer between the vaginal wall and bladder wall with adrenaline in normal saline 1:100,000. If patient is hypertensive, use plain normal saline. This facilitates dissection and reduces bleeding when the adrenaline-saline solution is used.

vi. The fistula is dilated, and size 14 or 12, or 10 or 8, 2- way Foley catheter depending on the size of fistula is inserted into the fistula tract and the balloon inflated with 5 mls of sterile water.

vii. Commensurate traction is applied distally on the catheter in the fistula to enhance access, purchase and exposure.

viii. The vaginal skin is incised elliptically around the fistula. Using sharp dissection with knife and slander scissors, the vaginal skin is carefully dissected from the bladder wall for a distance of 0.5–1.5 cm, to allow for tension free closure eventually, **Figure 6A**. Some authors recommend 1 cm towards the cervix and 0.5 cm laterally [37].

ix. Where possible separate the layer of tissue between the bladder and vagina (precervical fascia) from the bladder wall. This may be difficult in large and fibrotic fistulas. Use suture ligation with 5/0 polyglactin to control bleeding.

x. The fistula collar, **Figure 6B**, may or may not be excised depending on the size of the fistula. In large fistulas with repeated repair attempts, conservation is prudent. In the past some workers insist on total excision of fistulous tracts and fibrous tissue [43].

xi. Size 20, 2- way Foley catheter is placed suprapubically for drainage.

xii. Extra mucosal closure of the bladder is done, starting at each end and coming towards the center, with 5/0 poliglecaprone (Monocryl) on a 5/8 atraumatic needle, at 3–5 mm interval. Through – and - through bladder mucosal closure can be done with good result especially in large fibrotic fistulas [37], where tissues are not very pliable or bleeding mucosal edge [32]. The ureters can be avoided by conserving fistular collar in large fistulas and doing careful extra mucosal closure. In high fistulas near the cervix the bladder is usually closed transversely and in low fistulas near the urethra the first layer is sutured longitudinally [2, 32, 37]. There are no hard and fast rules about this, the bladder should be closed in the line of least tension [32].

xiii. The tightness of the repair is checked by instilling 200–300 mls of methylene blue normal saline solution into the bladder. More stitch is put at any leaking point, or the stitches removed, to start a fresh if the leakage is copious.

xiv. The precervical fascia is closed if possible or the first layer is imbricated by suturing the bladder muscularis layer together with 4/0 or 3/0 polyglactin 910, **Figure 6C**. The stitches of this layer are staggered between those of the first layer so that no stitch lies on top of each other.

xv. If the fistular is large or significant dead space exists, a graft is indicated. The bladder peritoneum can be mobilized or a Martius fat pad transpositional flap is raised and placed over the closed fistula [2, 3].

xvi. The vaginal skin is closed perpendicular to the bladder closure line, if possible, otherwise close according to easy approximation of edges. **Figure 6D**.

xvii. Repeat cystoscopy with intravenous indigo carmine to assess ureteric patency if available.

In Latzko technique, the fistulous tract is not excised. It is imbricated into the bladder with interrupted extra mucosal sutures on a small tapered needle [44]. The Latzko technique is versatile, simple and cost effective [45]. Many small and moderate sized vaults and high fistulas can be repaired with various versions of modified Latzko technique [46, 47].

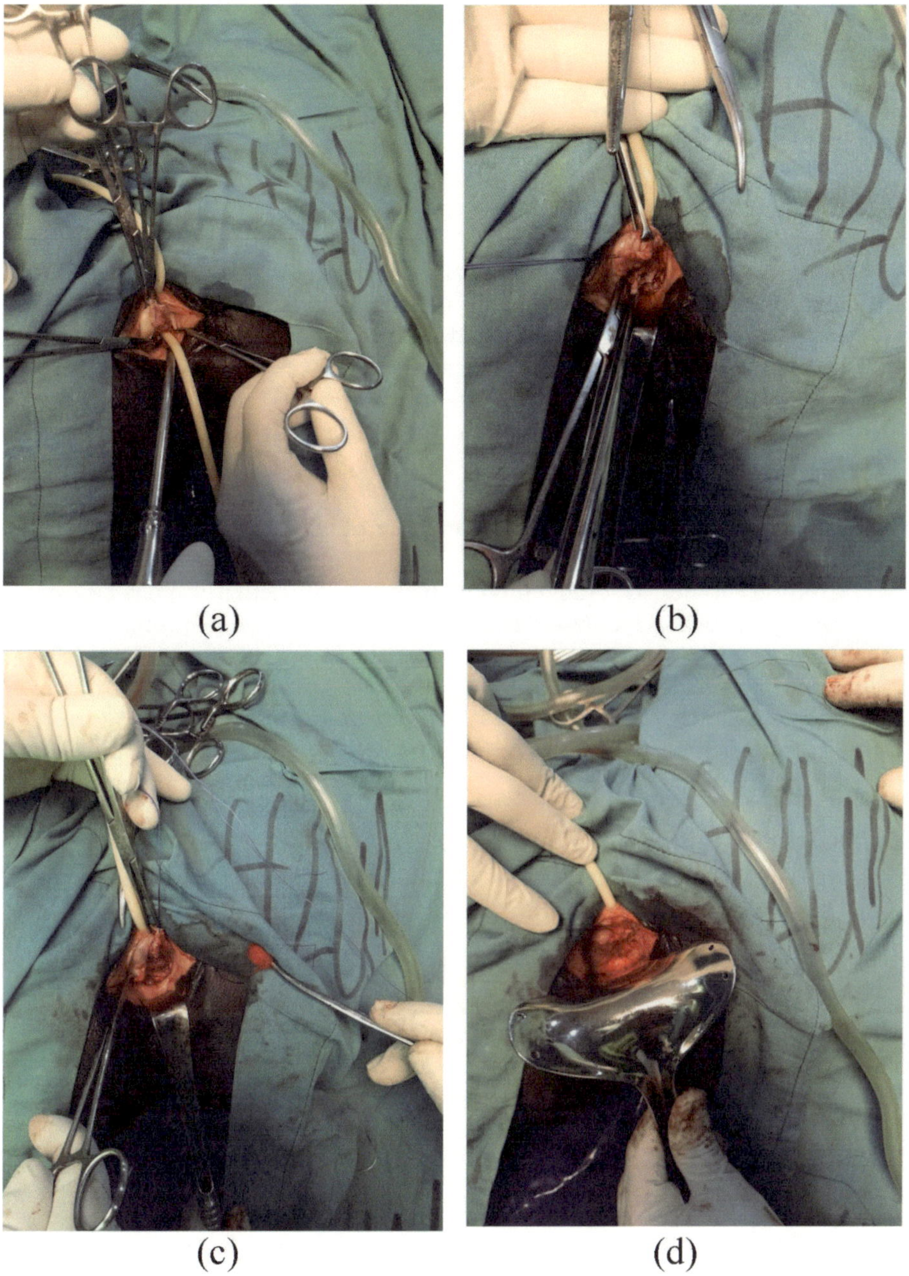

Figure 6.
(a) Vaginal wall is dissected off the bladder wall. (b) Dissecting out fistula collar. (c) Closed precervical fascia. (d) Closed vaginal skin.

The vaginal flap technique made popular by Zimmern et al. and Eilber et al., results in four-layer closure when the flap is used [48, 49]. It is well illustrated by Ganabathi K, Sirls L, Zimmern PE and Leach GC [50].

6.2.2.6 Abdominal approach in VVF repair

Extra peritoneal and intraperitoneal techniques of VVF repairs have been well discussed by Gabanathi K, et al. and Wein AJ et al. [51, 52].

7. Post-operative management of VVF repair

i. Presumptive intravenous antibiotics with 3rd generation cephalosporine in combination with metronidazole or tinidazole continued for 5 days is recommended, because of the peculiar setting of rural practice. Routine presumptive antibiotics regimen is not practiced in developed countries [32].

ii. Efficient and effective bladder drainage. Urine bags should be emptied hourly and recorded in a chart [37]. Debate on method of catheter drainage is still on. Advocates of single urethral catheter as Collins CG et al., Trancer ML and Leng WW et al., found it effective [40, 52, 53]. Suprapubic catheter drainage alone is advocated by Blaivas JG et al. and, Carr and Webster [54, 55]. Both suprapubic and urethral catheters drainage were favored by Wein AJ et al., Eilber et al. and others [2, 32, 37, 49–51].

iii. In transperitoneal technique, nil orally until bowel function returns.

iv. Urethral catheter is removed when macroscopic hematuria has cleared, usually about the 3rd day in the case of double catheter drainage, and leave the suprapubic for three weeks.

v. The catheter is spigoted at day 18 and bladder training is commenced: release urine hourly for 3 hours, then 2 hourly for 6 hours and thereafter 3–4 hourly from day 20. If all is well, catheter is removed on day 21.

vi. Patient is observed for 2 days for normal micturition and dryness. If she leaks urine, examination in the left lateral position is done, to ascertain whether urine is coming from the fistula or urethra.

vii. If she is leaking from the urethra, discharge and reassess at 6 weeks. If she is leaking from the fistula, recommence bladder drainage for 21 days. If she does not close, remove catheter and recommence salt (Sitz) bath.

viii. Counsel and work her up for future repair.

7.1 Adjuncts

- Anticholinergics to control bladder spasms, oxybutinine 5 mg twice or three times daily; Tolterodine 2 mg twice daily, and solifenacin 5 mg daily are useful.

- Loose vaginal gauze as wick drains and changed daily. Some authors use vaginal packs after abdominal approach [2], while others do not [32].

- Estrogen may be given to enhance vaginal skin [2, 32, 50]. Estrogen is rarely used in rural practice.

7.1.1 Postoperative counseling

- Sexual intercourse is forbidden for 3 months.

- Subsequent pregnancies shall be delivered by cesarean section.

7.2 Failure of VVF repair

Failure after repair may result from.

a. host factors as presence of foreign body, tissue ischemia, infection, metabolic diseases as diabetes mellitus, peripheral vascular diseases and rarely malignancy.

b. Surgical factors as undetected distal urinary obstruction, inadequate post-operative urinary drainage.

c. Surgical technique as inexperience, inadequate excision of devitalized tissues and scar tissue, use of inappropriate suture materials and lack of adherence to detailed measures in the principles of surgical repair of vesicovaginal fistula.

8. Complex vesicovaginal fistula

These include:

- Multiple vesicovaginal fistulas involving the urethra and intestine, associated with trauma of fall from heights, anterior posterior- compression fractures from road traffic accidents, and gun short injuries.
- Giant Vesicovaginal fistulas of more than 5 cm in diameter. Those associated with partial or complete loss of urethra, stress incontinence, narrow vagina and small bladder capacity.
- Those involving the cervix and lower uterine segments.
- Those complex fistulas are referred to fistula units in tertiary institutions and fistula centers. Elsewhere the author has emphasized the importance of sustaining the 2- way referral system in the practice of medicine [6]. It supports a good rural surgical practice.

9. Rectovaginal fistulas (RVF)

9.1 Etiology and clinical presentation

This is an abnormal connection between the rectum and vagina. The etiology, pathogenesis, clinical presentation and diagnosis of RVF have been discussed in the preceding sections and highlighted on **Tables 1** and **2**. RVF can be classified as low, mid and high vaginal fistula. Low is from the vaginal opening to the hymenal ring, mid from the hymenal ring to the external cervical os, and high from the external cervical opening to the vault of the vagina (area of the cul-de-sac) [32].

9.2 Management

Conservative management may be tried. Some resulting from penetrating and stab wounds responds to antibiotics, salt bath and fluid diet. Defunctioning colostomy has been performed for some cases. Obstetric RVF will require surgical correction after treating infection and resolution of inflammation.

Time of repair: A waiting period of 3–6 months is allowed, and salt bath continues before repair.

9.2.1 Surgical repair of RVF

A defunctioning sigmoid colostomy may be done.

Assessment under anesthesia as soon as possible to ascertain the location, size and state of the fistula, presence of sloughs, and edema. If the fistula is above 8 cm from the fourchette refer to higher center for repair from above. For mid and low fistulas, repairs can be undertaken from below. If there is associated VVF, it should be repaired first [37].

9.2.1.1 Low fistula

Spinal anesthesia, prophylactic antibiotics, supine lithotomy position, aseptic technique, transperineal, transvaginal or transanal approach may be used [32, 37]. The tissue around the fistula is infiltrated with adrenalin-normal saline solution as in VVF. An incision along the anterior anal sphincter border or transverse along the posterior fourchette is deepened and dissected proximally separating the vaginal wall from the perineal body, anal sphincter, anal and rectal walls, developing a reasonable dissection of the rectovaginal space proximally, distally and laterally. The fistula is excised, homeostasis achieved, extraluminal closure of the rectum is done using interrupted 3/0 polyglactin and imbricated with seromuscular layer incorporating the internal anal sphincter using interrupted 2/0 polyglactin. Vaginal wall is closed with 3/0 polyglactin. The external anal sphincter if disrupted is repaired end-to-end with interrupted polyglactin O.

9.2.1.2 Mid fistula

The transvaginal approach is preferred. The principles and techniques are the same. The fistula tract is dissected and excised, wide dissection of the rectovaginal space is done, layered closure of the rectum avoiding the lumen, and interrupted vaginal wall closure with 3/0 delayed absorbable suture.

9.2.1.3 Postoperative care

- Presumptive antibiotics for 5 days, since the wound is contaminated.
- Pain is controlled with pentazocine injection 30 mg 4–6 hourly for about 72 hours.
- Liquid diet for about 5 days, then low residue diet.
- Stool softener as lactulose suspension, without inducing diarrhea.
- Urethral catheter is left for 7 days.

10. Ureterovaginal fistula (UVF)

10.1 Etiology and clinical presentation

This is a pathological communication between the ureter and the vagina. Etiology includes surgical injuries especially hysterectomy [2, 56]. More cases of UVF are appearing in rural practice due to increasing rates of cesarean sections performed by unsupervised medical officers working alone. Other causes of UVF have been discussed by Payne CK and Raz S [56].

Vaginal urinary leakage after gynecologic or obstetric surgery is the commonest symptom. Urine may drain from incision wounds and wound drain. When urine collects in the abdomen or retroperitoneum, nonspecific symptoms of flank and abdominal pains, hiccups, fever, abdominal distension, ileus, localized fluctuance and tenderness may occur.

10.2 Diagnosis

Confirmation of the leakage as urine. Oral phenazopyridine hydrochloride (pyridium) is given. Brown coloration of the leakage confirms it is urine. Intravenous indigo carmine can be used. Dye test as described under VVF can be done. Staining of the gauze at the vault confirms UVF. Intravenous urogram (IVU) and micturating cystourethrogram (MCUG) can also be used. The MCUG will diagnose a bladder fistula, confirm or rule out ureteric reflux; while IVU shows the excretion function of the kidneys, site of contrast extravasation, dilatation of upper tract and contrast in the vagina. A postvoid film is needed to assess for a distal fistula. Once the diagnosis is made or suspected, refer the patient to a urologist.

11. Vesicouterine fistula (VUF)

11.1 Etiology and clinical presentation

An abnormal communication between the uterus or cervix and the urinary bladder. It is uncommon. The commonest cause is lower segment cesarean section [2, 5, 57]. Other causes include myomectomy [17], vaginal operative delivery, induced abortion and, dilatation and curettage. Presentation is the classical "Youssef's syndrome" of symptom complex: "menouria, cyclic hematuria associated with amenorrhea, secondary infertility and urinary continence" [58]. Diagnosis can be made by a combination of contrast cystogram with voiding cystogram and cystoscopy. Refer to a tertiary healthcare institution for multidisciplinary team management.

12. Urethrovaginal fistula (UrVF)

12.1 Etiology and clinical presentation

UrVF is an abnormal connection between the urethra and the vagina. The commonest cause in the developing world is obstructed labor followed by female genital mutilation as 'GISHIRI CUT in Northern Nigeria [8, 15, 37]. In the developed world it occurs as a result of vaginal surgery for incontinence, anterior colporrhaphy, vaginal prolapse and urethral diverticulum [2]. It is often associated with VVF [37]. It presents as urinary leakage from the vagina. A small fistula may produce minimal discomfort, while a large one leaks copiously. Distal small fistulas may be asymptomatic.

12.2 Diagnosis

The diagnosis is made clinically and confirmed by urethrocystoscopy if available or by micturating cystourethrogram.

12.3 Treatment

Treatment is by surgical repair. However, some workers recommend that distal urethral fistulas can be observed or managed with an extended meatotomy [59].

12.3.1 Operative repair

Spinal anesthesia, lithotomy position, aseptic technique is used. Size 16 urethral catheter is passed. The tissue around the fistula is infiltrated with adrenalin normal saline solution 1:100, 000 or plain saline. The fistula tract is encircled with incision. The vaginal skin is dissected free from the urethra all-round the fistula to about 5 mm. An inverted 'U' shaped incision is marked out on the anterior wall of the vagina with the base at the proximal margin of the encircled fistula. The area within the incision is infiltrated with the adrenalin saline solution and dissected off the periurethral fascia as a vaginal wall flap, to a reasonable distance not less than 2 cm. The edges of the fistula are mobilized, reflected over the fistula but not excised. It is closed with interrupted 5/0 monocry (poliglecaprone) or vicryl in the line of least tension. The periurethral fascia is closed perpendicular to the first as a second layer when possible. A Martius flap is raised and tunneled to the repair as an additional layer. The anterior vaginal wall flap is advanced over the closure and sutured with 4/0 vicryl to the distal margin of the wound. This repair technique is well illustrated by Rovner ES, and Leach GE et al. [2, 60]. The repair of UrVF may be very difficult due to relative lack of connective tissues in the mid and distal urethra. Interposition tissue flap is often indicated. Multiple and complex urethrovaginal fistulas should be referred to higher centers for multidisciplinary team approach.

13. Vesicointestinal (vesicoenteric) fistula (VEF)

13.1 Etiology and clinical presentation

This is a rare connection between the lumen of small bowel and urinary bladder. The etiology in the rural areas include penetrating and gunshot injuries to the lower abdomen and pelvis; and iatrogenic trauma. In the developed world, it is caused by diverticulitis, malignancy, Grohn's disease, trauma, foreign body and infection [2, 61].

Presenting symptoms include pneumaturia, fecaluria, debritic urine, lower urinary tract symptoms (LUTs), fever, chills, abdominal pain, hematuria, epididymitis, orchitis, and urine from the rectum [2, 61].

Once suspected, the patient should be referred to a higher center for multidisciplinary team management.

14. Enterovaginal fistula (EVF)

14.1 Etiology and clinical presentation

A rare abnormal connection between the small bowel and vagina. A complication of hysterectomy in the author's experience, **Table 2**. Elsewhere cases arising from Crohn's disease have been reported [62].

14.2 Treatment

Refer promptly and accordingly once diagnosed or suspected in rural practice.

15. Rectourethral fistula (RUF)

15.1 Etiology and clinical presentation

This distressing acquired abnormal communication between the urethra and rectum is seen in males. The author has encountered only seven cases in 28 years; 4 from gunshot **Figure 7**, two from stab injury and 1 iatrogenic endoscopic injury during endourology procedure, **Table 2**. Other causes in the literature are iatrogenic trauma during prostatectomy, cryotherapy, anorectal surgery, pelvic irradiation, urethral instrumentation, infection and Crohn's disease [2, 63]. The symptoms may include fecaluria, hematuria, LUTs, fever, malaise, urinary tract infection (UTI), nausea and vomiting [64].

15.2 Diagnosis

Diagnosis is by history, physical examination, urine microscopy and culture; high index of suspicion; and confirmed by retrograde urethrogram (RUG) and MCUG. Urethrocystoscopy and sigmoidoscopy may visualize the fistula.

15.3 Treatment

15.3.1 Conservative

Some will heal on conservative management [63, 64]. The author managed the RUF that resulted from iatrogenic trauma during a Direct Vision Internal Urethrotomy (DVIU) procedure with urethral catheterization continuous bladder drainage for 3 weeks, low residue diet and appropriate antibiotics cover.

15.3.2 Surgical repair

Surgical repair of RUF is beyond the scope of rural practice. Single and staged repairs with or without urinary and fecal (defunctioning colostomy) diversions have been described involving transrectal, transanal and transperineal approaches [64–69].

The York-Mason procedure is a transrectal approach requiring jack-knife prone position and skilled anesthesia. It has been found to be effective with low morbidity [70].

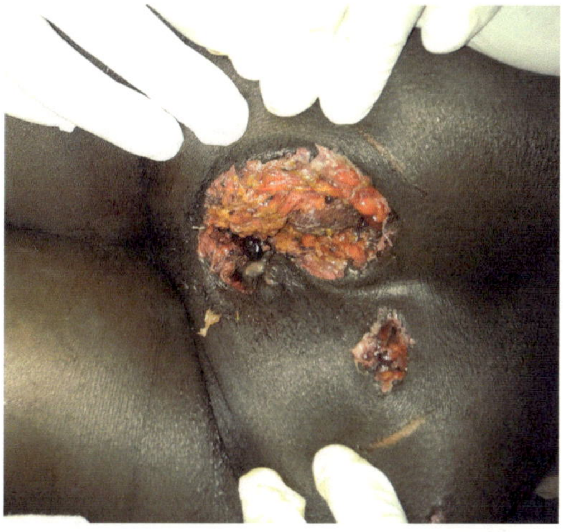

Figure 7.
Perineal gunshot injuries resulting in rectourethral fistula.

16. Vesicocutaneous fistula

16.1 Etiology and clinical presentation

An abnormal communication between the urinary bladder and the skin. The commonest variety is the type connecting the bladder and the skin of the lower abdomen or suprapubic region; **Figure 2**. This commonly follows prolonged or neglected suprapubic catheterization. Other sites encountered are perineum and upper thigh. Males are commonly affected. Other causes include gunshot and stab injuries, fall from heights and following pelvic surgery, **Table 2**.

It presents as urinary leakage through the skin.

16.2 Diagnosis

Diagnosis is clinical and confirmed by MCUG.

16.3 Treatment

16.3.1 Conservative

Removal or bypass of distal urethral obstruction will heal some.

16.3.2 Surgical treatment

Others will require surgical excision of fistulous tract, closure of urinary bladder in layers and wound closure may be primary or delayed depending on its state of cleanliness and contamination.

17. Urethrocutaneous fistula

17.1 Etiology and clinical presentation

This is an acquired connection between the urethra and skin. It commonly occurs on the penis, **Figure 8**.

In rural practice, it results commonly as circumcision mishap [71]. There are reported cases following surgery of urethral stricture and diverticulum; and hypospadias repair [72]. Others include paraurethral abscess, gunshot wounds and chronic inflammatory disease.

17.2 Diagnosis

Diagnosis is clinical.

17.3 Treatment

There is no standardized surgical repair technique for this condition. Each case should be individualized and treated according to its merit. Urethrocutaneous fistulas should be referred to the urologist.

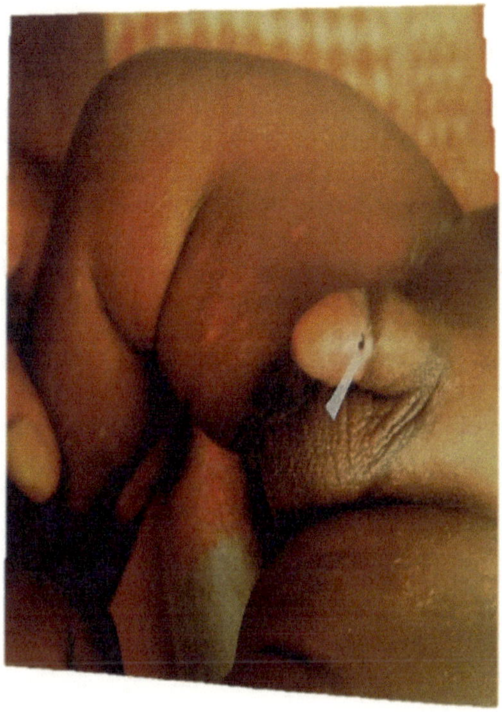

Figure 8.
Urethrocutaneous fistula complicating male circumcision.

18. Role of the rural practitioner and future research

The roles of the rural practitioner have not been clearly defined in the treatment and management of the genitourinary fistula patient. The following roles are suggested from this study. They should:

i. participate in the three preventive strategies mentioned in Section 5, and should participate in the treatment of the fistula from the beginning.

ii. Resuscitate and refer complex and recurrent fistulas promptly to centers with good fistula repair record. Sophisticated ones as UVF, VUF, VEF, EVF, RUF, vesicocutaneous and urethrocutaneous fistulas are beyond the scope of rural practice, and should be referred appropriately once the diagnoses are suspected.

iii. They may undertake the repair of simple fistulas after undergoing adequate training and exposure.

It will be worthwhile to determine the degree of involvement of rural practitioners in the treatment and management of genitourinary fistulas at present, and the impact on the burden of the disease when they are fully integrated.

19. Conclusion

Genitourinary fistulas which occur often in rural practice embarrass the patient and practitioner. The dearth of skilled medical personnel and trained fistula surgeons in the rural areas, made worse by brain drain, poor transport, education and health infrastructures complicate the burden of genitourinary disease. Thus, the patient will be most grateful to the rural practitioner who promptly guides and refers her to a good fistula surgeon who repairs her fistula successfully. The rural clinician should participate effectively in the preventive strategies, initiate treatment and care as soon as fistula occurs, refer complex and sophisticated ones, and may undertake repair of simple fistulas after adequate training and exposure. Good skill, dedication with passion, attention to the principles of fistula management and surgical treatment will achieve high repair success rate. More efforts in training the rural medical practitioner in fistula surgery, education of the girlchild and the public, deployment of more resources to improve social welfare infrastructures, the treatment and rehabilitation of victims, and regular frequent fistula treatment missions will reduce the prevalence of this condition. It is believed that the realization of these objectives will reduce the burden of genitourinary fistulas.

Author details

Chineme Michael Anyaeze[1,2,3]

1 Department of Surgery, Federal Medical Centre Owerri, Imo State, Nigeria

2 Surgery and Urology Unit, Six-C Specialist Clinic, Owerri, Nigeria

3 Mater Misericordiae Hospital, Afikpo, Ebonyi State, Nigeria

*Address all correspondence to: chinemema85@gmail.com

References

[1] Urogenital fistula. Wikipedia.en.m wikipedia.org. Accessed April 1, 2021

[2] Rovner ES., Urinary tract fistulae. in: Alan JW editor. Campbell – Walsh Urology. 10th/International ed; eds Kavoussi LR, Novic AC, Partin AW, Peters CA. Vol. 3. Philadelphia ELSEVIER SAUNDERS 2012 pp 2223 - 2261. ISBN 978-0-8089-2439-5

[3] Murphy M. social consequences of Vesico-Vaginal Fistula in Northern Nigeria. Journal of Biosocial science, vol. 13, issue 2, April 1981, pp. 139 – 150. Doi: https://doi.org/10.1017/s0021932000013304

[4] Lawson J. Vesico – Vaginal Fistula – A Tropical Disease. Trans R Soc Trop Med Hyg. Vol 83, issue 4, July – August 1989, pp 454 - 456, https://doi.org/10.1016/0035-9203(89) 90244 – 7

[5] Zacharin RF. A history of obstetrics vesicovaginal fistula. Aust N Z J surg. 2000; 70:851 - 854

[6] Anyaeze CM, Eke N, Anyanwu KK, and Enendu SE. Rural Medical and Surgical Outreach Mission: Experience of International College of Surgeons (The Nigerian National Section). 2018 Internationalsurgery.org/doi/abs/10.9738/INTSURG –D – 17 – 00131.1

[7] Cron J. Lessons from the developing world: Obstructed labor and the Vesico-vaginal fistula. MedGenMed. 2003 Aug 14; 5(3): 24.

[8] Elkins TE. Surgery for the obstetric vesicovaginal fistula: A review of 100 operations in 82 patients. Am J Obstet Gynecol. 1994; 170: 1108 - 1120

[9] Harrison KA. Child-bearing, health and social priorities: a survey of 22, 774 consecutive hospital births in Zaria, Northern Nigeria. Br J Obtet Gynecol. 1985; [suppl 5] 1 - 119.

[10] Wall LL. Obstetrics fistulas in Africa and the developing world: new efforts to solve an age-old problem. Women's Health issues. 996; 6:229 – 234

[11] Godwin WE, Scardino PT. Vesicovaginal and ureterovaginal fistulas: A summary of 25 years of experience. J Urol. 1980; 123:370 – 374

[12] SN Obi, BC Ozumba, AK Onyebuchi. Decreasing incidence and changing aetiological factors of vesico-vaginal fistula in south–east Nigeria. J Obstet Gynecol. 2008. Aug; 28(6):629 – 31. Doi: 10.1080/01443610802397686. PMID: 19003661

[13] DK Uprety, S Subedi, B Budhathoki, MC Regmi. Vesiovaginal fistula at tertiary care center in eastern Nepal. JNMA J Nepal Med Assoc. Jul – Sep 2008; 47[171]: 120 – 2

[14] Hilton P, Ward A. Epidemiological and surgical aspects of urogenital fistulae: a review of 25 years' experience in southeast Nigeria. Int Urogynecol J Pelvic Floor Dysfunct 1998;9(4): 189 - 94.doi: 10.1007/BF01901602. PMD: 9795822

[15] Danso KA, Martey JO, Wall LL, Elkins TE. The epidemiology of genitourinary fistulae in Kumasi, Ghana, 1997-1992. Int Urogynecol J Pelvic Floor Dysfunct. 1996. 7(3): 117 – 120. doi:10.1007/BF01894198. PMID: 8913827

[16] Priyadarshi V, Singh JP, Bera MK, Kundu AK, Pal DK. Genitourinary fistula: An Indian perspective. J Obstet Gynaecol India. 2016 June; 66 (3): 180 – 184. doi: 10.1007/s13224 - 051-0672-2.

[17] Okafor PI, Orakwe JC, Mbonu OO. Cyclical haematuria sequel to uterine myomectomy: A case report. West Afr J Med. 2002; 21(4): 341 - 342

[18] Ijaya MA, Rahman AG, Aboyeji AP, Olatinwo AW, Esuga SA, Ogah OK, Raji HO, Adebara IO, Akintobi AO, Adeniran AS, Adewole AA. Vesiocovaginal fistua: a review of Nigerian experience. West Afr J Med. 2010 Sep – Oct; 29[5]: 293 – 8 doi: 10.4314/wajm. v29i5.68247. PMID: 21089013

[19] PH Daru, JA Karshima, S Mikah, D Nyango. The burden of vesico-vaginal fistula in North Central Nigeria. J West Afr Coll Surg. 2011 April – Jun; 1 [2]: 50 - 62.

[20] Arrowsmith SD, Hamlin EC, Wall LL. Obstructed labor injury complex: Obstetric fistula formation and the multifaceted morbidity of maternal birth trauma in the developing world. Obstet Gynecol Surv. 1995;51: 568 - 574.

[21] Tahzib F. Epidemiological determinants of vesicovaginal fistulas. Br J Obstet Gynaecol. 1983; 90: 387 – 391

[22] Emembolu J. The obstetric fistula: Factors associated with improved pregnancy outcome after a successful repair. Int J Gynecol Obstet. 1992; 39: 205 - 212.

[23] Ekanem EI, Ekanem AD, Ekabua JE. Review of obstetrics genito – Urinary fistulae in the University of Calabar Teaching Hospital Calabar, Nigeria. Niger J Clin Pract. 2010; 13[3]:326 – 330

[24] Tancer ML. A report of thirty - four instances of urethrovaginal and bladder neck fistulas. Surg. Gynecol Obstet. 1993; 177:77 – 80

[25] Gerstenbluth RE, Goldman HB. Simultaneous urethral erosion of tension-free vaginal tape and woven polyester pubovaginal sling. J Urol. 2003; 170[2 pt 1]: 525 – 526

[26] Glavind K, Larsen EH. Results and complications of tension – Free vaginal tape (TVT) for surgical treatment of female stress incontinence. Int Urogynecol J Pelv Floor Dysfunct. 2001; 12 (6): 370 – 372.

[27] Carlin BI, Klutke CG. Development of urethrovaginal fistula following periurethral collagen injection. J urol. 2000; 164: 124

[28] Krissi H, Levy T, Ben – Rafael Z. Fistula formation after large loop excision of the transformation zone in patients with cervical intraepithelial neoplasia. Acta Obstet Gynecol Scand. 2001; 80: 1137 – 1138

[29] Abang M. Nigeria's Medical brain drain. Healthcare woes as doctors flee. www.aljazeera.com 8 Apr 2019.

[30] Imafidon J. One Way Traffic: Nigeria's Medical Brain Drain. A Challenge for Maternal Health and Public Health System in Nigeria. 2018. https://escholarship.org/uc/item/5q36r5xq

[31] Hutton JE Jr, Rich NM. Wounding and Wound Ballistics: Observations of Ballistic Behavior of Projectiles in Flight. In: McAninch JW (ed), Traumatic and Reconstructive Urology 1996. W. B. Saunders, pp 6 – 24. ISBN 0 – 7216 – 3886 – 4

[32] Adam R. Vesicovaginal, Urogenital and Rectovaginal Fistulas. In: Kovac SR, Zimmerman CW (eds). Reconstructive vaginal surgery. Philadelphia. LIPPINCOTT WILLIAMS & WILKINS. WOLTERS KLUWER HEALTH 2007, pp. 339 – 353.

[33] Domestic general government health expenditure per capital (US$) – Nigeria, Ghana, Kenya, Sub-saharan Africa. World Health Organization Global Health Expenditure data base (apps. who. Int/nha/database) data. Worldbank.org. Accessed Apr 27 2020

[34] Akinlusi F. Towards eliminating obstetric fistula in Nigeria. A time for

action. Be an Advocate For change. https://www.amchfoundation.com/towards-eliminating-obstetric-fistula-in-Nigeria/. Accessed April 11 2021

[35] Federal Ministry of Health, Nigeria. National Strategic Framework for Elimination of Obstetric Fistula in Nigeria, 2019 – 2023. 2019

[36] Nigeria|Fistula Foundation. Fistula. fistulafoundation.org. Accessed Apr 11, 2021

[37] Vesicovaginal Fistula (VVFs). In: King M, Bewes P, Cairns J, Thornton J [eds]; Primary Surgery vol. one. Non – Traumatic. Low – Priced ed. Oxford University Press. Oxford, Delhi, Kuala Lumpur, PP 228 – 291. ISBN 0-19-261694-3

[38] Arrowsmith SD. The classification of obstetric vesico – vaginal fistulas. A call for evidence – based approach. Int. J. Obstet Gynaecol. 2007; 99(1): 25 – 27. https://doi.org/10.1016/j.ijgo.2007.06.018

[39] Waaldjik K. Surgical classification of obstetric fistula. Int J Obstet Gynaecol.1995;49(2);161 – 163.

[40] Leng WW, Amundsen CL, McGuire EJ. Management of female, genito urinary fistulas: Transvesical or transvaginal approach? J. Urol 1998; 160: 1995 – 1999.

[41] Ogboli – Nwasor E. Drugs used in Total Intravenous Anaesthesia (TIVA). In: Total Intravenous Anaesthesia (TIVA) Made Easy. 2012. pp 11 – 23. ISBN: 978 – 125 – 843 – 8. Ahmadu Bello University Press Limited, Zaria, Nigeria.

[42] Rosen MA, McAninch JW. Wound closures and suture techniques in Reconstructive Procedures. In: McAninch J W (ed), Traumatic and Reconstructive Urology. 1996. W.B Saunders, PP 49 – 69. ISBN 0 – 7216 – 3886 - 4. Philadelphia London Toronto Montreal Sydney Tokyo.

[43] Sims JM. On the treatment of vesico – Vaginal fistula. 1852 Int J Urol. 1998; 9: 236 – 248. Doi:10.1007/BF01901610. PMID:9795830.

[44] Latzko W. Postoperative vesicovaginal fistulas, genesis and therapy. Am J Surg. 1942; 58: 211 – 228.

[45] Kieserman – Shmokler C, Sammarco AG, English EM, Swenson CW, Delancey JOL. The Latzko, a high value, versatile vesicovaginal fistula repair. International Continence Society 2018. Philadelphia Programme 532. Abstract 633.

[46] Ansquer Y, Mellier G, Santu Ui P, Bennis M, Mandelbrot L, Madelenat P, Carbonne B, Mathevet P. Latzko operation for vault vesicovaginal fistula. Acta Obstetricia et Gynaecologica. 2006; 85:1248 – 1251.

[47] Cardenas - Trowers C, Heusinkveld J, Hatch K. Simple and effective: transvaginal vesico – vaginal fistula repair with a modified Latzko technique. Int Urogynecol J. 2018 May; 29(5):767 – 769. doi: 10.1007/s00192 - 017-3471 - 8. Epub 2017 Sep 7. PMID: 28884350

[48] Zimmern PE, Hadley HR, Staskin DR, et al: Genitourinary fistulae. Vaginal approach for repair of vesicovaginal fistulae. Urol Clin North Am 12:361, 1985.

[49] Eilber KS, Kavaler E, Rodriguez LV, et al. Ten years' experience with transvaginal vesicovaginal fistula repair using tissue interposition. J Urol 2003; 169:1033 – 1036.

[50] Ganabathi K, Sirls L, Zimmern PE, Leach GE. Vesicovaginal Fistulas: Reconstructive Techniques. In: McAninch JW (ed), Traumatic and Reconstructive Urology. 1996 W. B. Saunders, pp 31 - 35.

[51] Wein AJ, Malloy TR, Carpiniello VL, et al. Repair of vaginal fistula by a

suprapubic trans-vesical approach. Surg. Gynecol Obstet 150:57, 1980.

[52] Collins CG, Pent D, Jones FB, Results of early repair of vesicovaginal fistula with preliminary cortisone treatment. AM J Obstet. Gynecol. 80:1005, 1960.

[53] Tancer ML. The post – Total hysterectomy (vault) vesicovaginal fistula. J Urol 123:839, 1980.

[54] Blaivas JG, Heritz DM, Romanzi LJ. Early versus late repair of vesicovaginal fistulas: Vaginal and abdominal approaches. J Urol. 1995; 153 (4); 1110 – 1112.

[55] Carr LK, Webster GD. Abdominal repair of vesicovaginal fistula. Urology. 1996; 48(1): 10 – 11

[56] Payne CK, Raz S. Ureterovaginal and related fistulas. In: McAninch JW (Ed), Traumatic and Reconstructive Urology. 1996. W.B Saunders, pp 213 – 247.

[57] Bhattacharjee S, Kohli UA, Sood A, Tripathy S, Gupta M. Vesicouterine fistula: Youssef's syndrome. Med J Armed Forces India 2015 July; 71 (suppl 1). S175 – S177. Doi: 10.1016/j. mjafi.2013.11.006. PMID:26265822.

[58] Youssef AF. Menouria following lower segment cesarean section: A syndrome. AM J Obstet Gynecol. 1957, 73:759 – 767.

[59] Lamensdorf H, Compre DE, Begley GF. Simple correction of urethrovaginal fistula. Urology. 1977 Aug; 10(2):152 – 3. doi:10.1016/0090 - 4295(77)90017 – 6. PMID:898457.

[60] Leach GE, Kobashi KC. Urethral diverticulum and fistula. In: Cordozo L, Staskin D (eds). Textbook of Female Urology and Urogynecology. London: Isis Medical Media; 2001.PP. 721 – 745.

[61] Basler D, Adekoya E. Enterovesical Fistula: Practice Essentials. In: Schwartz BF(ed) emedicine. medscape.com Dec. 24, 2020. Accessed Apr 19, 2021.

[62] Givel JC, Hawker P, Allan RN, Alexander – Williams J. Enterovaginal fistulas associated with Crohn's disease. Surg Gynecol Obstet 1982 Oct; 155(4): 494 – 496. PMID:6889768.

[63] Kumar S, Kekre NS, Gopalakrishnan G. Diagnosis and Conservative treatment of Tubercular Rectoprostatic Fistula. Ann R Coll Surg Engl.2006 Jan; 88(1):26. doi:10.1308/ 147870806X83242. PMC 1963633. PMID. 16460634.

[64] Thomas C, Jonas J, Jager Wetral. Incidence, clinical symptoms and management of recto-urethral fistulas after radical prostatectomy. J. Urol 183: 608 – 612. https://doi.org/10.1016/j, juro.2009.10.020.

[65] Burkowski TP, Chakrabarty A, Powell IJ et al. Acquired rectourethral fistula: Methods of repair. J. Urol 1995. 153: 730 – 733. https://doi.org/10.1016/ s0022-5347(01)67701-2.

[66] Dreznik Z, Alper D, Vishne TH et al. Rectal flap advancement – A simple and effective approach for the treatment of rectourethral fistula. Colorectal Dis 2003 Jan 10. 5: 53 – 55. https://doi.org/ 10.1046/j.1463 - 1318.2003.00400.x

[67] Gupta G, Kumar S, Kekre NS et al. Surgical management of rectourethral fistula. Urol 2008. 71: 267 – 271. Doi: https://doi.org/10.1016/j.urology. 2007. 10.042.

[68] Razi A, Yahyazadeh SR, Gilani MAS, Kazemeyni. SM, Transanal repair of rectourethral and rectovaginal fistulas. Urol J 2008 Spring; 5:111 – 114. PMID:18592464.

[69] Garofalo TE, Delaney CP, Remzi FH, Fazio VW. Rectal advancement flap repair of rectourethral fistula: A 20 – Year experience. 2003 Dis Colon 46 (6)

p 762 - 769. doi:10.1007/s10350 - 004-6654 - 6.

[70] Crippa A, Dall'Oglio MF, Nesrallah LJ, Hasegawa E, Antunes A, Srougi M. The York – Mason technique for recto-urethral fistulas. Clinics Vol. 62 No.6 Sao Paulo 2017. httsp://doi.org/10.1590/S1807 - 59322007000600007.

[71] Ahmed A, Mbibu, Dawam D, Kalayi GD. Complications of traditional male circumcision. Annals of Tropical Paediatrics (1999) 19, 113 – 117.

[72] Srivastava RK, Tandale MS, Panse N, Gupta A, Sahane P. Management of urethrocutaneous fistula after hypospadias surgery – An experience of thirty – five cases. Indian J Plast Surg. 2011 Jan – Apr; 44(1): 98 – 103. Doi: 10.4103/0970 – 0358.81456. PMCID: PMC3111134. PMID: 21713169

Section 3

Human Resources for Health Promotion

Chapter 4

Improving Human Resource for Health in Rural Northern Nigeria

Adetoro A. Adegoke, Godwin Y. Afenyadu,
Fatima L. Adamu and Sally Findley

Abstract

Inadequate number of health workers in rural areas is a major concern in many countries. It causes underutilization, prevents equitable access of health services, and is a barrier to universal health coverage. To increase the number and improve retention of health workers in rural areas, the World Health Organization (WHO) issued global recommendations to improve the rural retention of the health workforce. This paper presents the experiences of adopting and implementing the WHO recommendations in four states in Northern Nigeria. It highlights the results, challenges and lessons learnt with the implementation. We used an implementation research approach and evaluated the implementation at three stages: the pilot; full implementation; and immediate post exit. A total of 477 midwives were recruited and deployed to rural health facilities over a period of four years. Of these, 196 (41%) were in Jigawa, 126 (26.4%) in Yobe, 78 (16.4%) in Zamfara and 77 (16.1%) in Katsina. Midwives' retention rates increased gradually over the four years. In three (Jigawa, Katsina and Zamfara) of the four states, midwives' retention rates increased from 69.2% in Jigawa in 2013 to 98% in 2016; from 53.3% in Katsina in 2013 to 100% retention in 2016. Zamfara made the most progress with a poor retention rate of 42.8% in 2013 to 100% retention rate in 2016. In Yobe state, the retention rate of 47% in 2013 gradually increased to 100% in 2015. This however slightly dropped to 90% in 2016 as a result of the deteriorating security situation in 2015. Other effects of the initiative included: heightened determination of states to increase the production of indigenous midwives; reversal of policy directives that banned the recruitment of health workers including midwives; and to provide incentives such as safe and comfortable accommodation.

Keywords: Rural retention, universal health coverage, incentives scheme, skilled birth attendance, rural health workers, midwives

1. Introduction

The Maternal Mortality Ratio (MMR) in Nigeria is amongst the highest in the world (576 per 100,000 live births) [1]. Within Nigeria, the burden of MMR remains heaviest in the Northern part of the country with rates as high as 1549 and 1025 per 100,000 live births in the Northeast and Northwest zones respectively [2]. Most of these deaths occur in the rural areas where about 69–70% of the population lives. It is estimated that the MMR could be as high as 1,732 per 1000,000 live births amongst the rural population under longitudinal surveillance by the Nahuche Health and demographic surveillance system in Zamfara state [2].

The high mortality rates in Northern Nigeria are due to a multiple of factors such as gaps in the health system, socioeconomic factors, and cultural norms regarding practices during labor and childbirth [3]. The key to addressing these factors is access to culturally appropriate and quality maternal health care for antenatal care, family planning counselling, and skilled birth attendance, with availability of basic emergency obstetric care providing quality intrapartum and immediate postnatal care [4]. An adequate and equitable distribution of maternal health care workers is therefore key to reducing maternal mortality rates [3, 4].

Providing an adequate number of maternal health care workers in Northern Nigeria requires increasing the number of qualified midwives who are trained and willing to be sent to the rural clinics where they are most needed. The harsh working environment in the rural areas however, discourages midwives from going to and staying at rural health facilities [5]. Health facilities in the rural areas of Northern states are therefore understaffed with qualified midwives and are consequently largely dysfunctional. Even experienced midwives from these states are unwilling to be posted to the rural health facilities, leaving them largely staffed by Community Health Extension Workers (CHEWs) and young, inexperienced, unmarried midwives from Southern Nigeria who are undergoing their compulsory post-graduation clinical service as part of the national Midwives Service Scheme (MSS) [6, 7].

To attract, recruit and retain health workers in rural and underserved areas, the World Health Organisation (WHO) recommends an integrated set of incentive mechanisms. As shown in **Table 1**, the integrated bundle spans the

A. Education	A1. Students from rural backgrounds
	A2. Health professional schools outside major cities
	A3. Clinical rotation in rural areas during studies
	A4. Curricula that reflect rural health issues
	A5. Continuous professional development for rural health workers
B. Regulatory	B1. Enhanced scope of practice
	B2. Different types of health workers
	B3. Compulsory service
	B4. Subsidized education for return of service
C. Financial incentives	C1. Appropriate financial incentives
D. Professional and personal support	D1. Better living conditions
	D2. Safe and supportive working environment
	D3. Outreach support
	D4. Career development programmes
	D5 Professional networks
	D6 Public recognition measures

Source: WHO. (2010). Increasing access to health workers in remote and rural areas through improved retention: global policy recommendations. Geneva: World Health Organization; 2010.

Table 1.
WHO framework to attract, recruit and retain health workers (including midwives) in rural areas.

areas of education, regulation, financial rewards, and the improvement in the working environment and welfare of the health worker. It recommends wide stakeholder consultation in adapting this model to state-specific needs along with effective monitoring and evaluation of whichever package is adopted [8].

In 2011, four Northern Nigerian states with severe shortages of health workers met to begin adapting this WHO framework for their needs. These consultative meetings included Directors of State Primary Health Care Development Agency, Health Human Resources, State Ministry of Health (SMOH), Heads of Midwifery and Nursing training institutions, and a few midwives. During these meetings, these stakeholders conducted their own situational analysis to prioritize and contextualize the WHO recommendations on incentive mechanisms to attract, recruit, and retain female health workers. There was a broad consensus that the most critical shortage was for midwives, who were grossly inadequate in numbers and inequitably distributed. By the end of 2012, each state had developed an incentive package to produce, attract, recruit, and retain midwives in rural health facilities as shown in **Table 2**. They also developed implementation plans, which included routine monitoring and evaluation to feedback into the implementation process. The package developed by each state was called the Midwife Recruitment and Retention Scheme (MRRS). The developmental process has been described in an earlier publication [9].

In this paper, we describe the 2012–2016 MRRS implementation experience and results from each of the four Northern Nigerian states (Jigawa, Katsina, Yobe and Zamfara).

State	Proposed Incentive Package
Jigawa State	Payment of Midwife specific rural allowance
	Provision of safe and comfortable accommodation and water
	Provide safe working environment, equipment and logistics
	Providing priority access to continuous education
	Instituting public recognition and award scheme
Yobe State	Payment of midwife specific hardship allowance in addition to any existing allowance
	Provide safe and comfortable accommodation to improve living conditions
	Enhance the scope of practice of rural midwives
	Schemes to support continuing education and professional development of midwives in rural practice
Katsina State	Payment of midwife specific rural allowance
	Provision of safe accommodation, portable water and electricity
	Provision of supervision and mentoring support to MSS midwives
	Provision of permanent employment to non-indigenes
Zamfara State	Payment of midwife specific rural allowance
	Provision of accommodation with easy reach of MNCH facility
	Lift ban on recruitment of midwives to targeted rural health facilities providing MNCH services

Source: Afenyadu et al. [9].

Table 2.
Agreed state specific incentive package to attract, recruit and retain midwives at inception.

2. Methods

Study design: Each state used phased implementation research to assess the implementation of each of three implementation phases:

Phase 1: Pilot phase (2012–2013). The first phase focused on establishing all the elements of the incentive package. During this phase, additional modifications to the MRRS incentives may have been adopted, after reconciliation of the MRRS with the realities of political support, human resource (HR) policy, and budgetary funding availability in each state.

Phase 2: Full Implementation phase (2013–2016). During the full implementation phase, the Women for Health (W4H) programme supported the states to initiate the necessary HR policy reforms and provide the budgetary allocations necessary to roll out each state-specific package. Each state worked towards an effective implementation of the full complement of an incentive package carefully selected from the four broad intervention areas of Education, Regulation, Financial Incentives, and Professional and/or Personal support as outlined in **Table 2**. Implementation was also conditional on having midwives available to be recruited from anywhere in Nigeria, as well as rural health facilities being functional with the requisite logistics, supplies, and equipment. During 2013–2014, W4H provided some financial support to pay the salaries and rural allowances of the midwives posted to rural facilities per each state's MRRS incentive package. From 2015 onward, each state took over the responsibility for this financial support. They developed and initiated the roll out of sustainability plans by the end of this period.

Phase 3: Post-exit phase (2016–2017). W4H supported the continuing monitoring and evaluation of the implementation by the states.

Evaluation Methods: The evaluation was guided by the MRRS logic model shown in **Figure 1**. The evaluation used multiple methods, both qualitative and quantitative, with repeated measures of the outputs and outcomes throughout the study period.

2.1 Monitoring and evaluation activities

2.1.1 Establishment of State MRRS Implementation Committees

The State Implementation Committee (SIC) consist of key stakeholders including those from the State Primary Health Care Development Agency, SMOH, and the Local Government Areas (LGAs). The SIC engaged key decision makers,

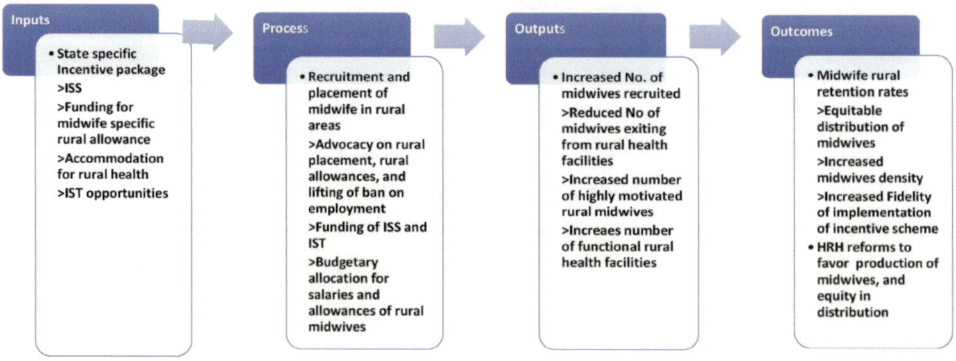

Figure 1.
MRRS Logic model.

gatekeepers, and centers of power, especially those responsible for policy decision-making and the management of the budgetary funds required to roll out the incentive packages. It also monitored and provided feedback on progress and challenges with the implementation process at several cross-state review meetings that were organized to facilitate cross-state learning and sharing of experience [10].

2.1.2 Assessment of state of readiness for full implementation at the end of the pilot phase

At the end of the pilot phase, each state team was facilitated to assess its readiness to implement its MRRS package by ranking the perceived status of selected determinants of readiness to cope with the initial implementation stage. These determinants were: cooperation and support of stakeholders (CS), team confidence (TC), management of fear and resistance to change (F&R), favorable (recruitment) policy environment (FPE), reporting and reviewing framework (RRF), availability of human resource (AHR), and availability of a funding stream (AF) [11].

Each member of the SIC ranked, by scoring each of the determinants from one to three, where three is the highest and one is the lowest. The scores by each member of the committee were then aggregated and averaged for each determinant. This helped to obtain a consensus position on the state readiness of each participating state. A radial graph that summarizes the status of the determinants in each state is shown in **Figures 2–5**. The graphs illustrate the extent to which each state is ready or able to cope with the initial implementation phase as determined by the status of the seven variables.

The assessment method depends on group judgment or consensus. In spite of standardizing the methodology and data tools, the variations within the group judgment or consensus from one state to the other limits, comparability between states. However, it aptly describes the status of readiness as perceived by each state and helped map out what determinants require more attention for a successful implementation.

2.1.3 Monthly collection of data on midwife retention

Data were collected monthly from each participating rural health facility on number of midwives at post at the beginning of the month at each rural facility in

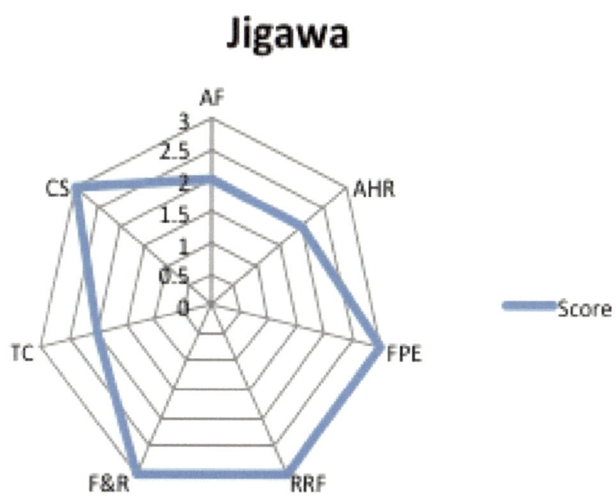

Figure 2.
Jigawa state-strongest supporting structures for change.

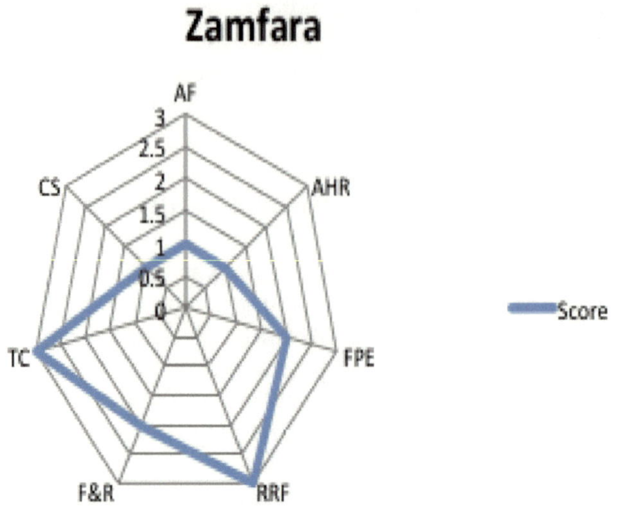

Figure 3.
Zamfara state-weakest supporting structures for change.

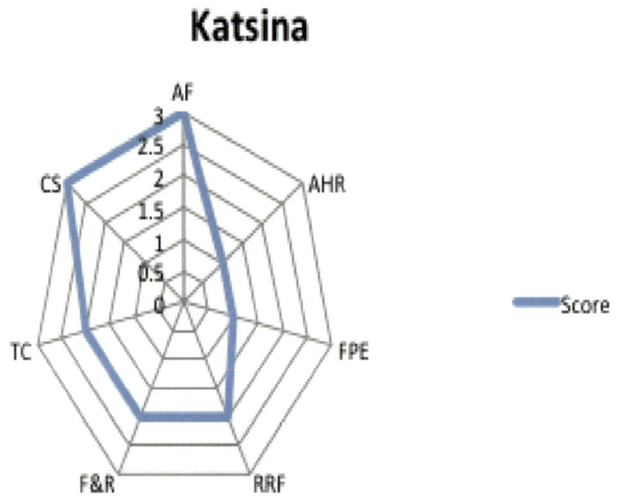

Figure 4.
Katsina state readiness.

the scheme (x), numbers of midwives posted that month (y) and the numbers exiting that month from the facility (z). After cleaning, quarterly retention rates were computed and feedback was provided to the state implementation teams. Percentage Retention Rates (PRR) values were calculated for each month as: $PRR = (x + y - z)/(x + y)$ x100%. These PRR were subsequently discussed at the quarterly cross-state review meetings, where outliers (very high or low) attrition or exit rates were interrogated for any lessons that might be learned for strengthening MRRS implementation.

2.1.4 Quarterly cross state review meetings

During implementation, a series of review meetings were held with the state implementation teams to track progress, discuss challenges encountered, share

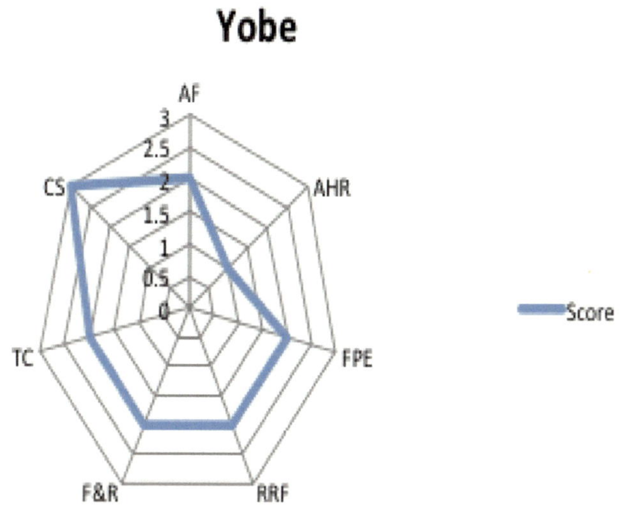

Figure 5.
Yobe state readiness. Legend: AF, Availability of funding stream (fiscal budget); AHR, Availability of Human Resource (Midwives); FPE, Favorable Policy environment; RRF, Reporting and Reviewing Framework; F&R, Management of fear and /or resistance to change and the complexities of change; TC, Team confidence; CS, Cooperation and support of stakeholders.

information on how such challenges were resolved or mitigated, and propose recommendations to strengthen the implementation of the incentive scheme.

2.1.5 Annual evaluation

An independent consultant was engaged each year to evaluate the MRRS scheme, guided by terms of reference relevant to the stage of implementation of the initiative across implementing states. The methods adopted included a survey of midwives, key informant interviews of selected key stakeholders at the community, LGA, and state levels.

2.1.6 Post-exit evaluation activities

Comparable to the annual evaluation, post-exit evaluations were conducted in 2016 to focus on sustainability of the results and steps taken to sustain the gains of the initiative.

Ethical approval: As this study was categorized under service evaluation, ethics committee approval was not needed because the study does not constitute research in Nigeria, where it was conducted. Written informed consent was however obtained from all participants to collect, analyze and publish the data.

3. Results

3.1 The Pilot Implementation Phase (2012–2013)

The pilot phase of the implementation was an opportunity to assess the complications of implementation and determine feasibility and readiness of the key stakeholders to support and fund the initiative. The phase was found to be associated with some hesitation by some policymakers, especially where the implementation of a particular component of the proposed incentive package meant reviewing existing state policies or providing additional budgetary funds.

3.2 Recruitment of midwives into the scheme

All four states in 2012 were well below the WHO global minimum standard of three midwives or nurses per 1000 women of reproductive age [12]. As shown in **Table 3**, Jigawa and Katsina had just under two midwives per 1000 women of reproductive age, and Yobe and Zamfara had only half (or less) as many. Across all states, 67% of the midwives' salaries were paid by the states. About 30% of midwives were supported by the federal MSS, which assigns newly graduated midwives to rural health facilities. Most of the MSS midwives came from states outside the Northern region, which already poses a retention challenge. This in part is due to cultural differences and the fact that the newly qualified midwives are young and may need to return to marry from their regions.

Production of midwives was severely constrained in all the states. At the inception of the W4H program, of the seven Nursing and Midwifery training institutions in the four states, none had full accreditation, three had provisional accreditation, and four were denied accreditation. A full accreditation status would allow the training institution to admit 100 students for training while a provisional accreditation meant that the training institution could admit 50 students. A denied accreditation, however, meant an embargo on student admission for training. Even though three of these training institutions had provisional accreditation, and could recruit 50 students per cohort per year, the training institutions were also experiencing high drop-out and low graduation rates. All these contribute to reduce number of health workers produced in the states.

In two of the states (Katsina and Zamfara), there was an embargo on employment of workers including midwives. In the remaining two states where employment was allowed, there was difficulty in getting midwives to recruit from within the state, due to inadequate production. These states were also unable to attract midwives from other states for recruitment. This is because midwives coming from other states preferred pensionable employment, but could only be offered non-pensionable contracts. Pensionable contracts were only available for indigenous health workers from the state. The recruitment into the rural MRRS was further encumbered by the lack of appropriate accommodation for the midwives in rural areas. Indeed, even if midwives were available, the scheme could only expand if functional rural health facilities with suitable accommodation were available. As

State	Population	Total Midwives	Midwife Density/1000 pop	Non-State Government sources
Jigawa	5,286,804	511	0.96	• MSS = 143 • Subsidy Reinvestment and Empowerment Programme-Maternal Newborn and Child Health (SURE-P MCH) =42
Katsina	6,500,000	581	0.89	• MSS = 144
Yobe	2,885,518	77	0.26	• MSS = 31 • SURE-P MCH = 1
Zamfara	4,064,012	202	0.50	• MSS = 89 • SURE-P MCH =5

Table 3.
2013 Midwife density in implementing states.

State	Category of Midwives			
	MSS	State government	SURE-P MCH	Total
Katsina	8	2	—	10
Yobe	14	1	—	15
Jigawa	18	3	3	24
Zamfara	12	1	—	13

Table 4.
Types of Midwives in the MRRS during the Pilot Phase.

shown in **Table 4**, across all states there were only 63 midwives enrolled in the MRRS (5% of the 1369 midwives in the states), and most of these had their salary support from the MSS.

3.3 Fidelity of implementation

The fidelity of implementation of the state specific rural incentive bundles is the extent to which the proposed contents of the rural incentive bundle had been implemented, calculated as an adherence ratio equal to the proportion of the components actually implemented out of the total proposed bundle of components. In addition, the status of implementation of each individual component of the state-specific incentive bundle was ranked by each SIC on a scale of 1 to 3: 1 = Not yet implemented (red), 2 = Partially implemented (yellow), 3 = Fully implemented (green).

As shown in **Table 5**, in the Pilot Phase (2013), no participating state could implement the full complement of its proposed incentive bundle to attract, recruit and retain midwives to work and live in health facilities in rural and underserved areas (Fidelity ratio < 1). Payment of midwife specific allowances was fully implemented in all states, although payment was irregular or in arrears, for example in Jigawa.

The components of the incentive bundles that could not be implemented during the pilot phase were largely those involving policy decisions by "power centers" who had little interest in those components, even if not fully voiced at the time of configuring the incentive package at the consultative meetings. These components included "decisions to lift the ban on employment," "enhancing the scope of practice of rural health workers (task shifting)," "granting preferential access to in-service training to midwives working in the rural health facilities," and the institutionalization of "public recognition and awards" for rural health workers, especially midwives.

These components require the support of those who control state political power and fiscal budgetary resources. Indeed, the ultimate decisions on health policy issues in the state were neither made by the technocrats or the directors responsible for the various departments of the health service (such as Human Resources, Nursing, and Policy and Planning), nor by the commissioner of health alone, but by the state governor.

The provision of suitable accommodation is capital intensive and was only partially implemented in most states. The SICs attributed the delay to the time required to present the bill of quantities (BoQ) and some bureaucracy associated with issuing contracts for the refurbishment of available accommodation. The BoQ, prepared by quantity surveyors, provided project specific measured quantities of the items of work identified by the drawings and specifications in the tender documentation. Preparing a BoQ requires that the design is complete and a specification has been prepared. Katsina and Jigawa states were yet to receive required

		Status of Implementation – Pilot Phase 2013		
State	**Bundle components**	**Fully**	**Partial**	**Not yet**
Jigawa State	Payment of ME specific allowance of N20,000 per month		[yellow]	
	Improve living conditions			[red]
	Provide safe working environment, equipment and logistics		[yellow]	
	Provision of safe accommodation within easy reach of facility & provision of water		[yellow]	
	Granting of preferential access to rural midwife to continuous education			[red]
	Public Recongition and award scheme			[red]
Yobe State	Improvement of living conditions of midwives working and living in the rural area		[yellow]	
	Enhanace the scope of practice for rural midwives (task sharing)			[red]
	Payment of midwife specific hardship allowance in addition to any existing allowance	[green]		
	Support continuing education and professional development of midwives living and working in the rural areas	[green]		
Katsina State	Payment of Midwife specific rural allowance	[green]		
	Provision of permanent employments		[yellow]	
	Provide supportive supervision and mentoring to MSS midwives	[green]		
	Provide safe accommodation znd portable water & electricity		[yellow]	
Zamfara State	Life ban on recruitment of midwives to targeted rural health facilities providing MNCH sevices			[red]
	Provide accommodation withi easy reach of MNCH facility		[yellow]	
	Payment of midwife specific rural allowance	[green]		
Legend				
[green]	Fully Implemented			
[yellow]	Partially implemented			
[red]	Unable to implement			

Table 5.
Fidelity of Implementation by the end of Pilot Phase.

funds to refurbish accommodation that would facilitate the planned expansion into additional health facilities due to unexplained bureaucratic bottlenecks.

3.4 Readiness to install incentive scheme to attract, recruit, and retain midwives in rural health facilities

At the end of the pilot phase, a state government was considered "ready to implement its midwife recruitment and retention scheme" if the following conditions were met:

- Availability of funds or willingness to contribute financially to the implementation of the initiative (AF)

- State government is demonstrably willing to invest in the production of midwives or take the pragmatic steps to make the human resource (midwives) available to service the scheme (AHR); A favorable state human resource for health (HRH) recruitment policy environment (FPE); Capacity to manage resistance or fear of change (F&R)

- Confident state implementation committee (TC); existing mechanisms for reporting and reviewing the implementation process (RRF); and the cooperation of relevant stakeholders (CS).

Across the four states, Zamfara, was the least prepared to cope with the complexities and challenges associated with the pilot phase. It scored 13 out of a maximum of 21 points. It was the most constrained with funding, had a ban on employment of health workers (including midwives), and was not getting optimal support and cooperation from some stakeholders.

In summary, the key challenges faced during the pilot phase of implementation were limited to no availability of midwives, an unfavorable HRH policy environment, and inadequate funding. The shortage of midwives in the states was linked to the low output of trained midwives from the state schools of midwifery, as well as the existing ban on employment in Jigawa, Katsina and Zamfara states. The policy of non-pensionable employment of midwives from the southern states of the country was counterproductive. As it made it difficult to attract midwives from other states to come and work in these four states. The provision of suitable accommodation for midwives posted to the rural areas and payment of midwife specific rural allowances require funding, which had budgetary implications.

4. The full implementation phase (2013 to 2015)

This phase was characterized by an expansion of the initiative, with intensified advocacy efforts to: increase availability and deployment of midwives to the targeted rural health facilities; improve the fidelity of implementation of the MRRS by working with all relevant stakeholders; pay rural incentive allowance; provide accommodation; provide supportive supervision; and provide opportunities for in-service training. It was also the stage for planning sustainability as implementation approached 2015.

During this phase, the W4H program supported the recruitment and posting of midwives to rural health facilities by providing funding for salaries and rural allowances with the understanding that the state governments would make the necessary policy reforms and budgetary allocations to take over the payment of salaries and rural allowances of these midwives and recruit additional ones. By the end of 2015, the W4H brought this financial support to an end and the period of full implementation was subsequently evaluated.

4.1 Progress made over the implementation period

4.1.1 Jigawa State

The Jigawa state government sustained the regular payment of salaries, rural allowances, and also provided accommodation for rural midwives over the implementation period. Although accommodations were provided, not all of them were fully furnished. The recruitment and placement of midwives in rural health facilities continued with additional numbers being recruited each year. By 2015, about 50 midwives were placed in 25 rural health facilities. This included the 18 midwives previously paid by W4H. However, non-indigenous midwives were given non-pensionable "contract" appointments instead of the preferred "permanent and pensionable" appointments (**Table 6**).

State	Bundle components	Status of implementation-Pilot Phase 2013			Status of implementation-ending 2015		
		Fully	Partial	Not yet	Fully	Partial	Not yet
Jigawa state	Payment of ME specific allowance of N20,000 per month		[yellow]		[green]		
	Improve living conditions			[red]	[green]		
	Provide safe working environment, equipment and logistics		[yellow]		[green]		
	Provision of safe accommodation within easy reach of facility & provision of water		[yellow]		[green]		
	Granting of preferential access to rural midwife to continuous education			[red]			[red]
	Public recognition and award scheme			[red]			[red]
Yobe state	Improvement of living conditions of midwives working and living in the rural area		[yellow]		[green]		
	Enhance the scope of practice for rural midwives (task shifting)			[red]			[red]
	Payment of midwife specific hardship allowance in addition to any existing allowance	[green]			[green]		
	Support continuing education and professional development of midwives living and working in the rural areas	[green]			[green]		
Katsina State	Payment of midwife specific rural allowance	[green]			[green]		
	Provision of permanent employments		[yellow]				[red]
	Provide supportive supervision and mentoring to MSS midwives	[green]				[yellow]	
	Provide accommodation and portable water and electricity		[yellow]		[green]		
Zamfara State	Lift ban on recruitment of midwives to targeted rural health facilities providing MNCH services			[red]			[red]
	Provide accommodation within easy reach of MNCH facility		[yellow]		[green]		
	Payment of midwife specific rural allowance	[green]			[green]		

LEGEND	
[green]	Fully implemented
[yellow]	Partially implemented
[red]	Unable to implement

Table 6.
Comparative Progress with implementation of state specific rural incentive package.

4.1.2 Katsina State

The Katsina state government regularly paid the monthly rural allowance to midwives over the period. It also took over the payment of the rural allowances and salaries of the 18 MRRS midwives originally recruited with the funding support from W4H. Available accommodations in rural health facilities were competitively allocated to health workers (including midwives) posted to rural health facilities and a rent allowance deducted from their salaries. There was therefore no special dispensation for midwives serving in rural health facilities. Less than 30% of midwives were offered accommodation. The state government was reluctant over the period to recruit MSS and the Subsidy Reinvestment and Empowerment Programme-Maternal and Child Health (SURE-P MCH) midwives who completed their training, due to a statewide embargo on employment. However, Katsina did try to recruit the new graduates from the Katsina midwifery training institution, most of whom are native to Katsina. In addition, the community midwifery program (an expedited program to train rural women and young girls as community midwives for rural health facilities) was up and running by 2015. The state government plans to post its graduates directly to rural health facilities in their respective LGAs (**Table 6**).

4.1.3 Yobe State

Yobe state absorbed the 19 MRRS midwives previously recruited with the support from W4H into its workforce. The state government regularly paid the midwives their rural allowance of N25,000 monthly, while some LGAs supplement this with N10,000 monthly. The rural allowance was paid to any other health worker working in the rural areas. The state government constructed, and in some cases, renovated health staff accommodations in the rural health facilities and some basic furnishing was also provided. A previous United Kingdom Department for International Development (UK-DFID) funded Maternal Newborn and Child Health project, the Partnership for Reviving Routine Immunisation in Northern Nigeria-Maternal Newborn and Child Health (PRRINN-MNCH) and the state government have equipped and refurbished health facilities in the state. The State governor gave approval for recruitment of 96 additional nurses and midwives, but there were no midwives from other states who wanted to come for employment in Yobe, as a result of the non-pensionable contract and the effect of the Islamic insurgency in the state.

There was inadequate support for supportive supervision of rural midwives by the state government over the implementation period. Training and mentoring opportunities for midwives also remained a challenge. The state also was unable to implement its proposed task-shifting and task-sharing policy as it was inconsistent with existing Federal policy (**Table 6**).

4.1.4 Zamfara State

By the end of 2015, the State governor approved and had taken over payment of the salaries of all the 32 midwives working in a total of 19 rural health facilities, spread over 11 LGAs where the midwives previously had been paid by W4H. Zamfara only paid its standard allowance that it pays to all rural health workers and abandoned the additional midwife-specific rural allowance. In addition, the majority of the newly recruited midwives continued to be posted to secondary health facilities, which may not necessarily be located in rural areas. The state also did not construct the accompanying accommodations for new PHCs. W4H either built, renovated, or worked with the facility health committee to provide the accommodation for midwives where there was no suitable accommodation. The rural midwives were provided supportive supervision by a supervisory team that was funded by some development Partners. However, this team went on supervision only when partner funds were available. There was ongoing advocacy by the SMOH to the legislature and traditional authorities on recruiting and retaining midwives in rural areas and making their salary more attractive (**Table 6**).

4.2 MRRS outcomes: progress with recruitment, deployment and retention of midwives to rural health facilities

Table 7 shows the pattern of recruitment and deployment of midwives across the four states. A total number of 477 midwives recruited and posted to rural health facilities in the study states over the period 2013–2016. Of these, 196 (41%) were from Jigawa, 126 (26,4%) from Yobe, 78 from Zamfara (16.4%), and 77 (16.1%) from Katsina. Fifty-nine (12.4%) of these midwives were recruited in 2013, 147 (31%) each in 2014 and 2015, and 124 (26%) in 2016. The proportion of midwives recruited and posted to rural Health facilities increased each year from 12.4–31% and declined moderately to 26%.

With the exception of Zamfara, all states showed a big increase in midwife recruitment from 2013 to 2014. Jigawa tripled its recruitment from 17 to 68 and

State	Year				Total
	2013	2014	2015	2016	
Jigawa	17	68	67	44	196 (41%)
Zamfara	15	18	36	9	78 (16.4%)
Katsina	12	28	13	24	77 (16.1%)
Yobe State	15	33	31	47	126 (26.4%)
Total	**59 (12.4%)**	**147 (31.0%)**	**147 (31.0%)**	**124 (26.0%)**	**477 (100%)**

Table 7.
Number of Midwives recruited and posted to Rural health facilities 2013–2016.

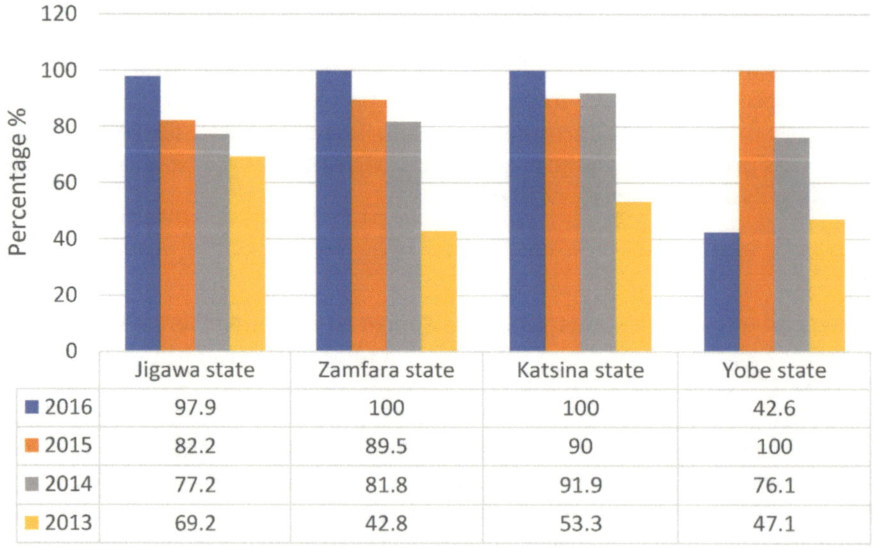

Figure 6.
Trends in Annual MW rural retention rates.

sustained this high level through 2015, but then dropped down to 44 in 2016, recruiting the most midwives (n = 196) of any state for the four-year period. Yobe recruited the second largest numbers of midwives, 126, showing steady increases in recruitment throughout the period. Katsina had small gains in recruitment for 2014–2016 over the 2013 numbers, and recruited only 77 midwives from 2013 to 2016. Zamfara recruited almost the same number of midwives as Katsina (n = 78), with the largest number in 2015, when 36 were recruited.

Midwife retention rates increased in all four states from 2013 to 2016 (**Figure 6**). In three states (Jigawa, Katsina and Zamfara), midwife retention rates increased steadily throughout the period 2013 and 2016: in Jigawa from 69.2–98%; in Katsina from 53.3–100%; and in Zamfara from 42.8–100%. In Yobe state, retention increased from 47% gradually to 100% in 2015, but then dropped slightly to 90% due to the loss of 27 midwives in the first quarter of 2016 due to deteriorating security measures following the insurgency activities of the Boko Haram terrorist group.

5. Discussion of findings and lessons learned

In spite of all the challenges encountered with its implementation, the MRRS has been a game changer in all the participating states. The key interventions implemented were: the provision of midwife specific rural allowance, ensuring regularity of payment of allowances, recruitment policy review on ban on recruitment of new health staff, provision of accommodation for staff posted to rural health facilities. Throughout the 2013–2016 period, all states increased the recruitment and retention of midwives, although more were recruited and retained in some states than others. A key cross cutting strategy for change was Advocacy on identifiable enablers for the retention of health staff in rural health facilities.

5.1 Advocacy for a favorable recruitment policy that targets rural health facility

Our implementation research showed the importance of a favorable recruitment policy environment, as exemplified in Jigawa state where progressive recruitment policies increased the number of midwives, particularly in targeted rural health facilities in the state. On the contrary, in the Katsina and Zamfara states, where there was an embargo on the recruitment of midwives amidst high maternal and newborn deaths, low recruitment of midwives, and poor access of the rural population to maternal care, progress in this regard has been significantly slow.

In advocating for reversing the ban on recruitment of health workers including midwives, we demonstrated to centers of power, the link between maternal and newborn health and access to trained midwives. This process was relentless, and response was slow as the restrictive policies were largely underpinned by budgetary constraints, particularly in the Katsina and Zamfara states. The process in Zamfara state for example illustrates the critical role of relentless advocacy appropriately targeted at "centers of power and decision making" [13]. Those targeted were state health commissioners, the Ministry of Local Government, the State House of Assembly Committee on Health, the state governor, and those who advise the governor. Two critical factors to ensuring sustainability of HRH interventions have been identified as the extent to which the chosen intervention was relevant to the need and health system context, and the extent of engagement of stakeholders in the design and identification of interventions [12]. Our study however shows that ensuring these critical factors at the design stage does not automatically translate to implementation as other nuances depending on the context will need to be taken into consideration. Evidence has shown that influencing a change in an existing policy can be difficult and complex. As it requires complex interactions and negotiations amongst a range of stakeholders, including politicians, interest groups, technocrats, advisers, bureaucrats, and a range of other actors. Especially in a diverse country such as Nigeria, gaining the support of the communities and the public and ensuring political will have been identified as essential factors that will result in policy change [14–16].

Presentations were made by W4H to the House of Assembly Committee for Health on the HRH situation in the state, the shortage of midwives and its effect on maternal mortality, the need to save lives and achieve universal health coverage. The importance of actively engaging stakeholders has been identified as a key factor to ensure increase access to health workers in rural areas in other studies [13, 17–19]. In addition, W4H initially paid for the recruitment and posting of 20 midwives to some selected rural health facilities in support of its advocacy on the need for the state to respond to the severe midwife shortage in peripheral rural health facilities. The subsequent withdrawal of that funding after the agreed number of years not only triggered the absorption of those midwives by the state government, but also the recruitment of additional midwives by the Commissioner of Health.

The engagement of the stakeholders in advocating for the recruitment and posting of additional midwives to rural health facilities drew more attention to strengthening the functionality of primary health care facilities. The heavy workload of the secondary facilities presents a dilemma to health service managers to allocate greater numbers of midwives to them. However, improving the health workforce situation in the PHC facilities will reduce the inequitable distribution of qualified midwives, making maternal health services available to the rural population and ultimately reducing the workload in the secondary facilities. The provision of quality services at the primary health level will reduce delays and complications, and the need to refer to higher level of care which will ultimately reduce the workload in the secondary health facilities. The Nigeria health system is decentralized into three levels with responsibilities at the federal, state and local government. All the three tiers are involved to some extent in all the major health system functions including financing, stewardship, governance and service provision [20]. As a result, the state oversees secondary health facilities while the LGAs oversee the primary health care facilities, it is therefore critical that the state and LGAs plan for the staffing of rural health facilities together such that they are strategically placed to reduce the need for the secondary health facilities to poach midwives from rural health facilities.

5.2 Other enablers of successful rural retention identified in the study

Similar to findings of other studies [21–23], other identifiable enablers of success of appropriate health staff recruitment policies included: regular payment of salaries and or rural allowances by state governments, providing "permanent and pensionable" employment to every midwife irrespective of their state of origin, provision of safe and comfortable accommodation, involvement of multiple state stakeholders in planning the initiative, and advocating for the creation of state budgetary space for meeting the cost of implementing the incentive package.

Providing "permanent and pensionable" employment to every midwife irrespective of state of origin.

Most State health staff recruitment policy offers non pensionable contracts to Nigerians from other states. This is a major policy bottleneck requiring pragmatic and prudent revision. It is difficult to navigate Nigeria's federal political structure on who gets pensionable employment, particularly if midwives from other states of the federation are willing to work in the rural health facilities of other states, at least until these states are graduating more of their own indigenes from their schools of midwifery. Perhaps some of the serious gaps in midwife availability could be mitigated if midwives from other states were offered pensionable employment. Unfortunately, the states that participated in this implementation were reluctant on providing pensionable employment to midwives from other states of the federation.

5.3 Availability of midwives

The MRRS initiative in the four states has also brought to the fore the need for them to put in place sustained strategies for the production of midwives, consistent with the efforts by W4H to increase student intakes and strengthen the capacity of state Nursing and Midwifery schools.

Huicho et al. [13] suggest that enhancing the attractiveness of working in a rural health facility can contribute to increased recruitment and retention, which may in turn have a positive effect on improving availability of health workers, and the quality of services. This framework assumes the availability of a supply of health workers who could be attracted by favorable contextual factors to accept placement in rural health facilities or underserved areas. This has not been the case in Northern Nigeria, because the production of midwives was severely constrained. While some of the states wanted to recruit additional midwives, the midwives were just not available from within the state or were constrained by the perceived unfavorable recruitment policies for non-native health workers. The logic that underpins the Huicho evaluation framework also assumes that availability of health workers naturally translates into improved quality of care and ultimately the improvement in the health status of the population. However, our evaluation shows that although the midwives may be available in the state, but they are not "available" for posting to rural facilities due to a variety of factors. The W4H MRRS initiative could directly provide funds to address some of these factors, such as a supplemental living allowance, but not all the incentive components that would make the rural areas attractive to the midwife (such as provision of comfortable accommodation as an example); interventions designed to increase availability of midwives (such as advocacy for the lifting of ban on recruitment, policy reforms to appropriately contract non-indigenous midwives); and their overall effect on midwife retention rates in the rural health facilities. Much of the advocacy implemented by W4H therefore targeted what could conceptually be described as "Centers of Power".

5.4 Advocacy targeting critical "Centers of Power" in leveraging policy change

A key lesson learned during the pilot phase that subsequently informed the full implementation phase was that a critical "center of power" that needs to be leveraged was located outside the health and health related departments. In Nigeria, policy decisions that had financial implications require the ultimate approval of the State Governor. The state governor's acceptance of the strategic response to the shortage and inequitable distribution of health staff was critical and also a potent enabler. In spite of the enthusiasm and commitment of state planning and finance officials and senior health managers to ensure that HRH issues were addressed, the state governor made the final critical decisions that could reverse the serious midwife shortages. The governor's office makes the ultimate budgetary decisions on HRH, including the recruitment of midwives, the provision of accommodation for midwives, and the payment of specific allowances to midwives. The office of the state governor is therefore a formidable ally in translating the proposed rural incentive package into reality. This factor from our experience made MRRS very successful in Jigawa state and had to be strategically worked at in other states. It also resulted in lifting the embargo placed on the recruitment of health workers (including midwives) by some of the states. The various SICs therefore discussed at cross-state review meetings and adopted strategies for effective advocacy to engender the support of political authorities.

5.5 Provision of health staff accommodation in rural health facilities

This is capital intensive and adequately responding to this was a challenge in all the states. The extent to which states responded to this has been already discussed but it will be prudent to have a policy to insist or negotiate the inclusion of staff accommodation in any contract for newly constructed rural health facilities, while LGAs seek funding through donor and other support to provide staff accommodation for existing rural health facilities.

5.6 Rural retention rates

The retention rate of midwives in rural areas significantly improved over the period of implementation, with the retention rates being doubled in some states (Jigawa and Katsina) and tripled in other states (Yobe and Zamfara). This suggests that the provision of safe and comfortable accommodations and the payment of rural allowances on a regular and sustained basis are key in leveraging higher retention rates in the Northern Nigerian context. Key interventions implemented across the four states were payment of rural hardship allowance, and improved living condition. These were linked to increased midwife retention rates across the four states. Retention rates increased to from 69.2–98% in Jigawa; from 53.3–100% in Katsina; from 42.8–100% in Zamfara; and from 47–90% in Yobe state between 2012 to 2016. This is in-line with findings from other African countries, discrete choice experiments in Kenya and South Africa suggest that hardship allowance and opportunities for further education are incentive preferences that could attract nurses to rural health facilities [24–28].

In spite of the state of emergency declared because of terrorist insurgency, Yobe was still able to maintain a retention rate of 90% with only a drop of 10% in 2016 at the height of the insurgency. This is a significant achievement considering the importance of strengthening health systems in conflict and post-conflict settings to help provide universal health coverage for all. In addition, health systems have to be responsive and resilient, especially in light of current outbreaks of epidemics and exacerbation of conflicts in many countries. Health workers in conflict settings face additional challenges that can compromise the sustainability of the healthcare delivery system. Studies from other conflict and post-conflict countries have identified the importance of financial incentives, sense of being of service to the communities, training opportunities, and religion as key factors that motivate health workers to continue to work in these difficult environments [28–33].

5.7 Immediate post implementation challenges

Following an immediate post MRRS implementation evaluation, a number of challenges were observed. Indeed, some of the persisting challenges to effective MRRS implementation after W4H withdrew all financial support to the initiative were the lack of a coordinated plan for continuing professional development for midwives working in rural health facilities, staff shortages, delay in paying allowances/salaries, insecurity in some areas due to the activities of bandits, as well as lack of working equipment and drug consumables [34–36]. Supportive supervision for rural midwives requires adequate funding to ensure regularity, as the status of funding for the integrated Supportive Supervision (ISS) did not significantly change since 2013 [37]. Persisting challenges also include lack of basic working equipment, drug consumable in some rural health facilities, poorly furnished accommodation (not comfortable), and poor security (caused by insurgency by Muslim militants) [38–40].

6. Conclusion

Adapting WHO recommendations on attracting, recruiting and retention of health workers in rural areas by the four states has been successfully implemented using an implementation research approach in Katsina, Yobe, Jigawa and Zamfara states of Northern Nigeria. In addition to the observed increase in recruitment and retention of midwives in rural health facilities over the period, the initiative additionally heightened awareness and determination by the implementing states to increase the production of midwives. Some of the states have moved away from the payment of midwife-specific rural allowance over and above that paid to all other health workers in rural areas to the payment of such an allowance to all category of health workers in rural and underserved areas. This is equitable, although it also de-emphasizes the focus on providing extra motivation to the midwife, a critical maternal health staff. On the other hand, this could be seen as a demonstration of the extent to which states have taken ownership of the initiative and adapted it to what works best for their particular circumstances.

Authors' contributions

AAA contributed to the study design, writing of the first draft of the manuscript, review of the manuscript at all stages and finalization. GYA designed the study and the writing of the first draft of the manuscript. FA participated in study design and reviewing the draft manuscript. SF participated in study design and reviewing the draft manuscript at all stages. All authors approved the final version of the manuscript.

Competing interests

We declare that we have no competing interests.

Author details

Adetoro A. Adegoke[1,2]*, Godwin Y. Afenyadu[3], Fatima L. Adamu[1,4] and Sally Findley[1,5]

1 Women for Health Programme, Kano, Nigeria

2 Health Service Delivery, DAI Global Health, London, UK

3 Heilbrunn Department of Population and Family Health, Mailman School of Public Health, Columbia University, New York, United States

4 Education for Women in Health, DAI Global Health, London, UK

5 Population and Family Health, Mailman School of Public Health, Columbia University Medical Centre, NY, NY, United States

*Address all correspondence to: ade.adegoke@gmail.com

References

[1] National Population Commission (NPC) [Nigeria] and ICF International. 2014. *Nigeria Demographic and Health Survey 2013*. Abuja, Nigeria, and Rockville, Maryland, USA: NPC and ICF International.

[2] Doctor HV, Olatunji A, Findley SE, Afenyadu GY, Abdulwahab A and Jumare A. 2012. Maternal mortality in northern Nigeria: findings of a health and demographic surveillance system in Zamfara State, Nigeria. *Tropical Doctor*. 42 (3):140-3. Epub 2012 Apr 27., doi: 10.1258/td.2012.120062

[3] Ujah IAO, Aisien OA, Mutihir JT, Vanderjagt DJ, Glew RH and Uguru VE. 2005. Factors Contributing to Maternal Mortality in North-Central Nigeria: A Seventeen-year Review. *African Journal of Reproductive Health*. 9, (3): 27-40.

[4] WHO. 2013. *WHO GUIDELINES on maternal, newborn, child and adolescent health: WHO Guidelines Review Committee Recommendations on maternal and perinatal health*. Available from <http://www.who.int/maternal_child_adolescent/documents/guidelines-recommendations-maternal-health.pdf>

[5] Ebuehi OM, Campbell PC. 2011. Attraction and retention of qualified health workers to rural areas in Nigeria: a case study of four LGAs in Ogun State, Nigeria. *Rural and Remote Health* 11: 1515. (Online), 2011.

[6] Abimbola S, Okoli U, Olubajo O, Abdullahi MJ, Pate MA. 2012. The midwives service scheme in Nigeria. *PLoS Med*. 2012; 9 (5): e1001211. doi: 10.1371/journal.pmed.1001211. Epub 2012 May 1.

[7] Adegoke AA, Atiyaye FB, Abubakar AS, Auta A, Aboda A. Job satisfaction and retention of midwives in rural Nigeria. *Midwifery*. 2015 Oct;31 (10):946-56. doi: 10.1016/j.midw.2015.06.010. Epub 2015 Jun 23.

[8] *WHO. Increasing access to health workers in remote and rural areas through improved retention: global policy recommendations*. Geneva: World Health Organization; 2010. Available from <http://whqlibdoc.who.int/publications/2010/9789241564014_eng.pdf>

[9] Afenyadu G, Adegoke A, Findley S (2017). Improving Human Resource for Health means retaining health workers: Application of the WHO Recommendations for the retention of health workers in Rural Northern Nigeria. *Journal of Health Care for the Poor and Underserved*. 29 (3) p1066-1086. (10.1353/hpu 2017.0098).

[10] Dieleman M, Gerretsen B and van der Wilt GJ. (2009). Human resource management interventions to improve health workers' performance in low and middle income countries: a realist review. Health Research Policy and Systems 2009, 7:7 doi:10.1186/1478-4505-7-7. Available from <https://health-policy-systems.biomedcentral.com/articles/10.1186/1478-4505-7-7>

[11] Fixsen DL, Naoom SF, Blase KA, Friedman RM and Wallace, F. 2005. *Implementation Research: A Synthesis of the Literature*. Tampa, FL: University of South Florida, Louis de la Parte Florida Mental Health Institute, the National Implementation Research Network

[12] *WHO 2010. World Health Statistics. World Health Organization, Geneva 27, Switzerland, ISBN 978 92 4 156398 7. Available from* <http://www.who.int/whosis/whostat/2010/en/index.html>

[13] Huicho L, Dieleman M, Campbell J, Codjia L, Balabanova D, Dussault G & Doleag C (2010). Increasing access to health workers in underserved areas: a conceptual framework for measuring

results. *Bull World Health Organ* 2010; 88:357–363 (doi:10.2471/ BLT.09.070920).

[14] Clavier C, De Leeuw E. (2013). Health promotion and the policy process. United Kingdom: Oxford University Press; 2013.

[15] Cullerton K, Donnet T, Lee A, Gallegos D (2016). Playing the policy game: a review of the barriers to and enablers of nutrition policy change. 2016;19 (14):2643–53.

[16] Christoffel KK. (2000). Public health advocacy: process and product. Am J Public Health. 2000; 90 (5):722–6.

[17] Nyoni J, Gbary A, Awases M, Ndecki P and Chatora R. (2006). *Policies and Plans for Human Resources for Health Guidelines for Countries in the WHO African Region.* WHO. Human Resource for Health Development Programme Division of Health Systems and Services Development. Brazzaville.

[18] Dormon F, Balen J, Schmidtke KA, Vlaev I. (2017). Healthworkers' motivation in low-and-middle income countries: A systematic review of the literature. *Medical Research Archives*. 2017 5, (8).

[19] Adeloye D, David RA, Olaogun AA, Auta A, Adesokan A, Gadanya M, Opele JK, Owagbemi O and Adeloye IA. et al. (2017). Health workforce and governance: the crisis in Nigeria. *Human Resources for Health*. 15:32 DOI 10.1186/ s12960-017-0205-4. Available from < https://human-resources-health. biomedcentral.com/track/pdf/10.1186/ s12960-017-0205-4>

[20] Nigeria Federal Ministry of Health (2004). Health Sector Reform Programme (HRSP): Strategic Thrust and Plan of Action 2004 – 2007. Abuja Nigeria. Federal Ministry of Health, 2004, 7.

[21] Grobler L, Marais BJ, Mabunda SA, Marindi PN, Reuter H, Volmink J. (2009). Interventions for increasing the proportion of health professionals practising in rural and other underserved areas. Cochrane Database Syst Rev (2009); 1: CD005314. PMID: 19160251.

[22] Wilson NW, Couper ID, De Vries E, Reid S, Fish T, Marais BJ. (2009). A critical review of interventions to redress the inequitable distribution of healthcare professionals to rural and remote areas. *Rural Remote Health.* 2009; 9:1060. PMID:19530891

[23] Dolea C, Stormont L, Braichet J-M. (2010). Evaluated strategies to increase attraction and retention of health workers in remote and rural areas. *Bull World Health Organ.* 2010, 88:379–385.

[24] Travis P, Bennett S, Haines A, Pang T, Bhutta Z, Hyder AA et al. (2004). Overcoming health-systems constraints to achieve the Millennium Development Goals. *The Lancet.* 364: 900–6. doi:10.1016/S0140-6736 (04) 16987-0 PMID:15351199

[25] WHO. (2006). *World health report 2006: Working together for health*. Geneva: WHO. 2006. 3.

[26] WHO. (2008). *World health report 2008: Primary health care, now more than ever*. Geneva: WHO. 2008.

[27] Wilson NW, Couper ID, De Vries E, Reid S, Fish T, Marais BJ. (2009). A critical review of interventions to redress the inequitable distribution of healthcare professionals to rural and remote areas. *Rural Remote Health*. 9: 1060. PMID:19530891.

[28] Buchan J, Couper ID, Tangcharoensathien V, Thepannya K, Jaskiewicz W, Perfilieva G, Dolea C. (2013). Early implementation of WHO recommendations for the retention of health workers in remote and rural

areas. *Bull World Health Organ*. 91:834–840 | doi: http://dx.doi.org/10.2471/BLT.13.119008.

[29] MacKinnon J, MacLaren B. (2012). *Human resources for health challenges in fragile states: evidence from Sierra Leone, South Sudan and Zimbabwe*. The North-South Institute. 2012.

[30] Bertone M, Samai M, Edem-Hotah J, Witter S. (2014). A window of opportunity for reform in post conflict settings? The case of human resource for health policies in Sierra Leone, 2002–2012. *Confl Heal*. 8:11.

[31] Witter S, Wurie H and Bertone MT. (2015). The Free Health Care Initiative: how has it affected health workers in Sierra Leone? *Health Policy and Planning*. 1–9.

[32] Wurie HR, Mohamed Samai M. and Witter S. (2016). Retention of health workers in rural Sierra Leone: findings from life histories. *Human Resources for Health*. 14 (3): 1-15. DOI 10.1186/s12960-016-0099-6. Available from <https://human-resources-health.biomedcentral.com/track/pdf/10.1186/s12960-016-0099-6?site=human-resources-health.biomedcentral.com>

[33] Witter S, Tulloch O. and Martineau T. (2012). *Health workers' incentives in post-conflict settings – a review of the literature and framework for research*. ReBUILD RPC research report. Pages 1- 11. Available from < https://assets.publishing.service.gov.uk/media/57a08a7be5274a31e0000614/rebuild_hwi_lit_review.pdf>

[34] Van Lerberghe W, Conceição, Van Damme W, Ferrinho P (2004). When staff is underpaid. Dealing with the individual coping strategies of health personnel. Towards a Global Health Workforce Strategy. Edited by: Ferrinho P, Dal Poz M. 2004, Antwerp: ITG Press, 411-420.

[35] Rowe AR, De Savigny D, Lanata CF, Victora C (2005). How can we achieve and maintain high quality performance of health workers in low-resource settings?. Lancet. 2005, 366: 1026-35. 10.1016/S0140-6736(05)67028-6.

[36] Haines A, Kuruvilla A, Borchert M. (2004). Bridging the implementation gap between knowledge and action for health. Bull World Health Organ. 2004, 82 (10): 724-732.

[37] Sennun P, Suwannapong N, Howteerakul N, Pacheun O (2006). Participatory supervision model: building health promotion capacity among health officers and the community. Rural Remote Health. 2006, 6 (2): 440

[38] Zurn P, Codjia L, Sall FL, Braichet JM. (2010). How to recruit and retain health workers in underserved areas: the Senegalese experience. *Bull World Health Organ* 2010; 88:386–9. doi: http://dx.doi.org/10.2471/BLT.09.070730 PMID:20461134.

[39] Dumont J-C, Zurn P, Church J, Le Thi C. (2008). *International mobility of health professionals and health workforce management in Canada: myths and realities*. Paris: Organization for Economic Co-operation and Development. Available from <http://www.oecd.org/canada/41590427.pdf>

[40] Grobler L, Marais BJ, Mabunda SA, Marindi PN, Reuter H, Volmink J. (2009). *Interventions for increasing the proportion of health professionals practising in rural and other underserved areas*. Cochrane Database Syst Rev. 1: CD005314. PMID:19160251 2.

Chapter 5

CRISPR Cas/Exosome Based Diagnostics: Future of Early Cancer Detection

P.P. Mubthasima, Kaumudi Pande, Rajalakshmi Prakash and Anbarasu Kannan

Abstract

Trending and Thriving, CRISPR/Cas has expanded its wings towards diagnostics in recent years. The potential of evading off targeting has not only made CRISPR/Cas an effective therapeutic aid but also an impressive diagnostic tool for various pathological conditions. Exosomes, 30 - 150nm sized extracellular vesicle present and secreted by almost all type of cells in body per se used as an effective diagnostic tool in early cancer detection. Cancer being the leading cause of global morbidity and mortality can be effectively targeted if detected in the early stage, but most of the currently used diagnostic tool fails to do so as they can only detect the cancer in the later stage. This can be overcome by the use of combo of the two fore mentioned diagnostic aids, CRISPR/Cas alongside exosomes, which can bridge the gap compensating the cons. This chapter focus on two plausible use of CRISPR/Cas, one being the combinatorial aid of CRISPR/Cas and Exosome, the two substantial diagnostic tools for successfully combating cancer and other, the use of CRISPR in detecting and targeting cancer exosomes, since they are released in a significant quantity in early stage by the cancer cells.

Keywords: CRISPR/Cas, exosomes, cancer, Cas12a, Cas13a, exosomal noncoding RNAs

1. Introduction

1.1 Cancer

Amongst the non-communicable diseases, cancer remains to be the major cause of morbidity and mortality globally. As per the GLOBOCAN index 2020, 19.3 million new cancer cases have been reported with around 10.0 million cancer deaths in 2020. Amongst the top 10 cancers, Lung cancer is considered leading cause of mortality with 18.0% of the total cancer deaths, followed by colorectal cancer with the death rate 9.4%, liver with the mortality rate of 8.3%, stomach with 7.7%, and female breast cancer with the death rate of 6.9% (**Figure 1**) [1]. Cancer, by definition is considered as a condition characterized with uncontrolled division of particular cell type in a definite site anywhere in the body as an aftermath of various triggering factors technically termed as Carcinogens, which have the ability to convert proto - oncogenes to Oncogenes causing cancer. Cancer cells can

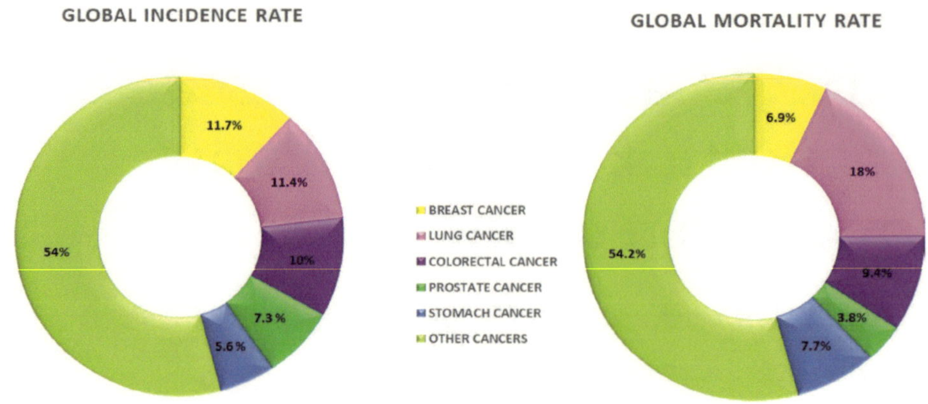

Figure 1.
Global incidence rate and death rate.

divert metabolites into anabolic pathways to support their rapid proliferation and to accumulate the cellular building blocks required for tumor growth and differ morphologically from other normal cells. It is reported that only around 5 – 10% total cancer is caused due to genetic defects such as *BRCA1* and *BRCA2* gene mutation in case of breast and ovarian cancer. Whereas, the other 90% is due to external factors such as exposure to potent carcinogens, lifestyle factors such as diet, stress, obesity, infections etc. [2–5].

WHO has broadly classified these carcinogens into physical (UV and other ionizing radiations), Chemical (alcohol, tobacco smoke, aflatoxins and various laboratory chemicals), Biological (Viruses such as Human Papilloma virus, hepatitis B virus, HIV etc., bacteria such as *Helicobacter pylori, Mycobacterium tuberculosis* etc., and parasites such as *Schistosoma haematobium*) and environmental (Air pollutants) factors [6]. The uncontrolled growth of cells when occur in a solid tissue such as in an organ or muscle are termed as tumors. All tumors not necessarily be cancerous, the tumors are further classified into benign tumors, which are noncancerous, devoid of spreading and malignant tumors, which are the cancerous ones that have the potential to spread to a distant organ via blood stream [7]. Cancer cells are known to invade adjoining parts of the body and spread to other organs to form the secondary tumor and this process is termed as metastasis, the primary cause of death from cancer.

Histologically, WHO has broadly classified cancers into following main categories viz.... Carcinoma (Cancer of epithelial tissue), Sarcoma (cancer of connective tissue), Myeloma (cancer of plasma cells of bone marrow), Lymphoma (cancer of lymphatic system), Leukemia (liquid cancer or cancer of blood), melanoma (cancer of pigment cells) and mixed types. Carcinoma accounts for around 180 – 90% of all cancer cases and are further sub divided into two categories such as Adenocarcinoma and squamous cell carcinoma [8, 9].

TNM (Tumor node metastasis) classification system, created in 1958 by the American Joint Committee on Cancer (AJCC) and the Union for International Cancer control (UICC) is yet another widely used system that classifies malignant tumor based on tumor spreading. It usually scores the size of the primary tumor (T), degree of spreading to the lymph node (N) and the presence of distant metastasis (M). Based on different combinations of T, N and M, cancer has been categorized into different stages 0 – IV for the aid of clinicians to establish the anatomic extent of infection. The stage 0 represents carcinoma in situ with the combination Tis, N0, M0 and are considered noncancerous but with the possibility of becoming one. Whereas, Stage I represents localized cancer with the TNM combination of T1-T2, N0, M0. Stage II is referred to locally advanced cancer with early stages and combination of T2-T4, N0, M0. While Stage III is characterized with locally advanced cancer, late stages with the combination T1-T4, N1-N3, M0, here the cancer would have been progressed with respect to the size of the tumor as well as it would have been spread to the adjacent lymph nodes. The stage IV is considered as the most severe stage, which is metastatic cancer with the combination, T1-T4, N1-N3, M1 [7, 10–12]. It is reported by that the above staging system is associated with severity of the disease and the survival rate of the patients, which is indirectly proportional i. e., higher the cancer stage so will be the severity of the disease and lesser will be the survival rate. For instance, 5-year survival rate of colorectal carcinoma at stage I is around 74% whereas, at stage IV it is only of 5% [10].

The signs and symptoms of cancer includes loss of appetite, extreme fatigue, pain in certain areas, persistent coughing, sudden loss of weight, blood in sputum, urine or stool, lumps on neck, breast, testicle etc. that does not hurt, changes in skin coloration, texture in certain areas etc. These fore said symptoms may not all ways point towards cancer, it could be due to any other pathological conditions too, but are the ones that should not be ignored [13, 14]. Currently there are several diagnostic tools in use for the detection of cancer such as laboratory testing of blood and urine for unusual blood count and for the detection of cancer biomarkers such as CA 125, CA 19-9, CA-15-3, CD117, CD19, CD 20, HE4, alpha-fetoproteins (AFP), bladder tumor antigen (BTA) etc. [15, 16]. Noninvasive Imagining tests includes CT scan, X-ray, mammography, ultrasound, Positron emission tomography (PET) etc. and more invasive method of biopsy which is considered as the golden standard for cancer diagnosis. However these diagnostics tools are not devoid of their own cons as most of them only detect cancer in its later stages leading to poor treatment efficiency [17].

The available treatment options for cancer includes surgical removal of solid tumor, Chemotherapy, Radiation therapy, Gene therapy, hormone therapy, immuno therapy, bone marrow transplantation, targeted drug therapy etc. Based on the severity, resistance of the cancer cells towards any of the above mentioned therapeutic options and in order to avoid cancer relapse, a combination of the fore said therapies will be used as an adjuvant therapy. For instance surgical removal in combination with chemotherapy and radiation therapy are practiced in order to avoid recurrence rate of the cancer [18].

1.2 Exosomes

Exosomes, the nanosized extracellular vesicles ranging 30 - 150 nm, are known to be secreted by all most all types of cells into the extracellular space and are present in all body fluids viz.... blood, tears, saliva, sputum, pleural fluid/effusions, cerebrospinal fluid (CSF), breast milk, amniotic fluid, semen, urine etc. [19, 20]. First discovered in the year 1983 by Stahl and Johnstone independently in reticulocytes, these extracellular vesicles were later termed as "Exosomes" by Rose Johnstone in the year 1987 [21–23]. The exosomes are reported to be encompass bimolecular components such as proteins, lipid, DNA, RNA (both coding as well as non-coding), metabolites and various enzymes etc. recapitulating the parent cell. Morphologically, exosomes are cup shaped extracellular vesicles where the central lumen composing the cargo of variety of fore mentioned biomolecules will be surrounded by the lipid bilayer structure. Accounting for the presence of these cargo, these nano scaled endocytic vesicles has engrossed plethora of attention amongst the scientific community around the globe, for its remarkable role as an efficient diagnostic tool [24–26].

The exosomes are known to be produced more in cancer cells than that of normal cells. The tumor derived exosomes are mainly involved in the cell–cell communication between cancer cells with both adjacent as well as distant cells as they gets secreted to the extracellular space and travel to a longer distant organ and tissue via blood stream facilitating cancer proliferation, Metastasis, drug resistance and immunomodulation. Apart from being involved in the dynamic crosstalk between the cells exosomes also proves to be an ideal drug delivery system with benefits such as specificity, safety and stability, since they are small and native to animals, they are able to avoid recognition and premature degradation by body's immune defense mechanism. In recent years, exosomes are emerging as a promising biomarker tool as they carry specific genetic information and influence tumor growth and progression [27, 28].

1.3 CRISPR/Cas

CRISPR (Clustered Regularly Interspaced Short Palindromic Repeats)/Cas (CRISPR associated endonuclease), a remarkable genome editing tool, has garnered plethora of interest of researchers in the field of modern gene therapy. Ever since the discovery of CRISPR locus in *E. coli* in the year 1987, several molecular biologists have shown tremendous interest and effort in characterizing and developing this wonder technique whereas, the noble prize for the development of this gene editing tool was bagged by Emmanuelle Charpentier and Jennifer Doudna in the year 2020 [29].

The CRISPR/Cas system is thought to be evolved from the prokaryotes such as bacteria and archaea as part of their adaptive immune system for combating viral infections. Precisely, they use a fragment of previously invaded viral genome called "spacer" as a source to memorize and defend any future attack by destroying the DNA from the similar viral particle, in association of Cas protein, which is an endonuclease enzyme, a molecular scissor to cut the double stranded DNA at a specific location on the target genome. It is reported that the CRISPR/Cas array is made of AT rich leader sequence, which is fenced by a set of Cas genes encoding the Cas proteins. The CRISPR/Cas is known to act through inducing site-specific DNA double stranded breaks and are known to surpass the other genome editing tools such as meganucleases, zinc finger nucleases (ZFNs), transcription activator like effectors (TALENs) etc., in being more precise, faster, efficient and inexpensive.

To brief out the conventional mechanism through which CRISPR/Cas executes their genome editing the following mechanism of gene editing pertaining to involvement of CRISPR/Cas9 has been described as follows, the CRISPR/Cas9 system is said to be RNA guided DNA targeting endonuclease system, which works through sequence specific manner. The mechanism of CRISPR/Cas9 based genome editing has been divided into three main stages viz.... I) DNA acquisition from the invading phage particle (adaptation). II) Biogenesis of CrRNA or CRISPR/Cas assembly formation and III) target DNA annihilation or interference of the target DNA and Insertion of desired gene sequence (i. e., either knock out or knock in). briefly, a small fragment or scrap of foreign invading genome termed spacer gets incorporated genomic CRISPR array and gets transcribed during the process of adaptation or in the 1st stage leading to the synthesis of crRNA, which in turn gets bound to Cas endonucleases enabling specificity towards the target.

The advantage of CRISPR/Cas system over the other gene editing platforms are, it has the property of multiplicity, simple, easy to prepare and use, as only 20 nucleotides in the guide RNA needs to be changed in order to retarget the Cas in CRISPR/Cas which in case of ZFNs and TALENs goes beyond 500-1500 base pairs. The CRISPR/Cas system can use multiple guide RNAs for targeting multiple target sites simultaneously in the same cell at the same time. This justifies the property of multiplicity of CRISPR/Cas system [29–35].

2. Types of CRISPR/Cas systems and their applications

Based on the type Cas protein involved and the complexity of components the CRISPR/Cas system is divided into two classes viz.... Class I and Class II and are further classified into six types which are in turn categorized into 22 sub types. The class 1 classification that comprises of type I, III and IV are characterized to be containing the involvement of multiple Cas proteins are whereas, class II classification are reported to comprise types II, V and VI where, only one effector Cas protein will be associated alongside the CRISPR array of processed guide RNA or in other words crRNA. Accounting for their nature of simplicity, the types involved under Class II Classification of CRISPR/Cas are reported to be the easiest in using for effective genome edited and manipulation of nucleic acids devoid of cells. Apart from being involved in gene editing the types of CRISPR/Cas systems derived from Class2 classification i. e., type II, V and VI are said to be instrumental in developing competent diagnostic platform of disease detection [36]. Brief representation of the fore said classification along with their application pertaining to class II CRISPR/Cas is as follows, **Figure 2**.

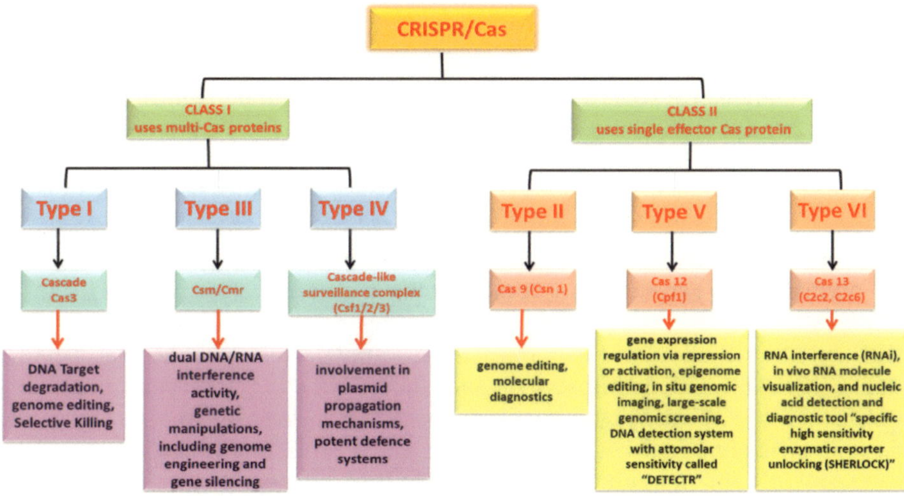

Figure 2.
Classification of CRISPR/Cas system with their emphasized application.

3. Exosomes in diagnosis

As mentioned prior in the introduction, exosomes are the nanosized form of extracellular vesicle of 30-150 nm size synthesized through a endosomal pathway via involvement of early, late endosomes and multi vesicular bodies (MVB) and are known to encompass several proteins lipids, nucleic acids etc. as their cargo. The exosomes are said to be involved in several biological processes such as, these are involved in cell–cell communication by the virtue of its cargo of fore mentioned compounds in the introduction both in physiological as well as pathological conditions. In pathological conditions including cancer, the cancer cell derived exosomes are reported to be synthesized or secreted in larger quantity than that from the normal cells, these cancer cell derived exosomes are considered key players in tumor growth and metastasis and are thought to be involved in stimulation of immune response. Apart from these, the exosomes are also suggested to be the part of dynamic cross talk between cancer cells and surrounding normal cells such as fibroblasts, endothelial cells, mesenchymal cells etc., and are considered to play an important role mediating resistance towards therapy [26, 27].

The biomarkers are any biochemical component of the body, whose presence can be used as an indication of certain pathological condition. A cancer biomarker are known to represent any molecule or a process that shows the existence of tumor or cancer in the body. Cancer exosomes are one such components, which in recent years have gained tremendous importance as a liquid biopsy tool as these exosomes are exact representation of their parent cell in terms of their cargo and reflects the altered state of the parent cell. The cancer exosomes are known to contribute to cancer progression via enhancement of intercellular transfer of their cargo within the tumor microenvironment. These minimally invasive biomarkers are more convenient over the conventional tissue biopsy involving surgery in being highly sensitive and specificity and are involved in early detection of cancer as these exosomes are required for the metastatic niche formation that can be accomplished by their release to the circulatory system from where they can be detected [26, 37, 38].

Isolation and characterization of exosomes are consider a very crucial step in diagnostics and biomarker development. Several techniques have been employed for an efficient isolation of these exosomes which includes classical ultracentrifugation (differential ultracentrifugation), precipitation based isolation (exosome isolation kits), using size exclusion chromatography, filtration based isolation, using immunomagnetic isolation method etc. Followed by their isolation these exosomes can be characterized for their number, size and zeta potential value by using instruments such as nano trafficking analysis (NTA), Dynamic light scattering (DLS), and for the morphological feature using SEM, TEM etc. [38–42].

The subsequent proteomic analysis of the isolated exosomes from the cancer cells have reported to shed light in identification of potent exosomal biomarker in several cancer types such as breast, lung, liver, prostate, ovarian, colorectal cancer, glioblastoma etc., the specific exosomal proteins includes surface proteins, Rab family GTPases, annexins, flotullin, exosome biogenesis proteins such as, Alix, Tsg101 and ESCRT complex. Several other exosomal protein includes, Tetraspanins (CD63, CD9, CD81, CD53etc.), Hsp90, Hsp70, EpCam etc. can serve as an efficient exosomal markers. A study by Rupp et al. Has reported the exosomal CD24 could serve as an efficient circulating biomarker for the detection of breast cancer. Several other exosomal protein biomarkers reported in breast cancer diagnosis are EDIL3 and fibronectin, for early breast cancer detection using ELISA, which can also serve as treatment response marker as the level of these two tremendously decreased after surgery. Likewise the expression of Survivin, a apoptosis inhibitor was found to be higher in prostate cancer exosomes compared to the normal. The urinary exosomes also do possess significant amount of biomarker such as PCA3, TMPRSS2: ERG in prostate cancer [38, 43–46].

Several recent studies have reported the development of numerous exosome-based diagnostic platform viz.... Exochip, which is a microfluidic device developed by Kanwar and team based on the exosomal tetraspanin protein CD63 where, the exosomes gets bound with CD63 antibody and a fluorescent reporter using which, the exosomes can be quantified. Another type of analytical technique used in exosome diagnostics is ExoScreen, the technique developed by Yoshioka et al., that utilizes CD9 and CD147 antibodies alongside photosensitizing beads. Apart from the above two, yet another exosome diagnosing tool was developed by Zhao and team called Exosearch chip which is a comparatively simpler technique which enables the quantitative isolation of exosomes by the virtue of immunomagnetic beads. The Exosearch technique was successfully used for the quantification of ovarian cancer exosomes using the exosomal markers CA-125, EpCam and CD24 [38, 47–49].

Apart from exosomal proteins, the use of techniques such as RNA-sequencing and DNA sequencing for the analysis of genomic data of cancer-derived exosomes have shed light on yet another exosomal component as an efficient biomarker use i. e., nucleic acid especially the ncRNAs including miRNAs and lncRNA. The exosomal miRNA are considered a most appropriate exosomal biomarker as they are quite stable against Rnase dependent degradation. Till date numerous exosomal miRNAs have been characterized as a potent tumor marker in several cancer conditions to name a few are, miR-21, miR-141, miR-220a, miR-200b, miR-203, miR-205, miR-214 in case of ovarian cancer as reported by Taylor et al. Other examples for exosomal miRNA biomarkers includes miR-31, miR-196a, miR-1246, miR-191, miR-451a, miR-483-3p, miR-16a etc. in case of pancreatic cancer have also been reported by several studies. Other ncRNAs accounting for exosomal long noncoding RNA, circular RNA have also been reported pertaining to the development of exosomal biomarkers for early cancer detection [38, 50–52].

4. CRISPR in diagnosis

Along with its extensive use in the field of genome editing, CRISPR/Cas system has expanded its wings towards diagnostics where it is mainly involved in detection of specific nucleic acid such as genomic DNA, non-genomic DNA, RNA, and pathogenic microbe genomes. This could have been accomplished due to their natural ability of efficient nucleic acid recognition and editing, have been demonstrated to be extraordinary tools for specific nucleic acid detection. The CRISPR diagnostics are reported to have influence the targeting efficiency of the CRISPR guide RNA either in the presence or absence of nucleic acid cleaving potential of the Cas nucleases. The basic principle of CRISPR based diagnostics is, here the CRISPR/Cas components are modified in such a way that, they will emit the color or fluorescence with response to their binding with the target nucleic acid sequence in certain pathological conditions. Based on the involvement of specific effector protein, several CRISPR based diagnostic tools kits have been developed which are mainly belonging to class II of CRISPR/Cas classification viz.... dCas9, SHERLOCK, SHERLOCK v2, DETECTR, HOLMES for an efficient detection of pathological conditions. A brief characterization, mode of action, application and advancement of these CRISPR tool kits in general and with respect to cancer will be discussed in this section.

Being the first effector protein to be characterized, Cas9 not only plays a vital role in genome editing, rather with minor modifications such as in dCas9, which is a nuclease-deactivated Cas9 (also termed as dead Cas9), it is also reported to be involved in nucleic acid detection as a simple and programmed detection tool. The dCas9 system is designed with modification in the basic activity of the conventional Cas9 protein in terms of deactivating the nucleic acid cleavage potential and only retaining the specific binding ability to target dsDNA. This was accomplished by inducing two point mutations H840A and D10A in the HNH and RuvC nuclease domain of the conventional Cas9 effector protein [36, 53].

Alongside classy Cas9, three more novel class 2 effector Cas proteins Cas12a (prior referred as Cpf1), Cas13a (prior referred as C2c2)and Cas14a have been showed to have more potent diagnostic properties and have become the latest interest of the scientific community. Unlike the Cas9 nuclease, the latter mentioned effector proteins have the property of "Collateral cleavage", the property in which they can induce cleavage of the nearby sequence, which is not complementary to the designed crRNA upon detection and binding to the target nucleic acid sequence. Precisely, the when crRNA along with its effector protein either Cas12a or Cas13a recognize and bind to their target nucleic acid sequence either DNA or RNA followed by their cleavage the activated effector protein also cleaves the nearby non targeted RNAs which does not emit the fluorescence until it is cleaved. With this, they offer a simple, fast, portable and reliable quantitative detection in diagnostics. It is this property of Cas12a and Cas13a, which has enabled effective tracing and detection of specific nucleic acid sequence, where the fluorescent ssDNA/ssRNA reporters are cleaved as a result of collateral cleavage.

Cas12a, which is previously referred to as Cpf1, are the variant of Cas effector protein which are RNA-guided, DNA-targeting enzyme, involved in type V of CRISPR/Cas classification. Unlike Cas9, these are reported to act or detect, bind and cleaves ssDNA. In contrast to this, Cas13a, which is previously referred to as C2c2 are RNA-guided targeting enzymes involved in type VI of CRISPR/Cas system and are specific for ssRNA. Based on the promiscuous Rnase ability of collateral cleavage of Cas12a as well as Cas13a several molecular diagnostic platforms have been developed in the recent years details of which will be discussed further [53–57].

As said before the collateral cleavage ability of Cas13a nuclease, lead to the development of a versatile *in vitro* nucleic acid detection platform named Specific High sensitivity Enzymatic Reporter UnLocking or simply abbreviated as SHERLOCK by Feng Zhang et al. in the year 2018, through technique of isothermal amplification along with recombinase polymerase amplification and T7 transcription, which has a wide spread application detecting viruses, pathogenic bacteria and in identifying tumor DNA mutation. Recent studies have reported the use of SHERLOCK in detecting two mutants BRAF V600E and EGFR L858R. An improved version of SHERLOCK, named SHERLOCKv2, was also came into existence with the ability to detect four viruses at the same time. Yet another CRISPR/Cas system involving Cas12a is also been found to be the basis of developing two more diagnostic tool (**Table 1**), named DETECTR (DNA endonuclease targeted CRISPR trans reporter) by Doudna et al. in 2018. The former has been found instrumental in diagnosing HPV + ve cervical cancer subtypes HPV 16 and HPV18 in both cell lines as well as clinical samples from the patients [53]. Apart from the above another diagnostic platform based on Cas12a has be developed called, one-hour low-cost multipurpose highly efficient system or simply HOLMES in the same year. Further experimentation focusing on the use of other Cas enzymes, Cas14 as well as CasX, which are Cas variants of type V CRISPR/Cas system alongside Cas12a. Development of newer diagnostic platform using these exceptionally smaller and compact RNA – guided nucleases made of 400-700 amino acids, targeting ssDNA are under progression for exploring their diagnostic potential as Cas14-DETECTR, yet another tool by Doudna and team [58, 59].

FEATURES	dCas9	SHERLOCK	DETECTR
Characteristics	cancer therapy by modifying DNA of target genes, stimulate tumor suppressor genes, knockdown oncogenes and tumor resistance pathways for targeted therapy	efficient, robust method to detect RNA and DNA, quick detection of infectious disease and involved in sensitive genotyping	genome editing tool based on its ability to stimulate genetic alteration in cells at sites of double-stranded DNA cut
Type of Cancer	Breast cancer, prostate cancer	Breast cancer	Cervical cancer
Target gene	AKT	EGFR L858R and BRAF V600E	HPV16, HPV18
References	[60]	[57, 61, 62]	[53, 59, 63]

Table 1.
Different CRISPR tools used for diagnosis of cancer malignancy.

5. Future of Exo CRISPR diagnostics

The two most important diagnostic markers Exosomes as well as CRISPR/Cas system and their features and advantages have been discussed thoroughly in the above sections. As mentioned before there are several exosome based diagnostic tools (ExoChip, ExoScreen, Exosearch) as well as CRISPR/Cas based diagnostic platforms (SHERLOCK, SHERLOCKv2, DETECTR and HOLMES) for the efficient diagnosis of the pathological conditions. Even though both of the fore said diagnostic platforms offers a greater advantage towards cancer diagnostics, these are not devoid of the cons pertaining to the exosomal detection, these are said to be in requirement of sophisticated sensing methodologies involving expensive equipments, and kits. On the other hand the CRISPR/Cas system, are in requirement of a efficient delivery in order to minimize the degradation by the systemic enzymes. With this insight, we hereby, suggest the use of a combinational technique made of both Exosomes and CRISPR where one can circumvent the drawback of other and becoming a full-fledged diagnostic platform.

In order to achieving efficient delivery of CRISPR/Cas system towards its target is an important step in the process of diagnostics and hence developing novel delivery system with higher efficiency and low immunogenicity and cytotoxicity is essential for the diagnostic applications. Off target effect of CRISPR system might lead to false acquisition of data for getting rid of which, the system has to be properly directed towards the target cell to achieve accuracy and efficiency. Different types of delivery system are available in present days this includes Adeno-associated viruses, Adenoviral vector, Lentiviral vector, Microinjection, electrophoresis, Lipid nanoparticle, cell penetrating peptides mediated and Gold nano particle mediated approaches [64]. Exosome, are reported to act as a promising carrier for CRISPR delivery, have an advantage over the other delivery system due to their natural biocompatible characteristics, high stability, low immunogenicity, and long circulation. Some exosomes can even have a high capacity to escape from degradation or clearance by the immune system [64, 65].

Recent advancement on this combinational approach has been reported by Yi He et al., and team where they have constructed a combinational tool called Aptamer-RPA-TMA-Cas13a Assay (ARTCA), a CRISPR/Cas13 based platform with modification for a significant detection of exosomal PD-L1 i. e., programmed cell death receptor, a promising biomarker for cancer immunotherapy monitoring, directly from the serum. This was accomplished by using an PD-L1 specific DNA aptamer which is further amplified by the aid of recombinase polymerase amplification (RPA) which is intern coupled with TMA (transcription-mediated amplification). By the aid of this tremendous diagnostic tool the expression level of PD-L1 in circulating tumor exosomes was constructed as reliable biomarker detection system. The same team have also reported the use of Cas12a for the construction of yet another CRISPR/Cas strategy, termed the apta-HCR-CRISPR assay, in order to detect nucleolin+ ve and PD-L1 + ve tumor derived exosomes [66–68]. With this we hereby, summarize the use of Exosome/CRISPR/Cas combo, where the exosomes can be effectively used for the delivery of CRISPR targeting the detection of specific nucleic acid or the array where the CRISPR/Cas system can be efficiently be targeted for the detection of exosomal biomarkers enlisted in the prior sections for early detection of cancer. The precise mechanism of Exosome/CRISPR/Cas system has been depicted in **Figure 3** where, the fore said combination can be used for both *In vivo* as well as *In vitro* diagnosis of tumor as picturized in **Figure 3A**. Here the exosomes derived from different sources can be used as a effective vehicle for site specific delivery of CRISPR/Cas detection system to avoid off target effect and false acquisitions. As depicted in **Figure 3B**, which is yet another possibility of using this

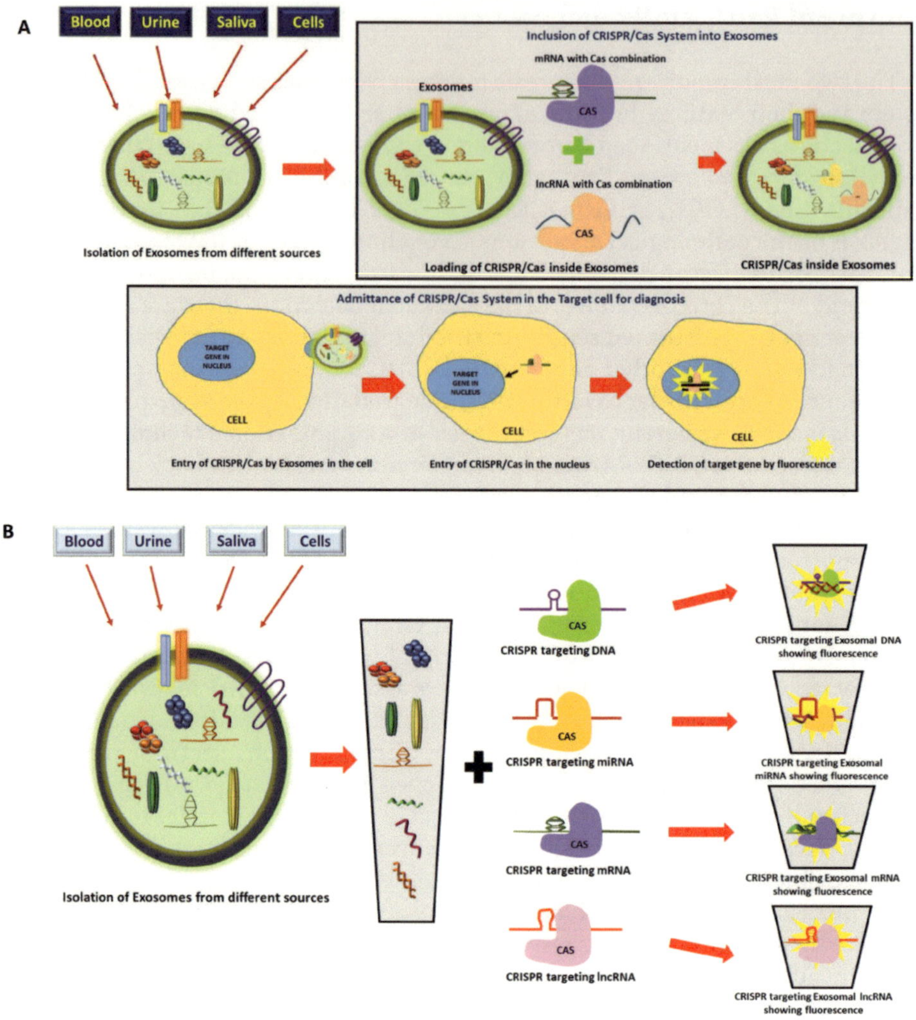

Figure 3.
Schematic representation of mechanism of action of exosome/CRISPR/Cas system for efficient cancer diagnosis. A) Exosome mediated delivery of CRISPR/Cas for effective detection of cancer. B) CRISPR/Cas based detection of exosomal biomarkers for early cancer diagnosis.

significant combination which can be optimized for *Ex Vivo* detection of cancer exosomal biomarkers that are secreted in early stages of cancer progression such as exosomal DNA, exosomal coding and noncoding RNAs (miRNA, lncRNA) and exosomal proteins. This can be beneficial for developing Exo CRISPR based early cancer detection kits.

6. Conclusion

It is generally stated, "The sooner, the better" which is more appropriate when it comes to diagnostics. If any pathological condition is detected in its earlier phases, the options for the effective treatment of that particular disease will be a lot more efficient than that of in the later phases. As mentioned in the fore said introduction, there are several diagnostic techniques available for the detection of cancer. Though these techniques offer a greater aid in the diagnosis of several pathological conditions including cancer, these are not devoid of the disadvantages in being pricey, time consuming and they do pose the threat to cause infections leading to worsening of the condition. For instance, in case of biopsies, even though it is considered the golden standard in the cancer diagnosis, they do have the threat in causing infections as, it is an invasive method. The threat of repetitive exposure to the radiations such as x-rays might also effect otherwise along with being useful in diagnosis of solid tumors.

As mentioned before the greatest drawback of the conventional diagnostic tools when it comes to cancer is, most of these techniques can only detect the disease in its later stages. Such as, in case of laboratory techniques, which uses of blood and urine for the presence of conventional biomarkers enlisted above, can be detected in the later stages when cancer has already become metastatic as these biomarker enters the blood stream in the later stages. This is where the role of exosomes comes into play as an efficient biomarker for early cancer detection as, there are several reports stating that the exosomes from the cancer cells are secreted more compared to the exosomes secreted from the normal cells, in order to aid in further spreading of the disease to the distant sites of the body. Moreover, these exosomes have unleashed the site for lesser - noninvasive method of diagnosis as it is present in all the body fluids enlisted in the introduction section.

Several research reports supports the use of CRISPR/Cas system for its substantial role in diagnosis. In recent years both exosomes as well as CRISPR/Cas per se has proven to be an excellent diagnostic aid. The CRISPR based diagnostics have unmatched advantages over the conventional diagnostic tools, and aided the researchers with its precision targeting efficiency, high specificity and single base specificity enabling early screening and detection of cancer susceptible genes and sensitivity towards the target nucleic acid and with its low time consuming and monetary costs. Here in this book chapter, we have summarized the possible combinatorial effect of these two tools, which might offer an additional competence. Detection of cancer in its early stages might be handy in improving the efficiency of its treatment and might reduce the possibility of cancer relapse as the recurrence rate is reported to be comparatively more in the later stages of cancer making it incurable.

Author details

P.P. Mubthasima[1,2†], Kaumudi Pande[1,2†], Rajalakshmi Prakash[1,2†] and Anbarasu Kannan[1,2*]

1 Department of Protein Chemistry and Technology, CSIR-Central Food Technological Research Institute, Mysuru, India

2 Academy of Scientific and Innovative Research (AcSIR), CSIR-Central Food Technological Research Institute (CSIR-CFTRI) Campus, Mysuru, India

*Address all correspondence to: anbarasu@cftri.res.in

† Equal contribution.

References

[1] Sung H, Ferlay J, Siegel RL, et al. Global Cancer Statistics 2020: GLOBOCAN Estimates of Incidence and Mortality Worldwide for 36 Cancers in 185 Countries. *CA Cancer J Clin*. 2021; 71(3):209-249. doi:10.3322/caac.21660.

[2] Zaorsky NG, Churilla TM, Egleston BL, et al. Causes of death among cancer patients. Ann Oncol. 2017;28(2):400-407. doi:10.1093/annonc/mdw604.

[3] Ames BN, Gold LS, Willett WC. The causes and prevention of cancer. Proc Natl Acad Sci U S A. 1995;92(12):5258-5265. doi:10.1073/pnas.92.12.5258Hulvat MC. Cancer Incidence and Trends. Surg Clin North Am. 2020;100(3):469-481. doi:10.1016/j.suc.2020.01.002.

[4] Anand P, Kunnumakkara AB, Sundaram C, etal. Cancer is a preventable disease that require major lifestyle changes. *Pharm Res.* 2008; 25 (9): 2097-2116. doi: 10.1007/s11095-008-9661-9.

[5] Blackadar CB. Historical review of the causes of cancer. *World J Clin Oncol*. 2016; 7 (1): 54-86. doi:10.5306/wjco.v7.i1.54.

[6] Malik MA, Sepehri Z, Shah ZA. Cancer: disease caused by alteration of genes. *Int J Basic Sci Med.* 2016; 1 (2): 37-39. doi: 10.15171/ijbms.2016.09.

[7] Carbone A. Cancer classification at the crossroads. *Cancers.* 2020; 12 (4): 980. http://doi.org/10.3390/cancers12040980.

[8] Akalin, A., Mu, X., Kon, M. *et al.* Classification of malignant and benign tumors of the lung by infrared spectral histopathology (SHP). *Lab Invest* **95,** 406-421 (2015). https://doi.org/10.1038/labinvest.2015.1.

[9] Sobin LH. The international histological classification of tumors. *Bull World Health Organization*. 1981; 59(6): 813-819.

[10] Rosen RD, Sapra A. TNM Classification. In: StatPearls [Internet]. Treasure Island (FL): StatPearls Publishing; 2021 Jan-. Available from: https://www.ncbi.nlm.nih.gov/books/NBK553187/.

[11] Brierley JD, Gospodarowicz MK, Wittekind Ch., editors. International Union Against Cancer (UICC). TNM Classification of Malignant Tumours, 8th edn : Chichester, UK Wiley Blackwell 2017.

[12] Hortobagyi GN, Edge SB, Giuliano A. New and Important Changes in the TNM Staging System for Breast Cancer. Am Soc Clin Oncol Educ Book. 2018; 38: 457-467. doi:10.1200/EDBK_201313.

[13] Scheel BI, Holtedahl K. Symptoms, signs, and tests: The general practitioner's comprehensive approach towards a cancer diagnosis. *Scand J Prim Health Care.* 2015; 33 (3): 170-177. Doi: 10.3109/02813432.2015.1067512.

[14] Koo MM, Hamilton W, Walter FM, Rubin GP, Lyratzopoulos G. Symptom signatures and diagnostic timeliness in cancer patients: A review of current Evidence. Neoplasia. 2018; 20(2): 165-174. Doi: 10.1016/j.neo.2017.11.005.

[15] Nagpal M, Singh S, Singh P, Chauhan P, Zaidi MA, Tumor markers: A diagnostic tool. *Natl J Maxillofac surg.* 2016; 7 (1): 17-20. doi: 10.4103/0975-5950.196135.

[16] Henry NL, Hayes DF. Cancer biomarkers. *Mol Oncol.* 2012; 6 (2): 140-146. doi: 10.1016/j.molonc.2012.01.010.

[17] Ferguson JL, Turner SP. Bone Cancer: Diagnosis and Treatment Principles. Am Fam Physician. 2018;98(4):205-213.

[18] Pucci C, Martinelli C, Ciofani G. Innovative approaches for cancer treatment: current perspectives and new challenges. Ecancermedicalscience. 2019;13:961. doi:10.3332/ecancer.2019.961.

[19] Chuanjiang He, Shu Zheng, Yan Luo and Ben Wang. Exosome Theranostics: Biology and Translational Medicine. *Theranostics*. 2018; 8(1): 237-255. doi: 10.7150/thno.21945.

[20] Doyle LM, Wang MZ. Overview of extracellular vesicles, their origin, composition, purpose, and methods for exosome isolation and analysis. *Cell*. 2019; 8 (7): 727. doi: 10.3390/cells8070727.

[21] Harding CV, Heuser JE, Stahl PD. Exosomes: looking back three decades and into the future. *J Cell Biol*. 2013; 200 (4):367-371. doi: 10.1083/jcb.201212113.

[22] Harding C, Stahl P. Transferrin recycling in reticulocytes: pH and iron are important determinants of ligand binding and processing. *Biochem Biophys Res Commun*. 1983; 113 (2): 650-658. doi: 10.1016/006-291x(83)91776-x.

[23] Pan BT, Johnstone RM. Fate of the transferrin receptor during maturation of sheep reticulocytes in vitro: selective externalization of the receptor. *Cell*. 1983; 33 (3): 967-978. doi: 10.1016/0092-8674(83)90040-5.

[24] Gurunathan S, Kang MH, Kim JH. A Comprehensive Review on Factors Influences Biogenesis, Functions, Therapeutic and Clinical Implications of Exosomes. Int J Nanomedicine. 2021;16:1281-1312. Published 2021 Feb 17. doi:10.2147/IJN.S291956.

[25] Willms, E., Johansson, H., Mäger, I. et al. Cells release subpopulations of exosomes with distinct molecular and biological properties. Sci Rep 6, 22519 (2016). https://doi.org/10.1038/srep22519.

[26] Huda MN, Nafiujjaman M, Deaguero IG, et al. Potential Use of Exosomes as Diagnostic Biomarkers and in Targeted Drug Delivery: Progress in Clinical and Preclinical Applications. ACS Biomater Sci Eng. 2021;7(6):2106-2149. doi:10.1021/acsbiomaterials.1c00217.

[27] Zhang Y, Liu Y, Liu H, Tang WH. Exosomes: biogenesis, biologic function and clinical potential. *Cell Biosci*. 2019;9:19. Published 2019 Feb 15. doi:10.1186/s13578-019-0282-2.

[28] Kalluri R, LeBleu VS. The biology, function, and biomedical applications of exosomes. *Science*. 2020; 367(6478):eaau6977. doi:10.1126/science.aau6977.

[29] Hille F, Charpentier E. CRISPR-Cas: biology, mechanisms and relevance. Phil. Trans. R. Soc. B. 2016; 371: 20150496. doi:10.1098/rstb.2015.0496

[30] Makarova, K., Wolf, Y., Alkhnbashi, O. et al. An updated evolutionary classification of CRISPR–Cas systems. *Nat Rev Microbiol*. 2015;13, 722-736. doi:10.1038/nrmicro3569

[31] Makarova KS, Haft DH, Barrangou R, et al. Evolution and classification of the CRISPR-Cas systems. *Nat Rev Microbiol*. 2011;9(6):467-477. doi:10.1038/nrmicro2577

[32] Hsu PD, Lander ES, Zhang F. Development and applications of CRISPR-Cas9 for genome engineering. *Cell*. 2014;157(6):1262-1278. doi:10.1016/j.cell.2014.05.010

[33] Rajat M. Gupta and Kiran Musunuru. Expanding the genetic editing tool kit: ZFNs, TALENs, and

CRISPR-Cas9. Review: *J Clin Invest*. 2014; 124(10):4154-4161. doi:10.1172/JCI72992

[34] Hiroko Koike-Yusa, Yilong Li, E-Pien Tan, Martin Del Castillo Velasco-Herrera & Kosuke Yusa. Genome-wide recessive genetic screening in mammalian cells with a lentiviral CRISPR-guide RNA library. *Nat Biotechnol*. 2014;32(3):267-273. doi:10.1038/nbt.2800

[35] Jinek M, Chylinski K, Fonfara I, Hauer M, Doudna JA, Charpentier E. A programmable dual-RNA-guided DNA endonuclease in adaptive bacterial immunity. *Science*. 2012; 337 (6096): 816-821. doi: 10.1126/science.1225829

[36] Liu Z, Dong H, Cui Y, Cong L, Zhang D. Application of different types of CRISPR/Cas-based systems in bacteria. Microb Cell Fact. 2020; 19 (1): 172. doi: 10.1186/s12934-020-01431-z.

[37] Zhang W, Peng P, Shen K. Role of Exosomal Shuttle RNA in Cell-to-cell Communication. *Zhongguo Yi Xue Ke Xue Yuan Xue Bao*. 2016; 38 (4): 480-483. doi: 10.3881/j.issn.1000-503X.2016.04.020.

[38] Soung YH, Ford S, Zhang V, Chung J. Exosomes in Cancer Diagnostics. Cancers (Basel). 2017;9(1):8. Published 2017 Jan 12. doi:10.3390/cancers9010008.

[39] Li P, Kaslan M, Lee SH, Yao J, Gao Z. Progress in Exosome Isolation Techniques. *Theranostics.* 2017; 7(3): 789-804. doi: 10.7150/thno.18133.

[40] Yu LL, Zhu J, Liu JX, Jiang F, Ni WK, Qu LS, Ni RZ, Lu CH, Xiao MB. A comparison of Traditional and Novel Method for the separation of Exosomes from Human Samples. *BioMed Research International*. 2018: 2018:36364563. doi: 10.1155/2018/3634563.

[41] Patel GK, Khan MA, Zubair H, Srivastava SK, Khusman M, Singh S, Singh AP. Comparative analysis of exosomes isolation methods using culture supernatant for optimum yield, purity and downstream applications. *Nat Sci Rep*. 2019; 9(1): 5335. doi: 10.1038/s41598-019-41800-2.

[42] Lobb RJ, Becker M, Wen SW, Wong CSF, Wiegmans AP, Leimburger A, Moller A. Optimized exosome isolation protocol for cell culture supernatant and human plasma. *Journal of Extracellular Vesicles*. 2015; 4(1): 27031. doi: 10.3402/jev.v4.27031.

[43] Rupp AK, Rupp C, Keller S, et al. Loss of EpCAM expression in breast cancer derived serum exosomes: role of proteolytic cleavage. Gynecol Oncol. 2011;122(2):437-446. doi:10.1016/j.ygyno.2011.04.035.

[44] Moon PG, Lee JE, Cho YE, et al. Identification of Developmental Endothelial Locus-1 on Circulating Extracellular Vesicles as a Novel Biomarker for Early Breast Cancer Detection. Clin Cancer Res. 2016;22(7): 1757-1766. doi:10.1158/1078-0432.CCR-15-0654.

[45] Khan S, Jutzy JM, Valenzuela MM, et al. Plasma-derived exosomal survivin, a plausible biomarker for early detection of prostate cancer. PLoS One. 2012;7(10):e46737. doi:10.1371/journal.pone.0046737.

[46] Nilsson J, Skog J, Nordstrand A, et al. Prostate cancer-derived urine exosomes: a novel approach to biomarkers for prostate cancer. Br J Cancer. 2009;100(10):1603-1607. doi:10.1038/sj.bjc.6605058.

[47] Kanwar SS, Dunlay CJ, Simeone DM, Nagrath S. Microfluidic device (ExoChip) for on-chip isolation, quantification and characterization of circulating exosomes. Lab Chip. 2014;14(11):1891-1900. doi:10.1039/c4lc00136b.

[48] Yoshioka Y, Kosaka N, Konishi Y, et al. Ultra-sensitive liquid biopsy of

circulating extracellular vesicles using ExoScreen. Nat Commun. 2014;5:3591. Published 2014 Apr 7. doi:10.1038/ncomms4591.

[49] Zhao Z, Yang Y, Zeng Y, He M. A microfluidic ExoSearch chip for multiplexed exosome detection towards blood-based ovarian cancer diagnosis. Lab Chip. 2016;16(3):489-496. doi:10.1039/c5lc01117e.

[50] Huang T, Deng CX. Current Progresses of Exosomes as Cancer Diagnostic and Prognostic Biomarkers. Int J Biol Sci. 2019;15(1):1-11. Published 2019 Jan 6. doi:10.7150/ijbs.27796.

[51] Zhou, B., Xu, K., Zheng, X. et al. Application of exosomes as liquid biopsy in clinical diagnosis. Sig Transduct Target Ther 5, 144 (2020). https://doi.org/10.1038/s41392-020-00258-9.

[52] Ariston Gabriel, A.N., Wang, F., Jiao, Q. et al. The involvement of exosomes in the diagnosis and treatment of pancreatic cancer. Mol Cancer 19, 132 (2020). https://doi.org/10.1186/s12943-020-01245-y.

[53] Zhu CS, Liu CY, Qiu XY, et al. Novel nucleic acid detection strategies based on CRISPR-Cas systems: From construction to application. *Biotechnol Bioeng*. 2020; 117(7): 2279-2294. doi:10.1002/bit.27334.

[54] Xu Y, Li Z. CRISPR-Cas systems: Overview, innovations and applications in human disease research and gene therapy. *Comput Struct Biotechnol J*. 2020;18:2401-2415. Published 2020 Sep 8. doi:10.1016/j.csbj.2020.08.031.

[55] Yao R, Liu D, Jia X, Zheng Y, Liu W, Xiao Y. CRISPR-Cas9/Cas12a biotechnology and application in bacteria [published correction appears in Synth Syst Biotechnol. 2020 Oct 12; 5(4): 328. *Synth Syst Biotechnol*. 2018; 3 (3): 135-149. Published 2018 Oct 3. doi:10.1016/j.synbio.2018.09.004.

[56] Jolany vangah S, Katalani C, Boone HA etal. CRISPR-Based Diagnosis of Infectious and Noninfectious Diseases. [published correction appears in *Biol Proced Online*. 2020 Nov 7;22(1):24]. *Biol Proced online.* 2020; 22; 22. Published 2020 sep 14. https://doi.org/10.1186/s12575-020-00135-3.

[57] Abudayyeh OO, Gootenberg JS, Essletzbichler P etal. RNA targeting with CRISPR-Cas13. *Nature.* 2017; 550 (7675): 280-284. doi: 10.1038/nature24049.

[58] Savage DF. Cas14: Big Advances from Small CRISPR Proteins. *Biochemistry.* 2019; 58(8): 1024-1025. http://doi.org/10.1021/acs.biochem.9b00035.

[59] Harrington LB, Brustein D, Chen JS, Paez-Espino D, Ma E, Witte IP, Cofsky JC, Kyrpides NC, Banfield JF and Doudna JA. Programmed DNA destruction by miniature CRISPR-Cas14 enzymes. *Science.* 2018; 362(6416): 839-842. doi: 10.1126/science.aav4294.

[60] Martinez-Escobar A, Luna-Callejas B, Ramón-Gallegos E. CRISPR-dCas9-Based Artificial Transcription Factors to Improve Efficacy of Cancer Treatment With Drug Repurposing: Proposal for Future Research. *Front Oncol*. 2021;10:604948. Published 2021 Feb 3. doi:10.3389/fonc.2020.604948.

[61] Mintz RL, Gao MA, Lo K, Lao YH, Li M, Leong KW. CRISPR Technology for Breast Cancer: Diagnostics, Modeling, and Therapy. Adv Biosyst. 2018;2(11):1800132. doi:10.1002/adbi.201800132.

[62] Gootenberg JS, Abudayyeh OO, Lee JW, et al. Nucleic acid detection with CRISPR-Cas13a/C2c2. Science.

2017;356(6336):438-442. doi:10.1126/science.aam9321.

[63] Chen JS, Ma E, Harrington LB, et al. CRISPR-Cas12a target binding unleashes indiscriminate single-stranded DNase activity [published correction appears in Science. 2021 Feb 19;371(6531):]. *Science*. 2018;360(6387):436-439. doi:10.1126/science.aar6245.

[64] Zhang S, Shen J, Li D, Cheng Y. Strategies in the delivery of Cas9 ribonucleoprotein for CRISPR/Cas9 genome editing. Theranostics. 2021;11(2):614-648. Published 2021 Jan 1. doi:10.7150/thno.47007

[65] Yang B, Chen Y, Shi J. Exosome Biochemistry and Advanced Nanotechnology for Next-Generation Theranostic Platforms. Adv Mater. 2019;31(2):e1802896. doi:10.1002/adma.201802896

[66] Y. He, Y. Wu, Y. Wang, X. Wang, S. Xing, H. Li, S. Guo, X. Yu, S. Dai, G. Zhang, Applying CRISPR/Cas13 to Construct Exosomal PD-L1 Ultrasensitive Biosensors for Dynamic Monitoring of Tumor Progression in Immunotherapy, Adv. Therapeut. 2020: 3 (10); https://doi.org/10.1002/adtp.202000093.

[67] Xing S, Lu Z, Huang Q, et al. An ultrasensitive hybridization chain reaction-amplified CRISPR-Cas12a aptasensor for extracellular vesicle surface protein quantification. Theranostics. 2020;10(22):10262-10273. Published 2020 Aug 13. doi:10.7150/thno.49047.

[68] De Jong, O.G., Murphy, D.E., Mäger, I. et al. A CRISPR-Cas9-based reporter system for single-cell detection of extracellular vesicle-mediated functional transfer of RNA. Nat Commun 11, 1113 (2020). https://doi.org/10.1038/s41467-020-14977-8.

Section 4

Maternal Mortality in Developing Countries: Case Study from Pakistan

Chapter 6

Maternal Mortality in Rural Areas of Pakistan: Challenges and Prospects

Muhammad Hanif, Siddra Khalid, Akhtar Rasul and Khalid Mahmood

Abstract

Pakistan is one of the countries in South Asia ranking high in maternal mortality rate. Though, a signatory of Agenda 2030, the country still lags behind considerably in achieving Sustainable Development Goals (SDGs). The ratio of maternal mortality is, even higher in rural areas of the country. Lack of health care facilities, education, malnutrition, poverty, high prevalence of violence against women in rural areas, and socioeconomic factors are some of the major contributing elements for elevated levels of maternal mortality and morbidity rate in Pakistan. By making inclusive policies at the national level to improve the reach of the rural population to healthcare facilities, educating women and eliminating gender-based disparities, introducing family planning interventions, accountability, and continuity of democracy are essentially needed to improve maternal health in Pakistan's rural areas. This chapter focuses on challenges to maternal health in rural areas and possible options to resolve these issues.

Keywords: Maternal mortality, Maternal mortality rate, Maternal mortality rate in Pakistan, maternal mortality ratio

1. Introduction

The maternal mortality rate is highest for Asia and it is even higher for South Asian countries including Pakistan. As per most recent stats around 295,000 women die during and following childbirth worldwide in a year. South Asia alone accounts for almost 1/5th of all these deaths (**Figure 1** and **Table 1**). It is regrettable to note that about 94% of maternal deaths occur in underdeveloped countries [3]. A most recent survey naming 'Pakistan Maternal Mortality Survey 2019' conducted by the National Institute of Population Studies funded by USAID shows considerable demographic variations in maternal mortality rates of women residing in rural and urban areas of Pakistan. The maternal mortality ratio in Pakistan is 186 deaths per 100,000 live births. The ratio is nearly 26% higher in rural areas as compared to urban areas [4]. In order to avoid complications, it is imperative to provide mothers with skilled care and safety during pregnancy, childbirth, and the postnatal period. There are various contributing factors including poverty, lack of education, gender-based inequalities, inadequate and poor quality of healthcare services, distant facilities, sociocultural values, malnutrition and violence against women, unfair distribution of resources, and political environment; can be termed as key indicators

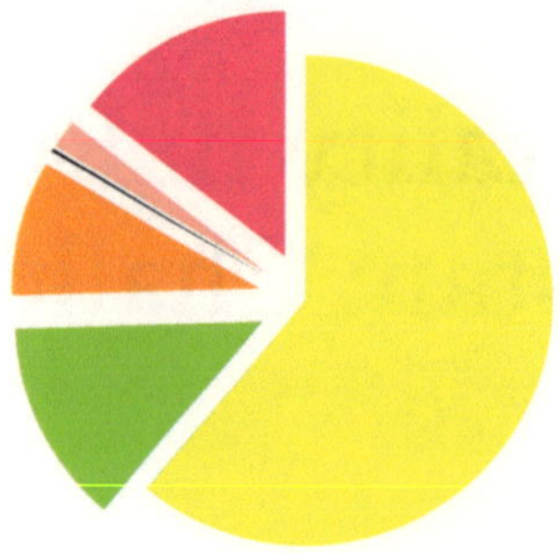

Figure 1.
The number of maternal deaths in the region of South Asia. Stats by the World Health Organization on maternal mortality trends 2000–2017 estimates that South Asia accounts for 57,000 maternal deaths.

Sr. No	Country	Number of maternal deaths	Percentage of maternal deaths	Maternal Mortality Ratio (per 100 K live births)
1.	India	35,000	61.03%	145
2.	Pakistan	8,300	14.47%	140
3.	Afghanistan	7,700	13.43%	638
4.	Bangladesh	5,100	8.89%	173
5.	Nepal	1,100	1.92%	186
6.	Sri Lanka	120	0.21%	36
7.	Bhutan	24	0.04%	183
8.	Maldives	4	0.01%	53

Table 1.
Trends of maternal deaths and MMR in the region of South Asia as per most recent stats (Year 2017) provided by the World Health Organization [1, 2].

for increased maternal death burden in rural areas. Moreover, having the Millennium Development Goals (MDGs) failed, now Pakistan is lagging far behind in achieving Sustainable Development Goals (SDGs). Domains of unmet SDGs include a reduction in child death, improvement in maternal health, and a greater number of births by skilled personnel [5]. This chapter concentrates on challenges to maternal health in rural areas alongside options and interventions to deal with these challenges.

2. Definitions

2.1 What is the maternal mortality ratio?

The maternal mortality ratio (MMR) is defined as the number of maternal deaths in a certain time duration of 100,000 live births. It is an indicator of the possibility of maternal death with relevance to the number of live births. It is a measure of the risk of maternal death as per pregnancy or one live birth [6, 7].

2.2 Maternal deaths

It is the total number of annual women death expressed per 100,000 live births because of complications during pregnancy and childbirth or inside the time of 42 days following the end of pregnancy, regardless of the length and site of pregnancy, in a specified period. It is important to note that it does not include the incidental or accidental occurrence of maternal deaths [6].

2.3 Live birth

It is defined as the removal or extraction of the whole conceived product from the mother, regardless of the period of pregnancy, which after the expulsion shows any sign of life such as breathing, a beating heart, pulsating umbilical cord, moving voluntary muscles (irrespective of the fact that the placenta has been detached or not) [6].

2.4 What is the maternal mortality rate?

The maternal mortality rate can be defined as the number of mothers who die per 1000 women [8].

2.5 Formula to calculate the maternal mortality rate

Below is given the formula (Eq. 1) to calculate the maternal mortality rate in a specific geographical area [9].

$$\text{Maternal mortality rate} = \frac{\text{Number of inhabitant maternal deaths}}{\text{Number of inhabitants live births}} \times 100{,}000 \quad (1)$$

2.6 Pregnancy-related mortality ratio

The pregnancy-related mortality ratio (PRMR) is defined as the number of pregnancy-related deaths per 100,000 live births [10].

3. Current scenario of maternal health in rural areas of Pakistan

Pakistan ranks fifth in the world according to population. Pakistan is an agriculture-based economy and recent stats show that 64% of the Pakistani population lives in rural areas [11]. According to the most recent report on the nationwide maternal mortality survey in Pakistan, MMR is 186. The report also indicates a considerably increased incidence of maternal deaths in the rural areas of Pakistan. MMR for urban areas of Pakistan is 158 while on the other hand MMR for rural areas is 199 which shows there a difference of 41 deaths per 100,000 live births [4].

4. Major issues associated with maternal mortality in rural areas of Pakistan

With a majority of the population living in the rural areas, there is a major difference in health care services provided to the people living in urban areas as compared to those living in distant regions. Here are some of the contributing factors in poor health conditions of women during the prenatal and postnatal era which subsequently result in elevated levels of maternal deaths in rural areas.

4.1 Lack of education in rural women population

Pakistani women, especially those belonging to rural Pakistan are lacking in education which in turn serves as a stimulus for increasing maternal mortality ratio. According to recent surveys, 62% of the rural women population of reproductive age is uneducated which is way more than the uneducated percentage of the urban women population. A 34% women population of childbearing age living in urban areas has no education. While in urban Pakistan the percentage of women of reproductive age, possessing secondary or higher education is 39%. Only 14% of the rural women population have secondary or higher education. In Sindh and Balochistan, 4 in every 5 women are uneducated. When compared to the urban Sindh population, 2 in every 5 women have an education of secondary or higher levels. It has been estimated that around 63% of the maternal deaths account for those women who had no education (**Table 2** and **Figure 2**) [4].

It is pertinent to mention here that Article 25A of the constitution of Pakistan states that the onus is on the state to provide free and compulsory education to individuals between the ages of 5–16. Article 25 also enables the state to make any special provisions to ensure women's protection and the children thereon [12]. School dropout rate because of distant educational centers, inadequate safety measures such as missing boundary walls in schools, gender-based inequalities, and poverty are the main causes of vast differences in the educational attainment of the women living in urban and rural areas. The spirit of article 25 of the constitution of Pakistan is to empower every individual irrespective of gender and regardless of the area where one lives. Women who have no education at all have higher maternal

Attributes	Women with no education		Provincial distribution of uneducated women
Residence	Rural	Urban	
Level of schooling	62.3%	33.6%	Total uneducated = 51.7%
Punjab	50.5%	27.2%	41.7%
Sindh	82.4%	36.5%	57.1%
Khyber Pakhtunkhwa	70.0%	48.5%	66.8%
Balochistan	80.4%	66.5%	76.2%

Table 2.
A comparison of ever-married women between the ages of 15 to 49 having no education in rural and urban areas of Pakistan according to Pakistan Maternal Mortality Survey 2019 [4].

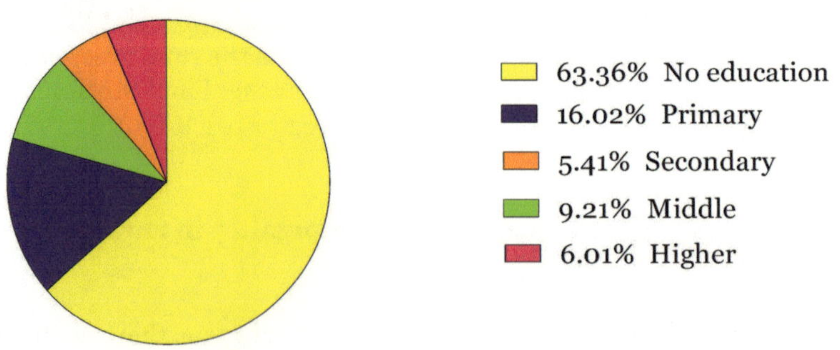

Figure 2.
Percentage distribution of educational attainment of deceased women who died three years before the Pakistan Maternal Mortality survey 2019 (Ages 15-49 yrs). Primary level education: Class 1–5, Middle-level education: Class 6–8, Secondary level education: Class 9–10, Higher level education: Class 11 and above.

mortality, malnutrition, children with stunted growth, and infant mortality rates. The disparities in educational infrastructure which the women face in rural areas are holding back them to showcase their full potential in all domains of life. There is a famous Chinese proverb, "If you are planning for a year, sow rice; if you are planning for a decade, plant trees; if you are planning for a lifetime, educate people."

4.2 Gender inequality

Women's reproductive behaviors are largely influenced by gender-based inequalities, by depriving them of their basic rights and self-sufficiency [13]. Pakistan ranks at number 151 out of 153 countries in Global Gender Gap Index which depicts Pakistan's bad standing in the global gender equality scenario [14]. It is a grim situation where almost 48% of the country's total population doesn't have equal opportunities in educational achievement, political participation, economic opportunities, and survival and health. A large chunk of the female population is deprived of basic healthcare facilities in rural areas of Pakistan. 69% of the total maternal mortalities occurring in Pakistan belong to women living in rural areas. When it comes to maternal health, the majority of the women don't have decisive powers even to seek healthcare facilities for themselves. Women's reproductive health, as well as maternal mortality rates, are largely dictated by their decision-making powers for their health [15]. Gender disparities directly predispose women to malnutrition, violence, delay in seeking healthcare, neglect, and ill-treatment during pregnancy, child marriages, and uncalled-for maternal mortality and morbidity. Some of the issues are explained in detail below.

4.2.1 Violence against women

Violence against women especially spousal violence has a negative impact not only on maternal health but also on antenatal care [13]. Vulnerability to all forms of violence—psychological, emotional, physical, verbal, and sexual—of rural women increases manifolds as they have no education, lack of skills and awareness to guard themselves. In many instances, domestic abuse is used to control and overpower women in rural areas. According to studies, spousal violence aggravates the risks associated with bad maternal health conditions. Women experiencing violence are likely to have more chances of pregnancy termination or lost pregnancies. In addition, in areas where healthcare facilities are already scarce, spousal violence contributes to decreasing the probability of maternal healthcare visits for antenatal care. In low-income countries like Pakistan, one in every ten women is subjected to spousal violence during the gestation period. Data shows that 24% of women experience less severe physical violence while 7.6% women population experience violence during pregnancy [16]. Women are more prone to domestic abuse in the case of female fetuses and in worst cases are even beaten to death [13]. This terrible reality further raises concerns for gender equality and equitable opportunities for maternal healthcare for women residing in remote areas.

4.2.2 Child marriages and honor killing

Rural women are victims of honor killing and similar crimes such as nose-cutting, acid attacks, burning, imprisonment, and forced or child marriages [17]. In a society with deeply ingrained social norms including killing girls in the name of honor and forcing them into early marriages result in exacerbation of the impacts of gender disparities. Pieces of evidence of child marriages remain high in the female population with no or low education residing in rural parts of the country. Women with early marriages i.e. before the legal age of marriage as per law are unlikely to utilize maternal health care services via trained medical staff. Hence they are more likely to have their children delivered at homes which are associated with the increased maternal mortality and morbidity rate. No denying the fact, high MMR correlates with early or child marriages which is essentially not as greater a concern for the neighboring countries like India, Bangladesh, and Nepal as it remains for Pakistan [18]. The majority of the women in Pakistan, let alone those living in the rural parts of the country, are generally vulnerable to old customs, and outdated cultural traditions which sometimes cost their lives.

4.3 Poverty

Poor health conditions of women in Pakistan especially those living in rural areas are essentially attributed to socioeconomic factors [8]. Pakistan is a developing economy with a population of 210million people, and the rural population is more prone to poverty and impoverishment. Recent trends show that 1/4th of the total population lives below the poverty line. With a majority of the people living in rural areas, 31% of the rural population is impoverished in comparison to 13% urban population [19]. A vast difference in the economic factors of rural and urban populations increases the reproductive health-related concerns in rural women. They are more vulnerable to undernourishment and their kids are more likely to be malnourished. Furthermore, poverty is a predisposing factor in seeking healthcare facilities before, during, or after pregnancy (**Table 3**). Women in impoverished households usually have higher fertility rates, more incidence of undergoing unsafe or traditional delivery practices performed by unskilled persons, and less evidence of following a family planning regimen. All these factors negatively impact the reproductive health of rural women and in turn, increases MMR for Pakistan.

4.4 Political instability in Pakistan

As per population, Pakistan ranks in 5th place in the world. Since the very first population census held in 1951, the population of the country has grown by more than 6-folds [20, 21]. Census is meant for the purpose to access and gather data about the individuals living in a country which enables the policy-developers to make policies and plan programs accordingly. Census is prescribed to be held in the country every ten years. Unfortunately, except for the second and the fourth census, none has been held according to the prescribed schedule. After 1951, the second census in Pakistan was carried out 1961. The third census was due in 1971, but it was held in 1972. The fifth census was to be organized in 1991, but it was

Economic status	Percentage of deceased women	Women with no education	Percentage of women seeking for treatment of pregnancy-related complications
Lowest wealth quintile	21.0%	91.2%	44%
Second wealth quintile	21.6%	73.8%	52%
Middle wealth quintile	21.4%	57.1%	52%
Fourth wealth quintile	18.4%	32.0%	56%
Highest wealth quintile	17.6%	13.7%	55%

Table 3.
Association of maternal mortality with economic conditions, educational attainment, and treatment-seeking behavior according to Pakistan Maternal Mortality Survey 2019.

conducted in 1998. And the most recent census in Pakistan has been arranged in 2017 [22]. Reasons for the delayed census are primarily political instability in the country. Pakistan has three times faced decade-long military rules. To date, none of the elected Prime Ministers in the country has ever completed a 5-years term. Additionally, the country has fought three major wars with India. Overcoming longs delay in census is a necessary element to curtail discrepancies in the health care infrastructure. Rural areas in Pakistan are deprived of necessary and essential healthcare facilities and so does the women living there. Many rural mothers die on their way to distant hospitals situated in cities. There is a dire need to ensure political stability and making long-term policies for the development of healthcare infrastructure in all areas of Pakistan. After all, health is wealth!

5. Towards finding solution

Since the day of inception, Pakistan has made very little progress towards improving key indicators of maternal health. Pakistan has been a signatory to many international conventions regarding improvement in maternal health and decreasing MMR. Despite various programs and efforts, the implementation regimen remains poor. Many disparities are prevailing between the rural and urban population and access to maternal healthcare services is one of them. Elevated levels of MMR in rural Pakistan are directly linked to a variety of factors such as compromised status of women in society, undernutrition, high-risk pregnancies, poor or delayed access to health care facilities, illiteracy, and poverty. Here are some options and interventions which are essential to improve maternal health in rural areas of Pakistan.

5.1 Women empowerment and gender equality

Women empowerment and gender equality contribute to a great extent in making women able to understand their own needs, a value in the family system, and a broader perspective in society as a whole. They can ask for their rights to access quality health care services and can better take care of themselves as well as their newborns. Moreover, to prevent maternal deaths and improving the wellbeing of rural mothers, this knowledge plays a fundamental role. Gender equality allows women to avail the lifesaving opportunities, taking all benefits from the public policies and programs which in turn uplifts the condition of maternal and neonatal health. Besides, equal participation of women in the healthcare workforce of rural areas is also crucial to curtailing MMR.

Pakistan has long remained hard on women and nonetheless, the situation is the same. Studies have shown that pregnant women living in rural areas of Pakistan are more victims of deprived mental health as compared to those of urban women [23]. The economic status of women, social relations and social conditions, and pregnancy-related concerns are major determinants of maternal mental health. Women in rural areas are more prone to subjugated roles, old customs and traditions, Watta Satta (exchange marriage of women from two families), and inheritance issues are some of the predominant causes of the depressed mental state of pregnant women in rural areas of Pakistan. Studies have suggested that depression is twice more common in rural mothers in comparison with urban pregnant women. On top of that, discussing or treating mental health issues is taken for granted in Pakistani society. A depressive mental state can have severe negative implications for the mother's health and the health of the kid and family associated with her [23]. Hence, investment in addressing social determinants of maternal health of rural women is of prime importance to reduce MMR and move a step forward in achieving SDGs.

Women consist of almost half of Pakistan's population [24]. For one, their participation is all the more important in the development and the progress of society. Countries, where women are empowered and getting equal opportunities, are quoted as instances of progress and prosperity. On the contrary, in Pakistan women, health care workers get targeted for the polio vaccine immunization program. This further poses a hindrance to the recruitment of women health care staff in high-risk rural districts. Consequently, the MMR for Pakistan especially in rural regions remains high.

Following are some key factors recommended by WHO to achieve essential goals to save women lives and to decrease maternal mortality by means for empowering women [25].

1. Reduction of the routine burden of physical labor on women in rural areas

2. Improving gender equality in relationships

3. Investing in the health-related literacy in women, and the overall community

4. Increasing and understanding the value of a girl-child and decreasing son preference

5. Abolishing harmful conventional norms and practices surrounding gestation and the postpartum period.

6. Eliminating child marriages

All aforementioned factors are equally necessary to improve maternal health and reduce the lifelong risk of maternal death and disability in rural Pakistan.

5.2 Political will and stability

Abraham Lincoln has said, "Democracy is the government of the people, for the people and by the people." Pakistan is a country with constitutional democracy. Respecting the constitution and understanding the letter and spirit of laws is indispensable for every citizen of the country. Where democracy goes from strength to strength, people are empowered. It also ensures the continuity of public programs and policies in the long run. Furthermore, the onus is on the policymakers to prioritize the health sector by allocating more budget to the health sector.

The recent ranking of Pakistan in the Open Budget Index 2019 is 93 out of 117 countries. Whereas the budget transparency score for Pakistan is 28 out of 100, which is way below the other South Asian countries. Budget transparency is an estimate of access of information of the general populace to the information about the central government's expenditure of public resources. It also estimates the involvement of the public in national budgetary concerns. Afghanistan, India, Nepal, Sri Lanka, and Bangladesh are ranking at better positions in comparison to Pakistan [26]. In 2017 Pakistan's expenditure on healthcare per capita was $42 and in 2018 it was $43 [27]. Pakistan is not at par with the developed economies in providing health security to all the citizens. Those living in distant areas are more affected by this grim reality. Rural women are reportedly seen to pay fewer maternal visits to the healthcare settings during and after pregnancy in contrast to urban women. Culturally and socially bound women living in rural areas need better healthcare facilities for themselves and their children. By taking into consideration suggestions from all the prominent stakeholders while planning and policymaking, creating long-term health-associated policies, and prioritizing a health-sensitive budget are vital factors to reduce MMR, improve human rights status, and obtaining success in Agenda 2030 (SDGs).

5.3 Success stories of exemplar countries and factor associated with achievement of low maternal mortality

A tremendous chance to learn how to reduce maternal mortality is knowing about the interventions and decisions from the exemplars who have achieved fairly low maternal mortality. A comparison of maternal mortality data of 1990 and 2013 (**Table 4**) shows that through the successful interventions—Bangladesh, China, Cambodia, Egypt, Nepal, Peru, Vietnam, Rwanda, and Lao PDR—have reduced almost 70,000 maternal deaths at a substantially faster pace [28]. Despite the enormous and individual political, social, and economic challenges; understanding that how these countries have got success in reducing child death and maternal mortality rates will be of great help to learn about the strategies, policies, and areas of investment and achieving desired outcomes in no time.

5.4 Recommendations for improving the status of maternal health in rural women in Pakistan

To reduce maternal mortality and morbidity in the rural Pakistan, there is a need to focus on the following aspects:

1. Increasing allocation of budget and funding in the health sector to the provinces (as per their needs) in NFC award (National Finance Commission) by a re-evaluation of healthcare infrastructure.

2. A collaboration of the center and provinces in integrating health with the economic progress and promoting the judicious distribution of resources.

3. Prioritizing women's reproductive health and investing more in maternal and child healthcare programs especially in rural areas of Pakistan.

4. Expanding the quality and quantity of primary healthcare services for maternal, neonatal, and child health care in remote and rural districts.

5. Introducing family planning programs and educating women and the community about the nutritional needs for maternal and neonatal care.

6. Spending in awareness campaigns and education of women to address social determinants of maternal mortality and morbidity in the remote areas.

7. Investing to strengthen the district healthcare information system, routine monitoring, accountability, and regular-evaluation of performance at district level health care centers and hospitals.

8. Investing in reachable, affordable, and quality education for women living in remote areas of Pakistan.

Sr. no	Countries	Reduction in Maternal mortality	Reduction in <5 child mortality	Successful interventions made by fast track countries
1	Bangladesh	66%	65%	Successful coverage of vital interventions (family planning, immunization, oral rehydration treatment in rural areas) Public-private partnership Gender equity Access to education for women Access to the latest information and communication technology Improving road networks
2	Cambodia	75%	57%	Timely access to immunization Developments in socioeconomic conditions Timely breastfeeding
3	China	80% (approximately)	80%	Successful coverage of vital interventions Strengthening healthcare workforce Access to water Access to sanitation
4	Egypt	69%	75%	Family planning Immunization Improving literacy rate Improving water access Improving access to sanitation facilities
5	Lao PDR	6.8%	56%	Strengthening coverage of vital immunization Preventing malaria Family planning Timely and exclusive lactation Improvements in socioeconomic status
6	Nepal	80%	66%	Increasing number of skilled birth attendance Integrating and prioritizing health in politics Improving education Improvements in transportation and communication Access to water and sanitization
7	Peru	65%	70%	Social progress Political will and stability Economic growth Addressing cultural barriers Increasing access to health care facilities by minimizing geographical barriers
8	Rwanda	22%	50%	Increasing healthcare workforce Improvements in healthcare infrastructure Improving access to healthcare centers Increasing access to education Prioritizing women political and economic involvement Addressing issues of malnutrition in women
9	Viet Nam	70%	60%	Prioritizing timely immunization Nutrition and child-survival regimes Skilled birth attendance Availability of contraceptives Access to clean drinking water Access to sanitation Increasing primary school enrollments

Table 4.
Successful interventions made by fast-track countries in curtailing maternal mortality rate and improving child health and survival rate. Data in the table shows a comparison of rapid reduction in maternal mortality and child mortality between 1990 and 2013 [28].

6. Conclusion

Maternal health is not only linked to a woman but also her kids and the family. Healthy mothers are a prerequisite for healthy children. And children are an asset for a country's future human capital. Mothers are directly involved in improving the nutritional outcome of this human capital. Women in Pakistan are dying because of many complications that are either avoidable or treatable. By bridging the gaps of gender-based inequalities, providing equal opportunities to all women in rural areas, social reforms, prioritizing a health-sensitive budget, promoting women education, long term policy development, and planning programs to improve maternal and child health, investing in bringing down disparities between urban and remote areas, health care system interventions at the district level, not only can help Pakistan in achieving the SDGs 2030 but also help in ranking the country higher in human development index. Whether these are rural or urban areas, at every level, all-inclusive regimens are required to achieve global goals to reduce the maternal death burden. As we grow, we grow up collectively!

Acknowledgements

Authors are very much thankful to Higher Education Commission (HEC) Pakistan for providing the financial assistance under the NRPU research project.

Conflict of interest

All the authors have no conflict of interest.

Notes/thanks/other declarations

Authors are very much thankful to you for the Dean faculty of Pharmacy, Prof. Dr. Muhammad Uzair, Chairman department of Pharmaceutics, Prof. Dr. Syed Nisar Hussain Shah, Associate professor department of statistics Dr. Muhammad Ahmad shahzad for providing the research facilities and survey based data.

Appendices and nomenclature

SDGs	Sustainable Development Goals
USAID	United States Agency for International Development
MDGs	Millennium Development Goals
MMR	Maternal mortality ratio
PRMR	Pregnancy-related mortality ratio
WHO	World Health Organization
NFC	National Finance Commission

Author details

Muhammad Hanif[1*], Siddra Khalid[1], Akhtar Rasul[2] and Khalid Mahmood[3]

1 Department of Pharmaceutics, Faculty of Pharmacy, Bahauddin Zakariya University Multan, Pakistan

2 Department of Pharmaceutics, Faculty of Pharmaceutical Sciences, Government College University, Faisalabad, Pakistan

3 Institute of Chemical Sciences, Bahauddin Zakariya University Multan, Pakistan

*Address all correspondence to: muhammad.hanif@bzu.edu.pk

References

[1] Maternal mortality ratio (modeled estimate, per 100,000 live births) 2019 [cited 2021 02-12]. Available from: https://data.worldbank.org/indicator/SH.STA.MMRT?locations=PK.

[2] Number of maternal deaths - South Asia 2019 [cited 2021 02-12]. Available from: https://data.worldbank.org/indicator/SH.MMR.DTHS?end=2017&locations=8S&start=2000&view=chart.

[3] Maternal mortality 2019 [updated 19 September 2019; cited 2021 10-02]. Available from: https://www.who.int/news-room/fact-sheets/detail/maternal-mortality.

[4] Pakistan Maternal Mortality Survey 2019: Key Indicators Report. Islamabad, Pakistan, and Rockville, Maryland, USA: NIPS and ICF.: National Institute of Population Studies (NIPS) [Pakistan] and ICF, 2020 2020. Report No.

[5] Adnan M, Mahmood H, Hassan M, Humayun A. Maternal Health Care Expenditure among Women in Rural Areas of Pakistan. Annals of King Edward Medical University. 2017;23(2).

[6] Mortality and burden of disease [cited 2021 10-02]. Available from: https://www.who.int/data/gho/indicator-metadata-registry/imr-details/26.

[7] Maternal Mortality and Pregnancy-related Mortality [cited 2021 10-02]. Available from: https://dhsprogram.com/Data/Guide-to-DHS-Statistics/Maternal_Mortality_and_Pregnancy-related_Mortality.htm#Pregnancy_related.

[8] Khan YP, Bhutta SZ, Munim S, Bhutta ZA. Maternal health and survival in Pakistan: issues and options. Journal of obstetrics and gynaecology canada. 2009;31(10):920-9.

[9] Maternal Mortality and Related Concepts. USA: National Center for Health Statistics, Services USDoHaH; 2007 Contract No.: 33.

[10] Maternal deaths [cited 2021 02-11]. Available from: https://www.who.int/data/gho/indicator-metadata-registry/imr-details/4622.

[11] Nasir Javed MK. 6th Population & Housing Census 2017 A Comprehensive Summary of Results. Unit TU; 2018.

[12] THE CONSTITUTION OF THE ISLAMIC REPUBLIC OF PAKISTAN. Eighth ed. Islamabad, Pakistan2018. p. 15.

[13] Rizvi N, Khan KS, Shaikh BT. Gender: shaping personality, lives and health of women in Pakistan. BMC women's health. 2014;14(1):1-8.

[14] Global Gender Gap Report. World Economic Forum, 2020.

[15] Jafree SR. The Sociology of South Asian Women's Health: Springer; 2020.

[16] Hassan S-U-N, Memon E, Shahab M, Mumtaz S. Utilization of maternal healthcare services in women experiencing spousal violence in Pakistan: A comparative analysis of 2012-13 and 2017-18 Pakistan Demographic Health Surveys. PloS one. 2020;15(9):e0239722.

[17] Country Policy and Information NotePakistan: Women fearing gender-based violence. In: Office UH, editor. UK2020. p. 1-68.

[18] Nasrullah M, Zakar R, Krämer A. Effect of child marriage on use of maternal health care services in Pakistan. Obstetrics & Gynecology. 2013;122(3):517-24.

[19] Farooq S, Ahmad U. Economic Growth and Rural Poverty in Pakistan:

A Panel Dataset Analysis. The European Journal of Development Research. 2020:1-23.

[20] U.S. and World Population Clock USA: U.S. Department of Commerce; 2021 [cited 2021 02-11]. Available from: https://www.census.gov/popclock/world.

[21] Pakistan's Population Challenge. Development Advocate of Pakistan. 2021 01-23.

[22] Population Census: Pakistan Bureau of Statistics; 2021 [updated 12-02-2021; cited 2021 02-12]. Available from: https://www.pbs.gov.pk/content/population-census.

[23] Zahidie A, Kazi A, Fatmi Z, Bhatti MT, Dureshahwar S. Social environment and depression among pregnant women in rural areas of Sind, Pakistan. JPMA-Journal of the Pakistan Medical Association. 2011;61(12):1183.

[24] Young Women in Pakistan – Status Report 2020 2020 [cited 2021 02-17]. Available from: https://asiapacific.unwomen.org/en/digital-library/publications/2020/11/young-women-in-pakistan-status-report-2020.

[25] Organization WH. Women's Empowerment and Gender Equality: Essential Goals for Saving Women's Lives. 2008. p. 4.

[26] Open Budget Survey 2019 2019 [cited 2021 02-13]. Available from: https://www.internationalbudget.org/open-budget-survey/country-results/2019/pakistan.

[27] Pakistan Healthcare Spending 2000-2021 [cited 2021 02-13]. Available from: https://www.macrotrends.net/countries/PAK/pakistan/healthcare-spending.

[28] Success Factors: Ten countries spotlighted for reducing mortality rates [press release]. Sandton Convention Centre, Johannesburg, South Africa: The partnership for maternal newborn and child health, 06-30 2014.

Section 5

Maternal and Child Health

Chapter 7

A Collaborative Health Promotion Approach to Improve Rural Health Delivery and Health Outcomes in Ghana: A Case Example of a Community-Based Health Planning and Services (CHPS) Strategy

Awolu Adam, Adam Fusheini and Daniel Dramani Kipo-Sunyehzi

Abstract

Rural health is a core component of public health but developing rural is a major public challenge, especially, in poor and resource-limited settings around the world. Poor rural healthcare, both access and quality is a strong contributory factor in poor health outcomes such as high maternal, under-five, and infant mortality rates in developing countries, particularly, in sub-Sahara Africa; as millions of rural folks including women and children face many challenges in accessing primary healthcare. This chapter will examine these challenges in rural communities that negatively affect health outcomes and create health disparities between rural and urban populations in Ghana. We will discuss how maternal and child health outcomes can be improved through collaborative rural health promotion. A case for collaborative rural health promotion efforts will be made in this chapter and a community-based health planning and delivery service (CHPS) model will be presented as an example of collaborative rural health promotion in Ghana.

Keywords: Rural, health disparity, Ghana, community-based, maternal/child, literacy

1. Introduction

Globally, the accessibility and availability of appropriate health services for people living in rural areas remain an ongoing issue of public health concern [1]. People living in rural areas experience inequitable access to basic, fundamental, primary, and specialty health care [2]. Thus, access constitutes and remains a major issue in rural health around the world [3]. The rural health literature identifies several and multiple issues related to rural peoples' access to health care services.

The issues range from transportation difficulties, low population density with a concomitant lack of associated social infrastructure to provide services, limitation of finances associated with low levels of income and employment, social isolation, inadequate funding, limited choice and availability of specialist physicians, poor quality professional care, and differences in cultural needs [2]. These issues are not unique or peculiar to any one country in the world. Rather, all countries have such difficulties in addition to communication, the challenge of shortages of doctors and other health professionals in rural and remote areas [3]. Thus, these go beyond health systems factors to include broadly the social determinants of health. This has implications on the health status and outcomes of those living in rural areas, as evidence exists to show that the health status of people in rural areas is generally worse than in urban areas [3] around the world.

While over the years, rural health issues have received attention worldwide, the COVID-19 pandemic outbreak has again highlighted the fact that the most vulnerable populations will likely feel the greatest impact. This includes people who live in rural and remote communities with less access to critical health services [4]. The case of Ghana is not different from this observation.

Ghana is a particularly interesting case because when compared to other countries in sub-Saharan Africa, the country can be said to have a well-developed health system [5]. Again, although in terms of physician, nursing, and midwifery personnel density, the country falls short of the World Health Organization's recommended minimum threshold of twenty-three doctors, nurses, and midwives per 10,000 population at almost one and over nine respectively, comparatively, Ghana performs satisfactorily to most other African countries [5, 6]. Life expectancy at birth for males was 63.8 years and 66.1 years for females in 2020, surpassing the average life expectancy on the continent (62 years and 65 years respectively) [7, 8]. Ghana has also gained the reputation as the first country in Sub-Saharan Africa with an operative nationwide health insurance scheme and a leader in universal health coverage (UHC) [9, 10]. This assures access to healthcare services for both those in the formal and informal sectors of the economy as well as the agricultural and rural populations in one national scheme [11, 12]. This is in addition to the implementation of the Community-Based Health Planning and Services (CHPS) program since the late 1990s and early 2000s as part of government policy and Ghana Health Service [GHS] strategy to bring basic health care to the doorstep of people living in rural and remote areas and other hard-to-reach communities.

Ghana has thus made progress since the introduction of the National Health Insurance Scheme [NHIS] in 2003, along with related policies in maternal and child health care [5]. For instance, according to the 2017 Maternal Health Survey [MHS], antenatal care [ANC] coverage by a skilled provider (doctor, nurse/midwife, or community health officer/nurse) improved from 96% in 2007 to 98% in 2017 [13], way above the sub-Saharan African region average. The neonatal, infant and under-5 mortality rates have also seen improvements for the same period. While the neonatal mortality rate was 25 deaths per 1,000 live births, the infant mortality rate was 37 per 1,000 live births and that of under-5 was 52 deaths per 1,000 live births [13]. In relation to maternal mortality ratio, it currently stands between 308 per 100,000 live births [14–16] and 310 per 100,000 live births [13]. At the health system level, nationally, there has also been an improvement in the doctor and nurse to population ratios. Between 2013 and 2017, ten years after the introduction of the universal health coverage (UHC) policy via a national health insurance scheme, the doctor to population ratio has improved from 1:9749 to 1:7374 with the total number of doctors increasing from 2,730 to 4,016 nationally. That of nurses has also improved from 1:2,172 in 2013 to 1:505 in 2017 with the total number of the nurse cadre workforce increasing from 12,245 in 2013 to 58,608 in

2017 [17]. The trend shows an incremental and steady improvement in the core indicators over the years. Thus, overall, Ghana has seen a marked improvement in the provision of healthcare for all of its citizens as demonstrated by the health indicators and outcomes that are comparatively better than most other African countries [5]. Despite the stated improvements in health indicators in several areas, there are still challenges and barriers, especially, in relation to healthcare access and utilization for those in the rural areas. This chapter focuses on the health disparity challenges of people living in rural areas of Ghana. Specifically, it explores how poor rural health care is a strong contributory factor for high maternal and infant mortality rates in the country. The next phase of the chapter discusses some of these challenges. However, before that we define some terms/concepts that are crucial to understanding rural health broadly and specifically in Ghana. The next section focuses on health disparities in rural and urban Ghana, the underlying causes and challenges while the last section discusses a major approach and strategy that has been adopted to deal with the rural health challenges in the country. This part also concludes the chapter.

2. Definition of terms

2.1 Collaborative health Promotion

There are different definitions of health promotion but one overarching goal cuts through all the various conceptualizations, that of improving the health of individuals, groups, and/or communities. According to the Ottawa Charter of 1986, health promotion is the process of enabling people to increase control over, and improve, their health [18]. The Joint Committee on Terminology for Health Education & Promotion also defined health promotion as any planned combinations of educational, political, environmental, regulatory, or organizational mechanisms that support actions of living conducive to individuals, groups, and communities [19, 20]. For this chapter, we define collaborative health promotion as health promotion policies, goals, strategies, and activities that do not emanate solely from the government but from the collaborative efforts and commitments of multidisciplinary and multi-agency teams including communities to promote health and prevent disease.

2.2 Defining rural and urban communities

In Ghana, the major marker of which community is rural or urban depends on the population of the specified community with localities of 5,000 or more people classified as urban [21]. According to the 2010 Ghana Housing and Population Census (GHPC), 50.9% of the population of Ghana live in urban communities while 49.1% live in rural communities. There are regional differences in urban and rural populations in Ghana. At the regional levels, Greater Accra and Ashanti regions had 90.5% and 60.6% of their population lived in urban communities. The Volta, Northern, and Upper West regions had 33.7%, 30.3%, and 16.3% of the populations living in urban areas in 2010 [22]. The designation of rural communities tended to classify those that were farther and distant from national, regional, municipal, and district capitals in the country. Again, this classification gave prominence to localities based on their population size, and also mostly characterized by bad road network, limited transportation choices, lack of well-equipped health facilities and qualified healthcare professionals, and largely agrarian. By definition, the localities are mostly reachable by feeder roads, which are often not motorable especially during extended rainy seasons.

2.3 Defining rural health

Defining rural health is a challenging venture as the term rural is not universal but relative. What is considered rural in one country or region within the same country may not be deemed the same in another due to different classifications of the constituents of rural. While some define rural by population size only as in the Ghana 2010 Population and Housing census [22], other countries use population in addition to distance or land area and infrastructure as well as socio-economic characteristics, as in the case of the United States Census Bureau [24]. In the context of this chapter, we would like to define rural health as the collective efforts, policies and programs geared towards the improvement of the health status of people living in geographically remote and smaller communities classified by a particular country or region to be a rural locality.

2.4 Health disparities between rural and urban populations in Ghana

Health disparities indicate the differences in the incidence, prevalence, mortality, and burden of diseases and other adverse health conditions that exist among specific population groups. Before discussing the challenges that rural health development and promotion are confronted with, it is important to highlight the indicators of health disparities between rural and urban populations in Ghana and around the world. Disparities exist when differences in health outcomes or health determinants are observed between populations [23]. The differences could be about availability and access to healthcare in terms of distance and cost, and health outcomes in terms of morbidity and mortality depending on different socio-demographic characteristics of different populations. Health disparity has been explained in different but similar terms to denote the lack of equity in access to healthcare and health outcomes. For instance, The Rural Health Information Hub (RHIhub) views health disparities as "differences in health status when compared to the population overall, often characterized by indicators such as higher incidence of disease and/or disability, increased mortality rates, lower life expectancies, and higher rates of pain and suffering" [24]. The U.S Department of Health and Human Services also described health disparities as preventable differences in the burden of disease, injury, violence, or opportunities to achieve optimal health that are experienced by socially disadvantaged populations [25].

Globally, there have always been and continues to be health disparities between developed and developing or rich and poor countries and sometimes the disparities within countries may be greater than disparities between developed and developing countries. These are witnessed among different racial or ethnic groups, between different socio-economic groups, sexual orientation, religious groups, and between rural and urban populations [26]. The focus of this chapter is rural health and so we will briefly discuss health disparities between rural and urban populations, especially in Ghana. In access to healthcare, for instance, rural and geographically isolated populations have limited access to qualified health professionals and health, well-equipped health facilities compared to people living in urban and metropolitan areas. In the United States (US), for instance, the National Center for Health Workforce Analysis (NCHWA) reported in 2014 that less than 8% of all qualified physicians and surgeons in the US chose to practice in rural settings [27]. The report also indicated that healthcare workers who are less educated and trained are living in rural areas. This trend is similar to the health workforce distribution in Ghana between rural and urban communities. The World Bank ranked Ghana as 14th in Africa for a doctor to population ratio with the doctor-population ratio being 0.1 per 1000 people [28] which is an improvement from previous years. The doctor to population ratio was 1:7374, 1:8481, 1:8808, 1:9043 and 1:9749 for 2017, 2016, 2015, 2014 and 2013 respectively [17]. The rural–urban differences were greater than the national ratios above. For example, the ratios for Greater Accra and Ashanti regions, which have larger proportions of their populations living in urban areas, were 1:3052 and 1:6,888 in 2017. On the other hand, Upper East, Western, and Upper West regions which have larger proportions of their population living in rural areas had doctor-to-population ratios of 1:26,489, 1:20,568, and 1:14,821 respectively in 2017 [17]. Huge differences also exist in the distribution of midwives in the country, where Greater Accra and Ashanti regions had 3,232 and 2597 midwives respectively while Northern which has almost 70% of its population in rural communities had 823 midwives [17] during the same period.

Not only access to healthcare but there are also disparities in health outcomes between rural and urban populations in Ghana. A few examples of these disparities in health outcomes cover mortality, malaria prevalence, and children's nutritional status. Under-5 mortality data from the 2014 Ghana Demographic and Health Survey (GDHS) showed regional differences in under-5 mortality with rural communities bearing the greatest burden of under-5 mortality. For instance, under-5 mortality was 75 deaths per 1,000 live births among children in rural areas compared to 64 deaths per 1,000 live births among children in urban areas [29]. The figures were 47 deaths per 1,000 live births in Greater Accra compared to 111 deaths per 1,000 live births in the Northern region. Infant mortality was also highest in the Upper West and Northern regions where two-thirds of their populations live in rural communities. In the same GDHS reported, malaria prevalence was higher among children 6–59 months in rural areas (38%) than children in urban areas (14%). On a regional basis, malaria prevalence was highest among children in the Northern region (40%) compared to Greater Accra (11%) region [29].

These are just a few examples to highlight the health disparities that exist between rural and urban communities in Ghana. There is, therefore, a justification for us to generalize that even though there is a remarkable improvement in the health sector; inequities exist in the health delivery system in Ghana, particularly, between rural and urban populations with rural populations bearing a disproportionate burden of poor health outcomes. These disparities do not occur in a vacuum but result from a constellation of factors that combine to create the disparities. The factors putting rural populations at a disadvantage of health disparities can include geographic isolation, lower socioeconomic status, higher rates of health risk behaviors, limited access to healthcare specialists and emergency care, and limited employment opportunities among others. Below, we discuss these factors under the bigger umbrella of social determinants of health.

2.5 Social determinants of rural health in Ghana

The health status of a particular community, locality, or group of people is not static but changes positively or negatively due to changes in the community or the lives of the people. In this section, we discuss various factors that contribute to the status of health of a group of people at a particular point in time and again focus on rural communities and populations in Ghana. These factors may be related to socio-demographic, economic, environmental, political, policy, and technological characteristics of the community or the group of people individually or a combination of these factors. These various factors are collectively referred to as social determinants of health by various health institutions and organizations. The WHO defined social determinants of health as 'the circumstances in which people are born, grow up, live, work and age, and the systems put in place to deal with illness [30]. These circumstances are in turn shaped by a wider set of forces: economics, social policies, and politics. In the Healthy People 2020 document, social determinants of health are defined as the 'conditions in the environments in which people are born, live, learn, work, play, worship, and age that affect a wide range of health, functioning, and quality-of-life outcomes and risks [31]. Evidence shows that social determinants of health contribute between 75–100% to health improvement and outcomes [32–36].

3. Access to healthcare challenges

3.1 Health insurance

As mentioned earlier, while the introduction of the NHIS and its related maternal health policies have contributed greatly to improving access to health services, especially, for the vulnerable including pregnant women, there is evidence to suggest coverage and utilization challenges for those living in rural and remote parts of the country. For instance, it was estimated that more than seven million people in Ghana had subscribed to the NHIS, corresponding to a coverage of 35% of the entire population in 2007. Concerns were, however, rife about the NHIS ability to carry along the poor, in particular, poor residents in rural areas [37]. In their study, Kwarteng and colleagues have also highlighted the low enrolment and coverage of rural residents by the NHIS that aims at protecting the vulnerable and poor from catastrophic health expenditure. They highlighted "the great disparities in NHIS enrolment against members of the poorest households, those without formal education and living in rural areas" [38]. Similarly, other researchers have demonstrated in a study spanning seven districts of the Upper East region that women of lower Socio-Economic Status, living in rural settings with no formal education among other conditions were less likely to register with the scheme [38, 39]. The researchers identified a number of factors militating against the willingness of those in the rural areas to subscribe to the NHIS. These include the absence and or inadequacy of health care facilities within reasonable reach of rural residents, which requires traveling longer distances at greater cost to access health care services unlike their urban counterparts [37, 38]. Additional disincentive to purchase insurance in their view is the associated high non-medical cost for rural residents and poorer households [38, 40, 41]. From these few studies, it can be said that in spite of the fact that the NHIS has improved access to care, inequalities in service usage still remain, particularly between those living in the rural areas and the urban centers. This view is corroborated by Van Der Wielen and colleagues, who argued strongly based on the findings from their study that the NHIS coverage although does increase healthcare utilization among rural older adults, inequalities remain. The poor are still at a great disadvantage in their use of health services overall and benefit less from enrolment for outpatient care [42].

3.2 Inequitable distribution of health professionals

The doctor and nurse to population ratios across regions and in rural communities as against metropolitan/urban areas are equally telling. While there is an upward trend and improvement over the years, the disparities and inequities are still wide and far apart for the rural dwellers. Between 2013 and 2017, the doctor to population ratios in the Greater Accra and Ashanti regions, the two largest urban areas in the country improved from 1:3,240 (total number of doctors = 1,356), to 1:3,052 (total number of doctors = 1583) and 1:9,280 (total number of doctors = 558), and 1: 6,888 (total number of doctors = 822) respectively [17]. The nurse to population ratio is also better in these two urban areas in comparative and population density terms as demonstrated below. While the Greater Accra region had a ratio of 1:1,904 (number of nurses = 3508) in 2013, this has dramatically improved to 1:530 (number of nurses = 9,124) in 2017. That of the Ashanti region has also seen similar improvements with the ratio declining from 1:2,244 (number of nurses = 2308) in 2013 to 1:548 (number of nurses = 10,332) in 2017 [17]. Conversely, the three most deprived northern regions (Northern, Upper East and Upper West) and the Volta Region, which are also largely rural, have not seen drastic improvement. The doctor to population ratios were 1:20,685 (total number of doctors = 131), 1:27,391 (total number of doctors = 40) and 1:38,692 (total number of doctors = 19) in 2013. While in 2017, it was 1:11,130 (total number of doctors = 269); 1:26,489 (total number of doctors = 47); 1:14,821 (total number of doctors (56) [17] respectively during the same period. For the nurse to population ratio, the following are particularly telling of what the challenges are in the rural areas. In 2013, the figures for the Northern, Upper East and Upper West were 1:1,170 (number of nurses = 1,067); 1:470 (number of nurses = 604); and 1:322 (number of nurses = 311). In 2017, the ratios were: 1: 479 (number of nurses = 6248); 1: 340 (number of nurses = 3,660); and 1: 308 (number of nurses = 2,69) [17] respectively. Besides, in the largely rural Volta Region, the ratios were quite alarming. While in 2013, the doctor to population ratio was 1:20,625 (total number of doctors = 111), this declined to 1:10,534 (total number of doctors = 242) in 2017. That of the nurse to population ratios were 1:988 (number of nurses = 785) in 2013 with an improvement in 2017 as the ratio stood at 1:542 (number of nurses = 4,700) [17]. However, even within the regions, there are large variations in these indicators between the urban and rural areas. This does not only pose serious challenges of health care access and utilization but also undermines efforts towards attaining universal health coverage through the NHIS, which is a policy goal of the national health policy.

3.3 Transportation challenges

The role of transportation in a society in terms of movement of people, services, and goods; and being an engine of economic growth cannot be over-emphasized. We believe that public transportation systems, transportation availability, and efficient transportation services have a critical link and impact on public health, especially primary and emergency health delivery systems. Road transportation is particularly important for the primary healthcare delivery system in Ghana and in the rural communities where most rural folks travel far distances to access primary healthcare. Unfortunately, the rural transportation system in Ghana is a major hurdle to access to healthcare. Many rural communities in Ghana have bad roads, poor transportation systems such as motor vehicles and buses and suffer the health, economic, and social consequences of poor road infrastructure. A large proportion of the rural population in Ghana depends on public transportation to travel, move goods, and seek or render services [43]. The poor road network in rural communities affects access to healthcare services especially for district hospitals and referral services that rural folks need to access, and this has been well-documented [43–46]. As a result of poor road infrastructure in rural areas, emergency services are not accessible for a greater proportion of the rural population. They are far fewer ambulance services and emergency cases can quickly escalate into poor health outcomes and death. For instance, in the Nanumba South District, for example, the major public referral hospitals are Tamale Teaching Hospital or Yendi Regional Hospital, which is 194 kilometers and 95.2 kilometers respectively from the district capital, Wulensi. In emergency cases, people struggle to get a means of transport and usually rely on motorcycles. There is a proliferation of motorcycle and tricycle taxis in rural communities and even peri-urban centers in the country popularly called Okada and motor (Abobo yaa) or "Yello Yello" in many parts of the country. These modes of transport have become the dominant and most common means of transport services in rural areas including bicycles and sometimes tractors with trailers. However, they are often not very safe and Okada was even banned in urban areas in Ghana in 2012 [43] although there are operating even in cities across the country.

Thus, on rural–urban transport system for healthcare, there is inequity in terms of accessibility to health facilities. Disparities exist in the distance travel to access healthcare services between rural and urban residents or dwellers in Ghana [21]. It is more worrying with rural women, most of whom lack means of transport and rely on their husbands or family relatives in times of emergencies. Studies show women in rural areas traveled 4 km more than their urban counterparts to reach a health facility like a hospital or clinic. The evidence shows that 56% of women bypassed the nearest hospital to reach their community with higher chances of human lives being lost in rural than urban areas in accessing healthcare services especially in terms of medical emergencies in Ghana [47, 48]. Therefore, poor road infrastructure and transportation systems are major challenges impacting rural health delivery in Ghana.

4. Lower socio-economic status (education, lack of employment, poverty)

In Ghana, those living in rural areas are unfavorably disadvantaged in relation to the social determinants of health, which evidence shows contribute between 75–100% to health improvement and outcomes [32–36]. A critical component of social determinants of health is socio-economic status of people, which varies depending on residence, educational attainment, and income levels. In the 2017 GMHS, it was reported that 95% of households in urban areas have access to an improved source of drinking water, compared to 81% of rural households. While only 18% of households in Ghana used improved toilet facilities, again the statistics were negatively stacked against rural households. Urban households were found to be more likely than rural households to use improved toilet facilities (22% versus 13%). Similarly, while more than three-quarters (79%) of Ghanaian households have electricity, the rural–urban disparities were clear with 90% of urban households having electricity as against 65% of rural households. The picture was not quite different with communication and information gadgets. Urban households were more likely than rural households to own a mobile telephone, radio, or television. Conversely, rural households were more likely than urban households to own agricultural land or farm animals [13]. The rural versus urban disparities were also observed in the area of education-an important determinant of good employment and health care access and utilization. Women in urban areas (65%) were reportedly more likely to be literate, compared to women in rural areas (41%) [13]. Meanwhile, evidence shows that being literate or educated is critical to making well-informed decisions on health, education or business. Literate women are better placed in terms of knowledge on healthcare services, decisions on the appropriate healthcare facility to seek care including family planning. This is crucial in efforts to bridge the gap between rural–urban in terms of inequities in health. It is clear from the foregoing that systemic barriers and challenges still exist that impede the quality of, and access to, healthcare for those living in the rural areas of Ghana despite the interventions in the form of the CHPS, the NHIS and others.

4.1 Poor health literacy

Health literacy is an important component of the social determinants of health and needs important attention from health education and health promotion professionals in their efforts to promote public and community health. In general, literacy, the ability to read, write, and understand can be a determinant of how individuals perceive their environment and how they conduct themselves in their daily lives. Specifically, health literacy can influence how individuals perceive health issues and how their health-seeking behaviors will be. There are many definitions of health literacy in the literature as the field of health literacy continues to develop and expand. Two definitions that are more widely accepted and we think are appropriate for the context in which we write this chapter are presented below. According to the Calgary Charter on Health Literacy, 'health literacy allows the public and personnel working in all healthcare-related contexts to find, understand, evaluate, communicate, and use health-related information'. Health literacy is also defined as the degree to which individuals can obtain, process, and understand basic health information and services needed to make appropriate health decisions [49]. It is therefore important to clarify that health literacy goes beyond being able to read and write to include conscious effort to seek information regarding health issues, understanding those pieces of information, and using the information to make positive health-related decisions. For instance, do individuals seek medical care immediately they feel changes in their physical or mental health? Do they understand the instructions from their healthcare providers? Moreover, do they adhere to treatment regimens provided by healthcare providers? These are important health literacy questions that health educators and healthcare providers need to find out about in their communities of service. Evidence shows that individuals and communities that have good or high health literacy levels are more likely to make more positive health-related decisions and engage in positive health behaviors resulting in positive health outcomes compared to individuals and communities with poor health literacy levels [24]. For instance, Berkman and colleagues in a systematic review republished reported that limited health literacy is associated with poor health status resulting from a lower likelihood of using preventive health services and a likelihood of wrong medicine usage [50].

Rural communities and people living in remote communities are likely to be more negatively impacted by poor health literacy compared to people living and working in urban communities. Thus, rural folks are at a greater risk of poor health literacy due to poor general literacy from lower educational status, and high poverty levels [24]. Many other studies in different parts of the world have reported poor health literacy in rural populations compared to urban populations [51–54]. Majority of studies have reported lower health literacy levels among rural populations compared to urban populations even though confounders were more responsible for the differences in health literacy levels [51–54].

Although health literacy has not been widely researched in Ghana, a few studies assessed its association with health outcomes on different health issues in the country; and the general picture is that there is a high level of poor health literacy. While we cannot discuss all the studies in this chapter due to the page limitation, it is important to mention a couple of them. For instance, in a study of health literacy about universal health coverage in Ghana, Amoah and Philips found that only a third of the study sample of 779 from both rural and urban communities reported sufficient health literacy and that poor quality of health status was associated with poor health literacy [55]. In another study, researchers assessed the association between health literacy and cholera in a predominantly low socioeconomic status community in Accra, the capital city. The researchers found a substantial gap in knowledge about environmental risk factors for cholera infection while reporting that high health literacy level was associated with the possibility to stay protected against cholera infection [56]. Lori and his colleagues also reported low health literacy among pregnant women in a qualitative study in an urban hospital in Ghana [57]. Again, almost half (49.1%) of the country's population live in rural areas as explained at the beginning of this chapter. This difference in health literacy between urban and rural populations in Ghana is a reflection of general literacy levels in the country. According to data from the 2010 Ghana Housing and Population Census (GHPC), literacy levels were 89.3% and 82.6% in the Greater Accra and Ashanti regions respectively, which have 90.5% and 60.6% of their populations living in urban areas respectively. However, literacy was 37.2% in the Northern region where 69.7% of the population was living in rural communities [22].

Health literacy, is, therefore, generally low and constitutes a major challenge in seeking and accessing healthcare and this can even be worse for rural populations in Ghana that already face a myriad of challenges in accessing healthcare. People living in rural communities may be more likely to develop chronic and non-communicable debilitating diseases than those living in metropolitan and urban areas. This is due to lack of regular health screenings, lack of awareness of the symptoms of diseases, and lack of knowledge of the importance of seeking healthcare early; and these diseases may develop into complications or advanced stages before being reported. For instance, as reported by Amoah and Phillips, even though the majority of their study participants subscribed to the national health insurance scheme, most of them had not accessed healthcare due to poor health literacy [55]. It will not be uncommon in rural communities in Ghana and among people with poor health literacy even urban communities to engage in medicine and treatment sharing, a phenomenon whereby one person shares his or her prescribed medication with a family member for similar symptoms. The same can be said about self-medication and a combination of herbal and orthodox medications. To help promote health literacy in Ghana as a whole and rural communities, in particular, we recommend prioritization of health literacy as a core mandate of institutions and policymakers so that health literacy can be incorporated into all health policy formulation and health program development and implementation strategies.

4.2 High risk sexual and reproductive health behaviors

People living in rural communities have characteristics that put their health at risk of negative health outcomes. They are likely to engage in certain behaviors that can jeopardize their health and this can be largely blamed on the low socio-economic characteristics described above. Examples of these include risky sexual and reproductive health behaviors, household size or total fertility rate and teenage parenthood.

In the 2014 GDHS, for instance, the total fertility rate for women in rural areas in the country was 5.1 compared to 3.4 among women in urban areas. The median age at first marriage for rural women was 19.2 years while it was 22.7 years for women in urban areas which means that women in rural areas marry 3.5 years earlier than their counterparts in urban centers in Ghana [29]. Women in the Northern region, which was then almost 70% rural, had a median age at marriage of 18.7 years, which was five years earlier than women in the Greater Accra region. Again, the percentage of women ages 15–19 who either were mothers or were pregnant at the time of the survey was 17 for rural women and 12 for women in urban centers. Both men and women in rural communities initiate sexual activity earlier than those in urban communities do. Thus, characteristics such as the desire for large family size, early marriage, and teenage parenting put the health and lives of women in rural communities at risk of pregnancy complications and maternal mortality and morbidity. Adolescent pregnancies and teen motherhood are major public health challenges in Ghana, especially in rural areas. The concern is that adolescent pregnancy and childbearing have profound educational, health, physical, mental, and psychological consequences on health, sexual and reproductive health. Adolescents who become pregnant and begin childbearing in many instances are less likely to graduate from high school, likely to have large families, live in poverty, and children born to them likely to have limited educational attainment [29]. The children of such teenage parents are then likely to fall into the cycle of less education, no employment skills, and poverty.

The place of birth for a pregnant woman and the one who assists in the delivery of the child, whether skilled or unskilled, can have serious health implications for both the woman and the child. Pregnancy complications coupled with unskilled birth attendance have the potential and have been linked to the incidence of maternal and infant mortality. However, research has shown that women in rural communities in Ghana continue to deliver babies outside of health facilities and a trained or skilled person does not attend many of the deliveries. For instance, data on childbirths in the GDHS of 2014 show that 90% of all births in urban areas took place in health facilities but only 59% of childbirths took place in health facilities among women in rural communities [29]. On a regional basis, the Greater Accra and Ashanti regions recorded 93% and 85.6% of institutional deliveries compared to 63% and 34.5% in the Upper West and Northern regions respectively. Other researchers have reported a similar trend of high home deliveries among rural women. Furthermore, they have investigated factors responsible for home deliveries in rural areas in Ghana and have identified health insurance issues, cultural and religious practices, low educational achievements, negative attitudes of nurses and midwives, poor knowledge about signs of delivery onset [58–62] among many others as key factors. Therefore, the above risky health behaviors and practices which are prevalent in rural communities more than in the urban areas as a result of a constellation of many socio-demographic and economic factors contribute to the high burden of disease and negative health outcomes affecting the quality of health of rural populations in the country.

4.3 Poor cultural competence among healthcare professionals

The relationship between healthcare professionals and healthcare services users or seekers and their communities is critical in ensuring that quality health services are rendered with the hope of achieving positive health outcomes. Ghana is a multi-cultural, ethnic, and religious society and so cultural practices and beliefs vary across the country. These beliefs, religious, and cultural heritage shape lifestyles and importantly people's perception of health and health-seeking behaviors. Each healthcare professional or support staff belongs to at least one of these different ethnic and cultural groups and enters the healthcare workforce with his or her inherent ethnic, religious, and cultural biases. Healthcare professional such as a doctor, nurse, midwife, or mental health counselor, holding on to their beliefs, ethnic and cultural traits against the ethnic, religious, and cultural backgrounds of healthcare service users may breed frustration, mistrust, and bad feeling, especially from the health service seeker. This in turn can negatively affect health-seeking behavior and health outcomes. Literature on issues related to attitudes and behaviors of nurses, midwives, doctors; and perceptions of patients about healthcare professionals and how these affect the health-seeking behaviors and health outcomes abound in Ghana and other developing countries. There is no doubt about the work ethic of healthcare professionals, especially nurses, midwives, and doctors in Ghana. Their contribution has led to improvement in health outcomes and status making the Ghanaian health care system one of the best and promising healthcare systems in Africa. However, negative attitudes and behaviors of some nurses, midwives, doctors, and other healthcare professionals towards mental health patients, pregnant women, people living with HIV, and culturally isolated people have been reported in the country [63–66]. These can have serious implications for health-seeking behaviors and health outcomes especially in rural communities in Ghana. Rural people may avoid seeking healthcare at health facilities for critical services such as mental health, pregnancy and childbirth, and malnutrition of children.

There is also the issue of confidentiality of personal health records and information of patients, which must be protected to the highest degree possible. In Ghana, there are codes of conduct for healthcare professionals including physicians, nurses, midwives, and auxiliary staff. There is also a bill of rights for patients and clients for healthcare institutions. These are usually posted on the walls in health facilities around the country. The questions are how many people in the rural communities, in particular, are aware of the code of ethics and bill of rights and how many can read and understand them? The presence of the code of ethics and bill of rights for healthcare professionals is not enough to ensure that culturally competent healthcare is delivered to the people. Unlike in the Western world where regulatory provisions are enacted and enforced such as the Health Insurance Portability and Accountability Act (HIPAA) of 1996, there is currently no such provision in Ghana.

Our observation is that there is a lack of cultural competency training in our health training institutions and for in-service training within the health delivery system. Thus, many healthcare professionals enter the healthcare industry without training in cultural competency and may have to learn from experience sometimes in a hard way of bad encounters. The 2002 Joint Committee on Health Education and Promotion Terminology defined cultural competence as "the ability of an individual to understand and respect values, attitudes, beliefs, and morals that differ across cultures, and to consider and respond appropriately to these differences in planning, implementing, and evaluating health education and programs and interventions' [19]. More practically, Perez and Luquis defined cultural competence as "a set of values, behaviors, attitudes, practices, and policies within an organization or program or among staff that enables people to work effectively with diverse groups" [67]. This is needed for healthcare professionals in Ghana and especially those who serve in the rural communities in the country. Many of the rural communities in Ghana do not have their people trained and stationed in the communities as nurses, for example, due to the low level of education described above, and so many nurses are posted to communities where they are total strangers. Cultural competency training is, therefore, very important for healthcare professionals in rural and traditionally setup communities. The importance of this is that being a culturally competent nurse, for instance, can significantly improve the quality of primary health delivery, which can then lead to positive health outcomes. Luquis and Perez asserted that "culturally and linguistically competent health services facilitate encounters with more favorable outcomes, enhance the potential for a more rewarding interpersonal experience, and increase the satisfaction of the individual receiving healthcare and disease prevention services" [67]. Cultural competency training needs to be prioritized by the Ghana Health Service and other healthcare institutions in the country for initial training and/or for annual or bi-annual in-service training.

4.4 Community-based health planning and services (CHPS) strategy and rural health in Ghana

To minimize the health disparities, bridge the inequities gap and to mitigate the challenges that bring about the disparities observed above between rural and urban populations, there have been concerted efforts from diverse stakeholders within local communities, national, and multinational levels, and from public and private individuals and entities. Although still facing many challenges in its implementation, the Community Health Planning and Services (CHPS) program being implemented in Ghana as a national health policy directive and strategy is a collaborative health promotion tool to improve rural health in the country. CHPS is defined as "a national strategy to deliver essential community-based health services involving planning and service delivery with the communities". Its primary focus is communities in deprived sub-districts and in general bringing health services close to the community [68]. The goal of the CHPS policy was to reach every community with a basic package of essential health services towards attaining universal health coverage and bridging the access inequity gap by 2020 [68, 69].

While we cannot fully cover CHPS implementation in this chapter, we provide a brief background about it and a summary of its major components for better understanding by readers. The CHPS concept was first piloted in Ghana in 1994 in Navrongo and with evidence of the concept steering community involvement in health services planning and delivery, it was adopted as a national strategy to improve healthcare access to deprived and geographically isolated localities in the country in 1999 [68, 69]. Ever since, CHPS has been implemented on a scale basis with the most recent remodeling and scale up launched in 2016. The CHPS strategy added a third service level, community (CHPS Zone), to the then district (hospital), sub-district (health center) levels thereby reaching more rural communities and populations in the country.

CHPS has two operational levels, which are the CHPS Zone and CHPS compound. CHPS zone is defined as a demarcated geographical area of up to 5,000 persons or 750 households in densely populated areas and maybe conterminous with electoral areas where feasible. CHPS compound on the other hand is an approved structure consisting of a service delivery point and community health officer (CHO) residential accommodation complex, both of which must be present [68]. The demarcated geographical area of up to 5,000 persons fits into the classification of a rural area by the Ghana Statistical Service [22]. The idea of the CHPS compound is to further reduce the distance of health services from smaller communities thereby increasing accessibility. Besides the leadership from GHS at national, regional, and district/municipal levels, CHPS direct implementation is carried out by CHOs, midwives if available, and community health volunteers (CHVs); and overseen by community health management committees (CHMCs).

The implementation of CHPS/CHPS+ is guided by four core policy directives according to GHS which include the duty of care and a minimum package of services, human resources for effective CHPS implementation, building and procurement of necessary infrastructure, and portfolio of financing for overhead and running cost of CHPS. The core package of services to be provided within the CHPS zone by the CHO and Community Health Volunteer (CHV) focuses predominantly on maternal and child health (MCH) and nutrition services.

5. Summary of the impact of CHPS national strategy on rural health in Ghana

The importance of CHPS and CHPS+ projects on rural health in Ghana cannot be over-emphasized. The policy guidelines for implementation of CHPS, the building of CHPS compounds in rural communities, and the training of CHOs, CHVs, and CHMCs have all resulted in improvement in health outcomes in rural communities in Ghana.

5.1 Improvement in primary health infrastructure in rural Ghana

As a result of the successes observed during the piloting and earlier implementation stages of CHPS, the concept was well accepted and efforts to make it a national health delivery system have led to remarkable progress in the development and procurement of infrastructure and equipment throughout rural and even urban areas around the country. For instance, by the end of 2018, the number of functional CHPS zones in the country was 5,987 according to the CHPS verification survey conducted in the country [70]. This was an increase from 4,400 in 2016 and from 3,951 in 2015 indicating a steady increase in infrastructure for CHPS over the years to reach a universal health coverage envisaged in the revised national CHPS policy of 2016. The large majority of these CHPS zones are in the rural areas of all the regions of the country. Apart from CHPS zones, there has equally been a remarkable increase in needed equipment and tools to facilitate the implementation of the program. Yeboah and colleagues have reported an extensive progress of CHPS in which the authors outlined various equipment procured for CHPS implementation. For example, the authors reported that the Japanese International Cooperation Agency (JICA) supported the CHPS program in the five Northern regions with the procurement of 30 vehicles, 1000 bicycles, and 300 motorcycles. The authors also reported that the World Bank through its maternal and child health and nutrition improvement project procured 56 vehicles, 1,000 bicycles, and 300 motorcycles to be distributed to CHPS zones throughout the country [71]. Again, this equipment in addition to medical supplies is geared towards improving delivery in rural areas in Ghana.

5.2 Improvement in access and service delivery in rural communities

The nationwide implementation has remarkably improved healthcare access and delivery for rural communities in the country. Access to services such as antenatal care (ANC), child welfare clinics, family planning (FP), outpatient admission, and skilled or health facility delivery in rural areas have increased through CHPS. For instance, according to the 2016 GHS annual report, CHPS contribution to outpatient admissions was 16%, 15.4%, 12.1%, and 11.5% in the Upper East, Upper West, Northern, and Western regions of the country respectively. In the same year, CHPS contribution to ANC services delivery was 34.7%, 27.4%, and 23.9% in the Upper West, Upper East, and Northern regions respectively. Again, in 2016, CHPS compounds served as skilled delivery places in Upper East, Upper West, and Northern regions with 11.8%, 8.1%, and 8.6% respectively [72]. These statistics are critical in improving maternal and child health in regions that have larger proportions of their populations living in rural communities. Without CHPS implementation, many of these services would have been missed and many of the deliveries would have taken place out of health facilities jeopardizing the lives of pregnant women and newly born or unborn babies.

5.3 Training and development of community health workers (CNOs) and community health volunteers (CHVs)

It is also important to recognize the workforce that has driven the progress achieved with CHPS implementation so far. The training and deployment of CHOs and CHVs in rural communities throughout the country is a remarkable improvement in rural health in Ghana. This is commendable because most of the rural communities are linked by feeder roads that can be difficult to ply; the communities have less or zero social amenities, and communication networks are poor in many rural areas. Accepting to serve in such deprived and geographically isolated areas is a call to duty. Over the years, the number of trained and deployed CHOs and CHVs has increased. For instance, 2,523 trained CHOs were operating across 5,062 functional CHPS zones with an active community health committee; and 19,411 active CHVs who support the CHOs in the implementation of CHPS [73]. Besides, support from sub-district, district, municipal, and regional levels are available to help facilitate the implementation; and training and deployment of the core human resources for CHPS implementation. However, the figures above are an indication of the commitment to strengthen capacity for the program so that health services will be closer to every rural community in the country.

5.4 Involvement of array of important stakeholders

Since its inception and throughout its policy initiation and implementation, CHPS and now CHPS Plus (CHPS+) has brought together important stakeholders with the goal of ensuring that effective and evidence-based approaches are adopted to bring critical primary health delivery to all parts of Ghana. The array of stakeholders cut across societies from the bottom up to the top hierarchy of health service consumers in the communities, health providers, healthcare professionals, political leaders, policymakers, and multi-national partners. Community members constitute the CHMCs and CHVs, district and municipal health directorates, district and municipal assemblies, regional health directorates, and GHS top management and Ministry of Health (MoH). Tertiary and research institutions are an integral part of the stakeholders driving CHPS strategy and implementation including the University of Ghana (UG), University of Health and Allied Sciences (UHAS), University for Development Studies (UDS), the Navrongo Research Center, and Mailman School of Public Health (MSPH) of Columbia University. International partners that have committed expertise and making an immense financial contribution to the implementation of CHPS and now CHPS+ include the World Bank (WB), USAID, JICA, the Korea International Co-operation Agency (KOICA), and Doris Dukes Charitable Foundation among others. The procurement of equipment and medical supplies by JICA and the WB presented above are examples of the financial commitments by the donor partners. The CHPS+ project was a five-year project (2016–2020) that was a collaboration between GHS and KOICA to strengthen the capacity of Ghana health systems in the Upper East Region at the cost of US$9 m. This project was a scale-up from the Ghana Essential Health Improvement Project (GEHIP), which was funded by Doris Duke Charitable Foundation and implemented in the four most impoverished districts in the Upper East Region from 2010 to 2015 [74].

Another component of the CHPS+ project was to scale up in the Northern and Volta regions selected as priority regions and funded by the Doris Dukes Charitable Foundation through the Mailman School of Public Health. It was a collaboration among Doris Dukes, MSPH, the Ghana Health Service Policy Planning, Monitoring and Evaluation Division (PPME), the universities (UG, UDS, UHAS), and community members. The main goal was to use the project to improve child survival and reduce under-five mortality in Ghana. Critical implementation components of this project included knowledge creation and utilization to improve child health, research into evidence-based approaches, health systems partnerships development, and development of learning platforms [75]. Two Systems Learning Districts (SLDs) were created in both the Northern and the Volta regions, which served as the centers of excellence for health systems strengthening to all other districts in the regions.

The importance of this array of stakeholders includes mobilizing resources for infrastructure and equipment, developing adequate and competent human resources, creating opportunities for communities to fully participate and share ownership of programs and initiatives concerning their health and wellbeing. Involving the universities is critical as research is earnestly needed to develop a comprehensive understanding of health behavior, the social determinants of health, development of evidence-based strategies to address health program implementation bottlenecks, and pave the way for effective and efficient implementation of CHPS+ so the universal health coverage envisaged can be achieved. For example, to understand the challenges of health delivery at the community level, professionals, and health system levels, researchers deployed a community scorecard in an explorative qualitative design in the two SLDs in the Volta Region. The researchers identified key bottlenecks that hindered the implementation of health services at levels of the community, healthcare professionals, and the health system [76]. Researchers also examined the importance of community involvement in the CHPS+ implementation as a strategy for improving health outcomes and found that overall acceptance of the CHPS+ strategy was 51.7% by participants in the two SLDs in the Volta Region and reported community involvement was low and needed to improve for Ghana to attain universal health coverage [63].

It can be seen from the above that great effort and commitment from all the stakeholders from the CHPS pilot in Navrongo through the implementation to the current CHPS+ project scale-up has been mobilized in the form of collaborative health promotion. Undoubtedly, the CHPS strategy has contributed greatly to the improvements in overall healthcare delivery in Ghana and rural communities across the country in particular. The report of the 2014 GDHS show improvements in major health indicators over the years from 2003 including reductions in infant, under-five, and maternal mortality in the country, increase in child immunizations, family planning uptake, children's nutrition, and reduction in mother-to-child HIV transmission among others [29]. For example, infant mortality in rural communities decreased from 70 deaths per 1,000 live births in 2003 to 46 deaths per 1,000 live births in 2014. During the same period, under-five mortality decreased from 118 per 1,000 live births to 75 deaths per 1,000 in rural areas [17]. Again, the maternal mortality ratio reduced from 254.8 deaths to 162 from 2003 to 2017 in the Northern Region; and from 256.2 to 139 deaths per 100,000 live births in the same period in the Volta Region [13]. We believe that CHPS implementation contributed to these positive outcomes. Studies have also shown that CHPS implementation has had a positive impact on maternal and child health services in rural areas [77], led to increased involvement of males in maternal and child health issues with positive health outcomes [78], and expanded primary healthcare in rural and deprived communities [79].

Notwithstanding the above contribution, CHPS implementation continues to face challenges throughout the country. The social determinants that cause the disparities in healthcare access and outcomes between rural and urban centers persist in the country and overcoming these challenges cannot be overnight but needs continuous collaborative health promotion efforts looking ahead. These challenges include financing and human resources [71], poor rural road infrastructure and transportation systems [44], and a host of other challenges.

In conclusion, although CHPS/CHPS+ implementation continues to face many challenges, by far the program has contributed to equitable healthcare service delivery in rural Ghana than any program ever implemented before it.

Author details

Awolu Adam[1*], Adam Fusheini[2] and Daniel Dramani Kipo-Sunyehzi[3,4]

1 Department of Family and Community Health, School of Public Health, University of Health and Allied Sciences, Ho, Ghana

2 Department of Preventive and Social Medicine, Dunedin School of Medicine, University of Otago, Dunedin, New Zealand

3 Legon Centre for International Affairs and Diplomacy, University of Ghana, Legon, Ghana

4 Center for Health Literacy and Rural Health Promotion, Accra, Ghana

*Address all correspondence to: awolu.adam74@gmail.com

References

[1] Brabyn L, Barnett R: Population need and geographical access to general practitioners in rural New Zealand. The New Zealand medical journal 2004, 117(1199):U996.

[2] Hopley M, Horsburgh M, Peri K: Barriers to accessing specialist care for older people with chronic obstructive pulmonary disease in rural New Zealand. Journal of Primary Health Care 2009, 1(3):207-214.

[3] Strasser R: Rural health around the world: Challenges and solutions. Family practice 2003, 20(4):457-463.

[4] Worley P: Why we need better rural and remote health, now more than ever. Rural and remote health 2020, 20(1):1.

[5] Asemota E: Better Care, Better Health: Optimizing Healthcare Provision inGhana. In: The Cornell Policy Review. UNICEF Ghana/Olivier Asselin; 2019.

[6] World Health Organization: Key Country Indicators-Ghana key indicators [https://apps.who.int/gho/data/node.cco.ki-GHA?lang=en]

[7] Statista: Average life expectancy at birth in 2020, by continent and gender (in years) In.: M. Szmigiera; 2021.

[8] Worldometer: Ghana Demographics [https://www.worldometers.info/demographics/ghana-demographics/]

[9] Agyepong IA: Universal Health Coverage: Breakthrough or Great White Elephant? The Lancet 2018.

[10] Fusheini A: Healthcare Financing Reforms: Ghana's National Health Insurance In: Health Reforms Across the World: the Experience of Twelve Small and Medium-sized Nations with Changing their Healthcare Systems. edn. Edited by Okma K, Tenbensel T. Singapore: World Scientific; 2020: 25-54.

[11] Fusheini A, Marnoch G, Gray AM: Stakeholders perspectives on the success drivers in Ghana's National Health Insurance Scheme - identifying policy translation issues. International Journal of Health Policy and Management 2017, 6(5):273-283.

[12] World Health Organization: Success Stories of Health Financing Reforms for Universal Coverage Ghana

[13] Ghana Statistical Service, Ghana Health Service, ICF.: Ghana Maternal Health Survey 2017: Key Findings. Rockville, Maryland, USA: GSS, GHS, and ICF; 2018.

[14] Konlan KD, Saah JA, Amoah RM, Doat AR, Mohammed I, Abdulai JA, Konlan KD: Factors influencing the utilization of focused antenatal care services during pregnancy, a study among postnatal women in a tertiary healthcare facility, Ghana. Nursing Open 2020, 7(6):1822-1832.

[15] World Health Organization: Trends in maternal mortality 2000 to 2017: estimates by WHO, UNICEF, UNFPA, World Bank Group and the United Nations Population Division. 2019.

[16] World Health Organization: World health statistics 2019: monitoring health for the SDGs, sustainable development goals. 2019.

[17] Ghana Health Service: The Health Sector in Ghana, Facts and Figures 2018. In.; 2018.

[18] Health Promotion: The 1st International Conference on Health Promotion, Ottawa, 1986 [https://www.who.int/teams/health-promotion/enhanced-wellbeing/first-global-conference]

[19] The Joint Committee on Terminology for Health Education & Promotion: Report of the 2000 Joint committee on health, education and Promotion terminology. American Journal of Health Education 2001, **32**(2):89-103.

[20] Gold RS, Miner KR: Report of the 2000 joint committee on health education and promotion terminology. Journal of School Health 2002, **72**(1):3-7.

[21] Ghana Statistical Service: 2010 population and housing census: national analytical report. In. Accra: Ghana Statistical Service; 2013.

[22] Ghana Statistical Service: 2010 Population and Housing Census. Summary Report of Final Results. In. Accra: Ghana Statistical service; 2012.

[23] Meyer PA, Yoon PW, Kaufmann RB: Introduction: CDC health disparities and inequalities report-United States, 2013. MMWR supplements 2013, 62(3):3-5.

[24] Rural Health Information Hub: Rural Health Disparities [https://www.ruralhealthinfo.org/topics/rural-health-disparities#causes]

[25] Community Health and Program Services (CHAPS): Health Disparities among Racial/Ethnic Populations

[26] Adolescents and School Health: Health disparities among youth [https://www.cdc.gov/healthyyouth/disparities/index.htm]

[27] National Center for Health Workforce Analysis: Distribution of U.S. Health Care Providers Residing in Rural and Urban Areas. In.; 2014.

[28] World Bank: World Health Organization's Global Health Workforce Statistics, OECD, supplemented by country data: Physician (per 1000 people) in Ghana. In.; 2021.

[29] Ghana Statistical Service - GSS, Ghana Health Service - GHS, ICF International: Ghana Demographic and Health Survey 2014. In. Rockville, Maryland, USA: GSS, GHS, and ICF International; 2015.

[30] World Health Organization: Social Determinants of Health [http://www.who.int/social_determinants/en/]

[31] Healthy Peole: Social Determinants of Health: Understanding Social Determinants of Health [https://www.healthypeople.gov/2020/topics-objectives/topic/social-determinants-of-health]

[32] Bunker JP, Frazier H, Mosteller F: The role of medical care in determining health: Creating an inventory of benefits. Society and health 1995: 305-341.

[33] Or Z: Determinants of health outcomes in industrialised countries: A pooled, cross-country, time-series analysis. OECD Economic studies 2000:53-78.

[34] Fusheini A: The Implementation of the National Health Insurance in Ghana (2003-2013): University of Ulster; 2013.

[35] McKeown T: The role of medicine: dream, mirage or nemesis? 1976. London: Nuffield Provincial Hospitals Trust, 180.

[36] McKeown T: The role of medicine: dream, mirage, or nemesis?, vol. 56: Princeton University Press; 2014.

[37] Sarpong N, Loag W, Fobil J, Meyer CG, Adu-Sarkodie Y, May J, Schwarz NG: National health insurance coverage and socio-economic status in a rural district of Ghana. Tropical medicine & international health 2010, **15**(2):191-197.

[38] Kwarteng A, Akazili J, Welaga P, Dalinjong PA, Asante KP, Sarpong D, Arthur S, Bangha M, Goudge J, Sankoh

O: The state of enrollment on the National Health Insurance Scheme in rural Ghana after eight years of implementation. International journal for equity in health 2020, 19(1):1-14.

[39] Akazili J, Welaga P, Bawah A, Achana FS, Oduro A, Awoonor-Williams JK, Williams JE, Aikins M, Phillips JF: Is Ghana's pro-poor health insurance scheme really for the poor? Evidence from northern Ghana. BMC health services research 2014, **14**(1):1-9.

[40] Mtei G, Makawia S, Ally M, Kuwawenaruwa A, Meheus F, Borghi J: Who pays and who benefits from health care? An assessment of equity in health care financing and benefit distribution in Tanzania. Health policy and planning 2012, 27(suppl_1):i23-i34.

[41] Onwujekwe O, Onoka C, Uzochukwu B, Hanson K: Constraints to universal coverage: Inequities in health service use and expenditures for different health conditions and providers. International journal for equity in health 2011, 10(1):1-9.

[42] Van Der Wielen N, Channon AA, Falkingham J: Does insurance enrolment increase healthcare utilisation among rural-dwelling older adults? Evidence from the National Health Insurance Scheme in Ghana. BMJ Global Health 2018, 3(1).

[43] Badu E, Owusu-Manu DG, Edwards DJ, Adesi M, Lichtenstein S: Rural infrastructure development in the Volta region of Ghana: Barriers and interventions. Journal of financial management of Property and Construction 2013.

[44] Atuoye KN, Dixon J, Rishworth A, Galaa SZ, Boamah SA, Luginaah I: Can she make it? Transportation barriers to accessing maternal and child health care services in rural Ghana. BMC health services research 2015, 15(1):1-10.

[45] Agbenyo F, Nunbogu AM, Dongzagla A: Accessibility mapping of health facilities in rural Ghana. Journal of Transport & Health 2017, 6:73-83.

[46] Agyemang-Duah W, Peprah C, Peprah P: Factors influencing the use of public and private health care facilities among poor older people in rural Ghana. Journal of Public Health 2020, 28(1):53-63.

[47] Nesbitt RC, Lohela TJ, Soremekun S, Vesel L, Manu A, Okyere E, Grundy C, Amenga-Etego S, Owusu-Agyei S, Kirkwood BR: The influence of distance and quality of care on place of delivery in rural Ghana. Scientific reports 2016, 6(1):1-8.

[48] Dotse-Gborgbortsi W, Dwomoh D, Alegana V, Hill A, Tatem AJ, Wright J: The influence of distance and quality on utilisation of birthing services at health facilities in Eastern Region, Ghana. BMJ global health 2020, 4(Suppl 5).

[49] Ratzan S, Parker R: Health Literacy. National library of medicine current bibliographies in medicine Bethesda: National Institutes of Health, US Department of Health and Human Services 2000.

[50] Berkman ND, Sheridan SL, Donahue KE, Halpern DJ, Viera A, Crotty K, Holland A, Brasure M, Lohr KN, Harden E: Health literacy interventions and outcomes: An updated systematic review. Evidence report/technology assessment 2011(199):1-941.

[51] Zahnd WE, Scaife SL, Francis ML: Health literacy skills in rural and urban populations. American journal of health behavior 2009, 33(5):550-557.

[52] Shrestha MK, Guo CW, Maharjan N, Gurung R, Ruit S: Health literacy of common ocular diseases in Nepal. BMC ophthalmology 2014, 14(1):1-8.

[53] Wang X, Guo H, Wang L, Li X, Huang M, Liu Z, Liu X, Wang K, Alamian A, Anderson JL: Investigation of residents' health literacy status and its risk factors in Jiangsu Province of China. Asia Pacific Journal of Public Health 2015, 27(2):NP2764-NP2772.

[54] Karim HA: Health literacy among rural communities: Issues of accessibility to information and media literacy. Jurnal Komunikasi: Malaysian Journal of Communication 2020, 36(1).

[55] Amoah PA, Phillips DR: Health literacy and health: Rethinking the strategies for universal health coverage in Ghana. Public health 2018, 159:40-49.

[56] Tutu RA, Gupta S, Busingye JD: Examining health literacy on cholera in an endemic community in Accra, Ghana: A cross-sectional study. Tropical medicine and health 2019, 47(1):31.

[57] Lori JR, Dahlem CHY, Ackah JV, Adanu RM: Examining antenatal health literacy in Ghana. Journal of Nursing Scholarship 2014, 46(6):432-440.

[58] Ganle JK, Mahama MS, Maya E, Manu A, Torpey K, Adanu R: Understanding factors influencing home delivery in the context of user-fee abolition in northern Ghana: Evidence from 2014 DHS. The International journal of health planning and management 2019, 34(2):727-743.

[59] Dankwah E, Zeng W, Feng C, Kirychuk S, Farag M: The social determinants of health facility delivery in Ghana. Reproductive health 2019, 16(1):1-10.

[60] Boah M, Adampah T, Jin B, Wan S, Mahama AB, Hyzam D, Akiti C: "I couldn't buy the items so I didn't go to deliver at the health facility" home delivery among rural women in northern Ghana: A mixed-method analysis. PloS one 2020, 15(3):e0230341.

[61] Akazili J, Doctor HV, Abokyi L, Hodgson A, Phillips JF: Is there any relationship between antenatal care and place of delivery? Findings from rural northern Ghana. Afr J Health Sci 2011, 18(1-2):62-73.

[62] Kotoh AM, Boah M: "No visible signs of pregnancy, no sickness, no antenatal care": Initiation of antenatal care in a rural district in northern Ghana. BMC public health 2019, 19(1):1-13.

[63] Kweku M, Amu H, Adjuik M, Manu E, Aku FY, Tarkang EE, Komesuor J, Asalu GA, Amuna NN, Boateng LA: Community involvement and perceptions of the community-based health planning and services (CHPS) strategy for improving health outcomes in Ghana: Quantitative comparative evidence from two system learning districts of the CHPS+ project. Advances in Public Health 2020, 2020.

[64] Osafo J, Knizek BL, Akotia CS, Hjelmeland H: Attitudes of psychologists and nurses toward suicide and suicide prevention in Ghana: A qualitative study. INTERNATIONAL JOURNAL OF NURSING STUDIES 2012, 49(6):691-700.

[65] Adjorlolo S, Abdul-Nasiru I, Chan HCO, Bambi LE: Mental health Professionals' attitudes toward offenders with mental illness (insanity Acquittees) in Ghana. International journal of offender therapy and comparative criminology 2018, 62(3):629-654.

[66] D'Ambruoso L, Abbey M: Midwives' Attitudes to Women in Labour in Ghana. 2008.

[67] Luquis RR, Pérez MA: Cultural competence and health education. Cultural Competence in Health

Education and Health Promotion 2008, 18:231.

[68] Ministry of Health: National Community-Based Health Planning and Services (CHPS) Policy. In. Accra: Ministry of Health; 2016.

[69] Ghana Health Service: Community-Based Health Planning and Services. Operational Policy. In: Ghana Health Service Policy Document No 20. 2005.

[70] Ministry of Health/Ghana Health Service: The CHPS verification survey/ Exercise. In. Accra; 2018.

[71] Yeboah BK, Letsa T, Mensah EA, Odame-Ankrah E: Progress of community-based health planning and Services in Ghana. Global Scientific Journals 2019, 7(12):1212-1228.

[72] Ghana Health Service: 2016 Annual Report. In. Accra: Ghana Health Service; 2017.

[73] Mwinnyaa G, Jones TC, Antwi P, Chan E, Phillips JF, Awoonor-Williams JK: Ghana's community health officers and community health volunteers. Health for the People: National Community Health Worker Programs from Afghanistan to Zimbabwe 2020:87.

[74] Ministry of Health: National CHPS+ Project launched [https://www.moh.gov.gh/national-chps-project-launched/]

[75] Mailman School of Public Health: CHPS+ [https://www.publichealth.columbia.edu/research/advancing-research-community-health-systems/chps]

[76] Kweku M, Amu H, Awolu A, Adjuik M, Ayanore MA, Manu E, Tarkang EE, Komesuor J, Asalu GA, Aku FY: Community-based health planning and services plus programme in Ghana: A qualitative study with stakeholders in two systems learning districts on improving the implementation of primary health care. PLoS One 2020, 15(1):e0226808.

[77] Alhassan RK, Nketiah-Amponsah E, Ayanore MA, Afaya A, Salia SM, Milipaak J, Ansah EK, Owusu-Agyei S: Impact of a bottom-up community engagement intervention on maternal and child health services utilization in Ghana: A cluster randomised trial. BMC public health 2019, 19(1):1-11.

[78] Adongo PB, Tapsoba P, Phillips JF, Tabong PT-N, Stone A, Kuffour E, Esantsi SF, Akweongo P: The role of community-based health planning and services strategy in involving males in the provision of family planning services: A qualitative study in southern Ghana. Reproductive health 2013, 10(1):36.

[79] Phillips JF, Awoonor-Williams JK, Bawah AA, Nimako BA, Kanlisi NS, Sheff MC, Asuming PO, Kyei PE, Biney A, Jackson EF: What do you do with success? The science of scaling up a health systems strengthening intervention in Ghana. BMC health services research 2018, 18(1):1-10.

Section 6

Healthcare Workers Safety

Chapter 8

The Prevalence of Low Back Pain and Evaluation of Prevention Strategies among the Electrophysiology and Catheterization Laboratory Community (Physicians, Nurses, Technicians) in Rural Hospitals

Khalid Sawalha, Nicholas Beresic, Shoaib Khan and Gilbert-Roy Kamoga

Abstract

Musculoskeletal disorders, such as low back pain, are a common and costly problem in today's workforce. Employees who work in a rural hospital's electrophysiology (EP) or catheterization lab (Cath lab) appear to be especially susceptible to injury. This increase in risk has been attributed to a shortage of physicians, less community-based resources available to hospital staff, and the forward-flexed postures EP/Cath lab professionals maintain for extended periods of time while working in the operating room. Traditionally, exercise and physical activity routines, health education, and continued management support have been promoted as low cost/low risk interventions to address low back pain. However, the extent to which hospital policy and culture enable these prevention strategies to be implemented is unknown. Thus, the objective of this study was to determine the prevalence of low back pain in rural EP/Cath laboratories and the significance of exercise and physical activity routines, health education, and continued management support as low back pain prevention strategies in the rural EP/Cath lab community.

Keywords: low back pain, rural hospitals, healthcare workers safety

1. Introduction

Hospital workers are highly susceptible to musculoskeletal disorders due to the regular lifting, positioning, and transporting of patients, combined with a fast pace work environment and a general collective temperament of putting their patients' health before their own [1]. Upon closer review, the EP/Cath lab subset of the rural hospital workforce appears to be especially susceptible to the specific musculoskeletal disorder of low back pain. This has been attributed to the sustained forward-flexed postures they commonly maintain while working in the operating room [2], combined with a shortage of rural physicians and less community-based resources available to rural hospital staff as compared to their urban counterparts [3]. As a strategy to address this dilemma, exercise and physical activity routines, health education, and continued management support have been broadly promoted as cost-effective programs which are powerful enough to improve the health of the workforce, yet also produce a positive return on investment [4]. In theory the implementation of these low cost/low risk programs is a sound strategy based on evidence-based guidelines. The American College of Physicians strongly recommends nonpharmacologic treatments for chronic low back pain, including exercise and mindfulness-based stress reduction, because the benefits clearly outweigh the risk [5]. In practice, though, limited time and the inability to incorporate the program into everyday work routines have been found to be the two main reasons why these worksite-based fitness programs have failed to produce significant findings [6]. To overcome these barriers, hospital management must concurrently have the social, financial, and strategic investments in place which complement and support these specific wellness interventions to realize significant and lasting reductions in musculoskeletal disorders [7]. Unfortunately, the extent to which these investments have been made by hospital management, and thus perceived effective by the EP/Cath lab workforce, is unknown. Thus, the objective of this study was to determine the prevalence of low back pain in rural EP/Cath laboratories and the significance of exercise and physical activity routines, health education, and continued management support as low back pain prevention strategies in the rural EP/Cath lab community.

2. Methods and data collection

Those individuals who worked in the EP/Cath laboratories of two rural hospitals in the state Arkansas were eligible to participate in the study. A convenience sample design was used, and all research data were collected through the electronic transmission of a Qualtrics survey. The survey included three general sections: Nordic Musculoskeletal Questionnaire (NMQ), demographics/applicable work practice details, and low back pain prevention strategies. The first section featuring the NMQ was used to calculate the prevalence of musculoskeletal symptoms within the study population. The NMQ was developed for the analysis of musculoskeletal symptoms, [8] and has been validated and applied to a wide range of occupational groups, including nursing [9]. Additionally, the validity and reliability of the NMQ was assessed to be moderate to high and its use appropriate for epidemiological research related to musculoskeletal disorders [10]. The second section on demographics/applicable work practice assessed height, weight, gender, age, number of years worked in an EP/Cath lab setting, number of hours per week in a lead apron, and percentage of average shift spent standing in the lab. The third section on low back pain prevention strategies assessed exercise and physical activity routines, health education, and continued management support. These questions were developed through the examination of peer-reviewed journal articles, scientific posters, and government websites which promote specific behaviors or actions that had the potential to prevent or reduce low back pain [11].

A total of 45 participants were invited to participate in the study. Upon receiving IRB approval, the survey was sent to the work email address of all study participants. Data were deidentified and summarized using Microsoft Excel. Analysis showed fifteen individuals either selected they did not want to participant in the study or did not complete the survey in its entirety and thus, were omitted from the final data set. Ultimately, a total of 30 completed surveys were included in the final data set for analysis.

3. Results

The first section of the survey featuring the NMQ assessed the prevalence of musculoskeletal symptoms in nine different regions of the body. The largest group, 18 (60%), stated they experienced pain in the lower back (L4 to S1) spinal level, while 12 (40%) reported no low back pain. Among the 60% of respondents who have experienced low back pain, eight (26.67%) had trouble in the last week and six (20%) were prevented from doing their normal work (at home or away from home) (**Table 1**).

Region of Body	**Recorded "Yes" (n = 30)**
Neck	46.67%
Trouble in the last 12 months	14
Prevented from normal work	1
Trouble in the last 7 days	4
Shoulders	40.00%
Trouble in the last 12 months	12
Prevented from normal work	2
Trouble in the last 7 days	4
Elbows	13.33%
Trouble in the last 12 months	4
Prevented from normal work	1
Trouble in the last 7 days	1
Wrists/Hands	13.33%
Trouble in the last 12 months	4
Prevented from normal work	1
Trouble in the last 7 days	1
Upper Back	36.67%
Trouble in the last 12 months	11
Prevented from normal work	1
Trouble in the last 7 days	3
Lower Back	60.00%
Trouble in the last 12 months	18
Prevented from normal work	6
Trouble in the last 7 days	8
Hips/Thighs	26.67%
Trouble in the last 12 months	8
Prevented from normal work	3
Trouble in the last 7 days	2
Knees	23.33%
Trouble in the last 12 months	7

Region of Body	Recorded "Yes" (n = 30)
Prevented from normal work	2
Trouble in the last 7 days	4
Feet/Ankles	30.00%
Trouble in the last 12 months	9
Prevented from normal work	1
Trouble in the last 7 days	5
Per Person Mean and SD	4.57 ± 4.03

Table 1.
Nordic musculoskeletal questionnaire number of recorded "Yes's".

4. Discussion

When we compare our study to a sample of Radiologic Technologists study who similarly wear lead aprons[1], the current study showed a higher overall pervasiveness of low back pain (60% to 47.62%) but less low back pain symptoms on the short-term basis (33.33% to 26.67%). Despite these discrepancies, low back pain was found to be the most prevalent musculoskeletal symptom recorded in both studies. Another significant finding in this study is the data showed an increase in the prevalence of low back pain once five years of service in an EP/Cath lab setting has been completed (58–61%) (**Table 2**). To provide a sense of comparison, Goldstein, et al. in (2004) likewise reported an upward trajectory in the prevalence of low back pain among Interventional Cardiologists as the number of years of service increased [12].

Finally, the top two prevention strategies reported by those with low back pain were "regularly complete at least 150 minutes per week of moderate-intensity aerobic physical activity" and "if a worksite-based fitness program will be offered to you at your department, will you be interested on joining it for at least a year" (**Table 3**).

	Total	LBP	No LBP
Number	30	18	12
Height (inches)	67.30 ± 5.47	67.28 ± 5.54	67.33 ± 5.61
Weight (pounds)	196.17 ± 31.79	194.44 ± 36.58	198.75 ± 24.16
Gender (% male)	46.67	44.44	50.00
Age	40.93 ± 11.92	38.67 ± 9.93	44.33 ± 14.20
Years working in EP/Cath lab setting	9.53 ± 9.79	8.22 ± 6.60	11.50 ± 13.36
under 5	12	7	5
5–10	8	6	2
11–16	4	2	2
17–20	4	3	1
21 or more	2	0	2
Hours per week in lead apron	18.13 ± 10.45	16.17 ± 10.53	21.08 ± 10.02
% of shift spent standing in lab	60.50 ± 24.96	59.44 ± 26.51	62.08 ± 23.50

Table 2.
Demographics/applicable work practice details stratified by the presence or absence of low Back pain (LBP).

Prevention Strategy	LBP (n = 18)	No LBP (n = 12)
Currently participate in early morning fitness program	6	5
Yes: Includes strength training exercises	6	4
Yes: Includes stretching exercises	5	5
Yes: Overall do you do your fitness program regularly	5	4
Worksite-based fitness program currently offered to dept	4	5
Yes: Occurred on company-time	0	0
Yes: Each class included exercises targeting the various muscle groups of the body	4	5
Yes: Customized around dept's specific needs, preferred communication methods, and resources available to the employees to help create a sense of ownership	2	1
If a worksite-based fitness program will be offered to you at your department, will you be interested on joining it for at least a year	10	1
Yes: How often to hold class (days/week)	3 Responses: Daily 6 Responses: 3x 1 Response: 1x	1 Response: Daily
Yes: How long to hold class (minutes)	2 Responses: 10–15 6 Responses: 15–20 2 Responses: Other	1 Response: 10–15
Yes: Led by a faciliator or instructor	7	1
Ergonomic-related topics discussed during team meetings	0	1
Yes: Includes discussion on poor posture(s)	0	1
Yes: Includes discussion on stress management	0	1
Yes: Includes discussion on active coping strategies	0	1
Yes: Strategies developed to overcome limited time to stretch	0	1
Yes: Strategies developed to overcome lack of regular breaks	0	1
Yes: Strategies developed to overcome requirement to keep the body in a sustained forward-flexed posture during surgery	0	1
Regularly complete at least 150 minutes per week of moderate-intensity aerobic physical activity	10	3
Regularly complete stretching exercises	6	6
Regularly complete strength training exercises two or more days/week	8	4
Yes: Systematically change number of sets, reps, or weight used in strength training program	7	4
Yes: Know how to engage the deep core muscles	7	4
Hospital management believes improvements in physical conditioning will help to prolong career	6	5
Low back pain and other musculoskeletal symptoms periodically evaluated	0	0
Functional Movement Screen or another validated screening tool periodically used to identify faulty movement patterns or muscular imbalances	1	2

Table 3.
Prevention strategies completed by EP/Cath lab physicians, managers, and technicians stratified by the presence or absence of low Back pain (LBP).

As motivation to exercise appears to be high, interestingly no responses were recorded when asked if their worksite-based fitness program occurred on company time or if low back pain and other musculoskeletal symptoms were periodically evaluated. In addition, only one response was recorded when asked if ergonomic-related topics were discussed during team meetings. These findings suggest it is the cultural norm of the EP/Cath lab community to believe it is the personal responsibility of the employee rather than shared responsibility of the employee and hospital (EP/Cath lab) management to address the widespread low back pain present in the workforce, personified by only 36.67% of respondents reporting "hospital management believes improvements in physical conditioning will help to prolong career."

5. Conclusion

The primary goal of this study was to illustrate the prevalence and generalized characteristics of back pain among EP and Cath laboratories in rural hospital settings. Conclusions that may be drawn from this study are the prevalence of low back pain demonstrated within this study were consistent when compared to available studies, low back pain is a common condition among EP and Cath lab employees, and several low cost/low risk preventative strategies for reducing musculoskeletal symptoms in the workforce are not currently being completed by those who participated in the study.

Author details

Khalid Sawalha[1*], Nicholas Beresic[2], Shoaib Khan[1] and Gilbert-Roy Kamoga[1]

1 Internal Medicine Department, White River Health System, Batesville, Arkansas, United States

2 University of North Carolina, Chapel Hill, North Carolina, United States

*Address all correspondence to: ksawalha@aol.com

References

[1] Occupational Safety and Health Administration. (2013). *Caring for our caregivers: Facts about hospital worker safety*. Retrieved from https://www.osha.gov/dsg/hospitals/documents/1.2_Factbook_508.pdf

[2] Johnson, D. (2012). *Efficacy of a novel thoracopelvic orthosis in reducing lumbar spine loading and muscle fatigue in flexion: A study with weighted garments* (Doctoral dissertation). Retrieved from https://deepblue.lib.umich.edu/bitstream/handle/2027.42/91450/danijohn_1.pdf%3Bsequence=1

[3] Jaret, P. (2020, February 3). *Attracting the next generation of physicians to rural medicine*. Retrieved from https://www.aamc.org/news-insights/attracting-next-generation-physicians-rural-medicine

[4] Goetzel, R., Roemer, E., Liss-Levinson, R., & Samoly, D. (2008). *Workplace health promotion: Policy recommendations that encourage employers to support health improvement programs for their workers*. Retrieved from http://citeseerx.ist.psu.edu/viewdoc/download?doi=10.1.1.460.912&rep=rep1&type=pdf

[5] Qaseem, A., Wilt, T., McLean, R., Forciea, M., & Clinical Guidelines Committee of the American College of Physicians. (2017). Noninvasive treatments for acute, subacute, and chronic low back pain: A clinical practice guideline from the American College of Physicians. *Annals of Internal Medicine, 166*, 514-530. https://doi.org/10.7326/M16-2367

[6] Christenssen, W. (2001). Stretch exercises: Reducing the musculoskeletal pain and discomfort in the arms and upper body of echocardiographers. *Journal of Diagnostic Medical Sonography, 17*(3), 123-140.

[7] Gartley, R., & Prosser, J. (2011). Stretching to prevent musculoskeletal injuries: An approach to workplace wellness. *AAOHN Journal, 59*(6), 247-252. https://doi.org/10.1177/216507991105900603

[8] Kuorinka, I., Jonsson, B., Kilbom, A., Vinterberg, H., Biering-Sørensen, F., Andersson, G., & Jorgensen, K. (1987). Standardised Nordic questionnaires for the analysis of musculoskeletal symptoms. *Applied Ergonomics, 18*(3), 233-237. http://dx.doi.org/10.1016/0003-6870(87)90010-X

[9] Crawford, J. (2007). The Nordic musculoskeletal questionnaire. *Occupational Medicine, 57*(4), 300-301. doi:10.1093/occmed/kqm036

[10] Lenderink, A. & Zoer, I. (2012). Review on the validity and reliability of self-reported work-related illness. Retrieved from http://www.hse.gov.uk/research/rrpdf/rr903.pdf

[11] Beresic, N. (2019). *Examining low back pain prevention strategies in the electrophysiology and catheterization lab* (Doctoral dissertation). Retrieved from, http://libres.uncg.edu/ir/uncg/f/Beresic_uncg_0154D_12712.pdf

[12] Goldstein, J., Balter, S., Cowley, M., Hodgson, J., & Klein, L. (2004). Occupational hazards of interventional cardiologists: Prevalence of orthopedic health problems in contemporary practice. *Catheterization and Cardiovascular Interventions, 63*(4), 407-411. doi:10.1002/ccd.20201

Section 7

Preventive Strategies and Measures

Chapter 9

A Comparative Study of the Efficacy of Community Health Clubs in Rural Areas of Vietnam and Zimbabwe to Control Diarrhoeal Disease

Juliet Waterkeyn, Victor K. Nyamandi and Nguyen Huy Nga

Abstract

The Community Health Club (CHC) Model in Makoni District, Zimbabwe operated 265 CHCs with 11,600 members from 1999 to 2001 at a cost of US$0.63 per beneficiary per annum. A decade later, 48 CHCs were started in three districts in Vietnam with 2,929 members at a cost of US$1.30. Hygiene behaviour change was compared using a similar survey of observable proxy indicators in both projects, before and after intervention. In Vietnam there was a mean of 36% change in 16 observable proxy indicators ($p > 0.001$) which compared positively with Makoni where there was a mean of 23% hygiene change in 10 indicators ($p > 0.001$). In Vietnam, 8 Health Centers reported a reduction of 117 cases of diarrhoeal diseases in CHC communes, compared to only 24 in non-CHC communes in one year; in 8 Health Centers in Makoni, Zimbabwe, a reduction of 1,219 reported cases over a 2–9 year period was reported, demonstrating the efficacy of CHC both in African and Asian context. We suggest that regular government data of reported cases at clinics may be a more reliable method than self-reported diarrhoea by carers in clustered-Randomised Control Trials, which have surprised practitioners by finding negligible impact of WASH interventions on diarrhoea in rural communities.

Keywords: community health club, hygiene behaviour change, sanitation, Vietnam, Zimbabwe

1. Introduction

This study provides a comparison between the first Community Health Club (CHC) pilot project in Makoni District, Zimbabwe in 2000 [1, 2] to the first a pilot project of a 'classic CHC' intervention in Vietnam which was researched and presented in conference proceedings in 2010 but not published [3]. Our interest is to establish if these two interventions can be considered efficacious in the prevention of diarrhoea in Community Health Club households in two very different settings.

1.1 Replication of the community health club approach

In the past 20 years, over 3,000 Community Health Clubs have been started in 12 countries in Africa reaching over 2.5 million people [4] but in SE Asia, only in Vietnam. Although CHCs have been replicated at a small scale in many countries, only in Zimbabwe and Rwanda have they gone to scale throughout the country [5]. In Zimbabwe most Non Governmental Organisations (NGOs) now use CHC as a standard means of mobilising community in Water and Sanitation Programmes and this method has been endorsed in both the Water Policy and the Sanitation Policy for the country and Ministry of Health is the custodian of this initiative though the Environmental Health Department. In Rwanda the government has taken a lead in coordination of all NGOs into a single National Community Based Environmental Health Promotion Programme (CBEHPP) in which CHCs have been started in all villages throughout the country [6]. A recent systematic review of studies reporting the effect of Community Health Clubs on behaviour relating to drinking water usage, sanitation, hand washing and clean kitchen hygiene [7] demonstrated a strong pattern of community response and a significant change in a wide raft of safe hygiene in virtually all such programmes conducting the 'Classic CHC' training as originally conceived [1]. However, this study is the first to compare CHC in Africa to a similar CHC pilot project in South East Asia.

1.2 Community health clubs in Zimbabwe

Makoni District in Zimbabwe was the first site internationally to field test the concept of a Community Health Club in 1994, and by 1999 an organisation called Zimbabwe AHEAD had been started to replicate and scale up the approach throughout the country.

Community Health Clubs are defined as a voluntary group of men and women, of all ages, education and income level, who are dedicated to improving the health and hygiene facilities and practices of all members so as to alleviate all preventable diseases and manage public health within the given catchment of the club. CHC are usually supported technically by Environmental Health Technicians (EHTs) responsible for public health who are usually based at Rural Health Centers who supervise voluntary community facilitators in at least 20 health promotion sessions every week for at least six months. The process of training has been well documented in the training manual [8].

1.3 Replication in Vietnam

In 2009, The Ministry of Health in Vietnam was looking for a hygiene behaviour strategy to galvanise communities into changing their high risk behaviour, as several approaches including PHAST [9], Community Led Total Sanitation (CLTS) [10] and Social Marketing [11] had already been tried in some areas but had not succeeded in reaching the last percentile. There was at this time much debate as to the most cost-effective methodology to achieve permanent hygiene and sanitation behaviour change.

As CHCs had not been used in S.E Asia at that time, there was some concern that with higher living standards in Vietnam, the CHC Approach could be too basic for rural Vietnamese. However, the level of literacy in women at 92% and in men at 96.1%, in Vietnam [12] was not much higher than in Zimbabwe which was 87.2% literacy for women and 94.2% for men in 2010 [13]. At the time, the national average for rural water supply household coverage in Vietnam was 83% whilst rural household sanitation was only 55%, of which only 18% of latrines in rural areas met

	Zimbabwe	Vietnam
National water supply household coverage	79%	83%
National rural sanitation coverage	24%	55%
Literacy in women / men (2010)	87.2% / 94.2%	92% / 96.1%
Number of Provinces	1	3
Number of Districts	1	3
Size of intervention area in hectares	802,800	225,100
Population in whole district (2003)	358,733	444,488
Households in whole district	65,225	98,775
% Households with CHC in whole district	17%	3%
Number of intervention wards /all	21/35	7/70
Number of CHC	265	48
Number CHC members	11,450	2,939
Number of beneficiaries	63,700	13,258
Average no members /CHC	43	68
Households in intervention ward/commune	38,181	10,824
Estimated % CHC coverage of households in intervention wards	30%	21% and 36%
Average Size of household	5.6	4.5
Period of intervention (1–2 years)	1999–2000	2009–2010
Number of health sessions held (I year)	3,731	960
Number of latrines built in 2 years	2,400	441
Cost per beneficiary per year	US$ 0.63	US$1.30

Table 1.
Demographic comparison between CHC intervention in Zimbabwe and Vietnam showing scope of project.

government standards of hygiene [12, 14]. Again, this compares to Zimbabwe where rural sanitation was estimated at 25% and rural water supply at 79%. Whilst the two cultures of Zimbabwe and Vietnam appear quite different, the demographic level are not dissimilar (**Table 1**).

2. The interventions

2.1 Makoni District, Zimbabwe

By the year 2000 there were 265 CHCs in 21 out of 35 wards of the district with 11,600 CHC members, involving an estimated 63,700 beneficiaries, calculated by the average of 5.6 family benefitting from improved hygiene in each family. During the period under review there had been 3,731 health promotion sessions held by 14 EHTs. Subsidies for VIP latrine construction at that time resulted in 2,400 VIP latrines being constructed in 2 years, which was considered remarkable given the total for the country was only 8,000 in 1998. No water component was included in the project, but the district was higher than the national average with 676 functional boreholes and 839 family wells [12]. The project was completed in 2000 when most donors withdrew from Zimbabwe for political reasons, and the CHC were largely left to their own resources, except those which continued with income generating activities started in a later programme [2].

Wards	Start Year of CHC	Spread of CHC	All h/holds	CHC members
Ruombwe	1995	80%	2,224	1,777
Nyamidzi	1996	113%*	1358	1540
Tikwiri	1998	68%	753	516
Mutanda	1998	43%	1186	513
Dumbamwe	1998	78%	939	730
Sangano	1998	20%	1558	309
Inyati Mine	2000	9%	2900	253
Chiduku	2000	NA	NA	NA

**Over 100% indicates more than one CHC member per household in the CHC.*

Table 2.
Spread of CHC in wards where health centers have provided reported cases of diarrhoea.

2.2 Adaptation of the CHC approach in Vietnam

The pilot CHC project was started in three Provinces of Northern Vietnam, Son La, Phu Tho and Ha Tinh with 48 CHCs with 2,393 members. An active health club of committed members was established in every village to manage environmental health and encourage community hygiene through non risk practices. Village Health Workers already part-employed with Ministry of Health were trained to conduct the sessions. The period of intervention was similar in both countries being from 18 months to 2 years with 20–24 sessions completed in a six-month period of weekly training.

2.3 Comparative scope and spread of the two interventions

The scope of the programme in Zimbabwe was five times larger than the pilot project in Vietnam. However, although the size of each CHC *appears* larger in Vietnam with a mean of 68 members compared to the Zimbabwean CHC with 43 members, those in Vietnam counted *all* members at registration but with no indication if they attended or not, as membership cards were not used. In Zimbabwe, only the *active* members who completed training were counted as members; if all registered members were counted the mean would be around 80 members. Also, the CHC density (spread) is high in Makoni with 21 out of 35 wards in the district with CHC, whereas in Vietnam only in 7 out of 70 communes had CHC. In Vietnam the two communes had a spread of 21% CHC households in Son La and 36% in Ha Tinh, whilst that of Phu Tho was not calculated. The mean coverage in Makoni was 30% but this ranged from 9% coverage in a new area such as Chiduku, to 113% in Nyamidzi where all households were in a CHC, some with more than one per households as a CHC Members. **Table 2** above shows the % spread in the 8 wards where data was collected from local Health Centers.

3. Methods

3.1 Objectives

This study seeks to compare outcomes from the Vietnamese pilot project and compare it to the Makoni CHC pilot project, in five measures: improved knowledge, hygiene and sanitation behaviour change, reduction in disease, cost-effectiveness and stakeholder perceptions.

3.2 Data collection

3.2.1. Data Collection in Zimbabwe

A case/control study was conducted in Zimbabwe in three districts, of which one of the districts was Makoni. The standard indicators used to measure hygiene and sanitation behaviour change included a spot observation of 17 indicators taken in 25 randomly selected CHCs, and within each CHC a random sample of 382 CHC members. These indicators were observed before and after in the CHC intervention villages and in the 113 households of non CHC members, in control villages using similar empirically observable proxy indicators to quantify changes in hygiene facilities and standards of cleanliness. There was no self-reported behaviour. Full details of data collection and analysis are fully described elsewhere [1, 2].

3.2.2. Data collection in Vietnam

3.2.2.1 Quantitative

- A household survey was carried out twice (pre and post) in each of the three Districts. As every household was surveyed in every village, there was strong statistical validity. Each enumerator was meant to survey 100 respondents, but when there were not enough CHC households, they also surveyed non-CHC households and the respondents were not differentiated in the data. Therefore, these statistics may show a combined level of CHC and non CHC, and the rate of change within the CHC membership may therefore be higher than shown [3].

- Secondary data was collected from 8 clinics in CHC areas and 5 clinics in non-CHC areas by the Ministry of Health and provided for analysis. The number of reported cases for Diarrhoea, Dysentery and Food Poisoning (DD & FP) in 2009 was collected and compared to those in 2010.

3.2.2.2 Qualitative data

- Structured interviews were done with key informants which included district officials and nurses from Ministry of Health and village leaders [3].

- A spot observation of a sample of six CHCs in action was done and six individual homes were visited, one in each of the Community Health Clubs.

3.3 Analysis of data

In Vietnam, analysis of data from each Province of the base line and post line survey was done by Ministry of Health officials and provided to one of the authors in excel for her interpretation. All data was cleaned and in this process it was decided to discard data from two of the districts (Phu Tho and Son La) because the standard household survey had been adapted by each district, which made comparative analysis difficult. Therefore, only data from Ha Tinh is used because it could provide raw data for the full base line and post intervention survey that could be checked. In this district a survey of 7,187 base line respondents, and 1,200 post intervention respondents was undertaken, and used to ascertain levels of knowledge and behaviour change. It was converted into SPSS statistics package and standards test of Chi square used to compare data sets [15].

3.4 Sources of bias and confounding

Some interviewer bias can be expected, as the data from the household survey in both Zimbabwe and Vietnam was collected by the same Village Health Workers who facilitated the project. However this was triangulated in spot checks using observable indicators which could be verified empirically.

The statistics collected from the Health Centers both in Zimbabwe and Vietnam are considered impartial as reported cases were not influenced by the objective of this research. The data was collected and analysed by each district by Ministry of Health and presented in their annual reports. National statistics also show a gradual trend in improvement of most communities in Vietnam over the previous five years (NTP2) [12]. Therefore, to identify the impact of only the CHC training we compared CHC with non CHCs areas as a control for clinical reported cases.

Ministry of Health statistics in Health Centers were taken to track the pattern of disease in wards or communes where CHCs were operational in both countries despite the fact that these figures may not reflect the true burden of disease, as only the most critical cases will be reported. This is not critical to this research as it is the pattern not the extent we are interested in examining. In Zimbabwe, the two wards where there were large hospitals were not used because the catchment of patients was referred from other areas and therefore could not be attributed to the CHC training.

In Vietnam, the CHC Pilot project was not the only health promotion being done in these districts during this one year period. In Ha Tinh, a Unilever Programme using extensive Social Marketing techniques promoting handwashing with soap was running concurrently for one year in all communes, including the CHC communes. Therefore, to avoid confounding and to measure the impact of *only* the CHC, we have only sited findings from topics which were not included in Unilever Information Education and Communication (IEC) material.

4. Results

4.1 Vietnam

The results for Vietnam are provided in five measures: improved knowledge, hygiene and sanitation behaviour change, reduction in disease, cost-effectiveness and stakeholder perceptions.

4.1.1 Improved knowledge

The spot observation done in two CHC per Province provided ample anecdotal evidence of the popularity of the CHCs, with high levels of attendance with an average of 68 people at each session.

The Vietnamese showed a strong interest in health education and although basic knowledge of hygiene was high, it did not seem that the training was pitched too low for their level of education. Two questions were asked to establish difference in health knowledge: the causes and prevention of diarrhoea and how to make Sugar Salt Solution (SSS) a homemade recipe to treat dehydration. Whilst the former was well-known due to Unilever programmes and showed little difference before and after the training (94%), knowledge of how to make SSS, was increased by 42% (**Figure 1**) and is more reliable an indicator as this was not taught in the Unilever programme.

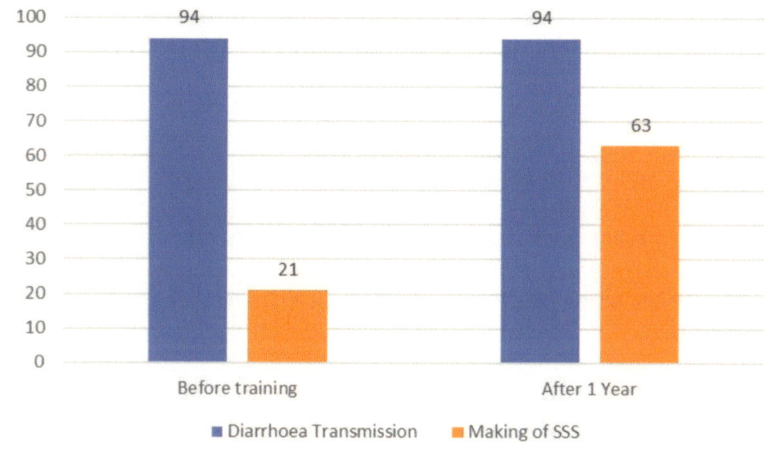

Figure 1.
Improved knowledge in Ha Tinh, Vietnam, after one year of health promotion using two indicators (2009–2010).

4.1.2 Hygiene and sanitation behaviour change

4.1.2.1 Hygiene in the home

Of the three provinces we chose to use Ha Tinh with 12 CHC and almost 900 CHC members as it provided the most reliable information on levels of hygiene behaviour change as summarised in **Figure 2** below. Across 17 indicators, only one indicator, the use of bednets, i.e. 'protection from mosquito' showed no significance at all, as it was 100% in both pre and post intervention survey. In the other 16 indicators, all practices showed compositive behaviour change of 36% (the mean of all 16 indicators) after one year: 'safe water source' and 'drinking water treated', which had

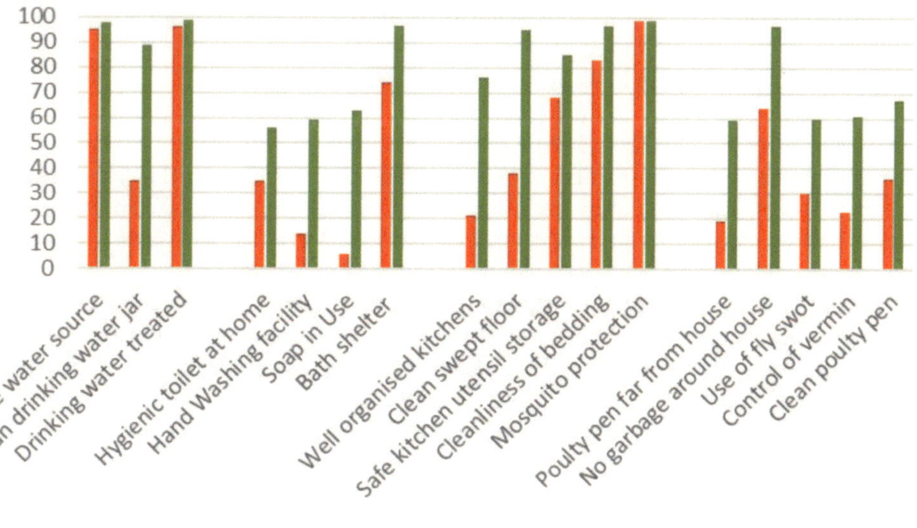

Figure 2.
Prevalence of observed proxy indicators of safe hygiene in CHC members after one year of health promotion, in 2 communes Ha Tinh District, Vietnam. (2009–2010).

been advocated by previous WASH projects were significant at $p > 0.05$; the other 14 indicators, not used in previous projects, were highly significant ($p > 0.001$).

- Hand washing facilities improved by 45% (from 14–59%)
- use of soap improved by 53% (from 6–63%)
- Safe storage of water increased by 54% (from 35–89%)
- 89% households had a combined measure of safe drinking safe (source, storage and treatment)
- The coverage of toilet increased from 35–56% after a year, with 265 new pit latrines, 7 covered pit latrines, 71 new composting latrines, and 71 with a septic tank (414 in total).
- Safe storage of kitchen utensils improved by 23% (from 68–85%)
- 'Well organized kitchens' (plates and food stored safely) improved 55% (from 21–76%).
- Clean swept floors increased by 57% (from 38–95%)
- Cleanliness of bedding improved by 14% (from 83–97%)
- Clean compound surrounded the house improved by 33% (litter decreasing from 36–3%)
- fly control increased by 30%, with 60% of people owning and using a fly swot to kill flies
- homes practicing some form of vermin control increased by 42%, from 23–61%

4.1.2.2 Speed of sanitation behaviour change

Community Health Club records were used to analyse the speed of adoption by the CHC members. At base line there was 99% open defecation in Ha Tinh (**Figure 3**). When a survey was taken only one month into the training when CHC members had attended 1–4 sessions, open defecation had decreased to 84%, with 13% now practicing cat sanitation and 3% having constructed a permanent latrine.

By the second and third month when between 5 and 12 sessions had been attended, open defecation had plummeted to only 2% with a massive uptake of 87% practicing cat sanitation, with 10% constructing permanent latrines and 1% having a temporary latrine.

By the time more than 20 sessions had been done, it was found that 49% had constructed a permanent latrine and 50% were still using cat sanitation with 1% having a temporary latrine.

Thus in 5 months Zero Open Defecation (ZOD) had been achieved.

4.1.3 Reported cases of diarrhoea, dystentry and food poisoning

Diarrhoea, Dysentery and Food Poisoning (DD & FP) are listed together as one category in reported cases in Health Centers in Vietnam. The communes selected

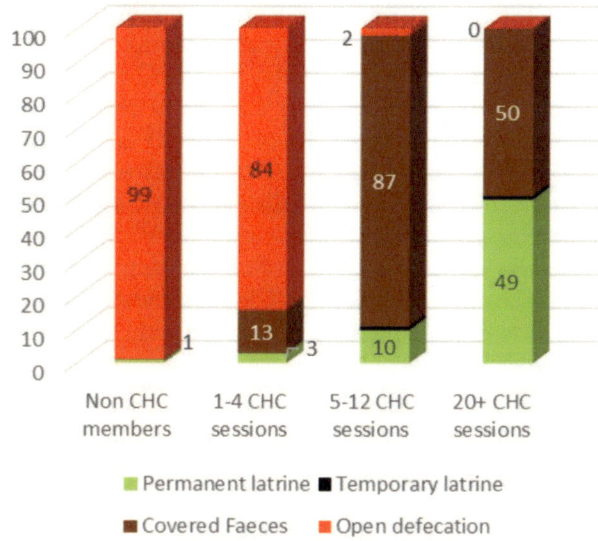

Figure 3.
Uptake of safe sanitation correlated with number of health sessions attended in community health clubs in one year in Ha Tinh District, Vietnam, (2009–2010).

for CHC were in most cases, the more challenging areas as shown by higher DD & FP at baseline (**Figure 3**, *above*). The data from all three provinces showed the same pattern of reduction in areas where Community Health Clubs were fully operational, all with a downward trend in reported cases. In total there were an estimated 459 saved cases in CHC Communes.

The Community Health Club communes showed a sharp decline in reported cases of DD & FP from a total of 171 cases to 17 cases in one year, saving an estimated 154 cases, a mean reduction of 61 cases in each commune from 2010 to 2011. By contrast, control communes with no CHC, reduced in DD & FP reported cases from 99 to 75, only 24 down from the previous year (**Figure 4**).

Of the non-CHC Control communes, only Pi Toong in Son La decreased in DD &FP, whilst in the two other non-CHC Communes Thach Vinh and Thach Dai reported cases of DD & FP *increased* in reported cases, despite the fact that in the latter a Social Marketing campaign was being conducted. In Son La Province, with a

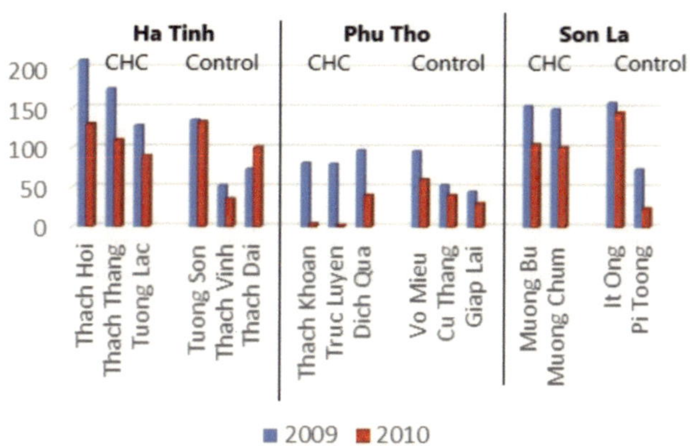

Figure 4.
Reduction of reported cases of diarrhoea, dysentery and food poisoning (DD & FP) in 7 CHC communes in Vietnam after one year of health promotion activity (2009–2010).

higher density of 12 CHC in 55 villages in the catchment of the Health Centre, there were no other public health programmes, therefore we attribute the decrease in DD & FP to the CHC intervention.

However, the data could not determine if there were fewer reported cases at Health Centres due to successful prevention of DD & FP by safe hygiene, or due treatment at home using SSS, but either way these numbers show some positive effect. Nurses interviewed from the Health Centres attributed the decrease in cases to the CHC training and maintain that patients were more able to distinguish between when it is necessary to come to the clinic for treatment and when they can treat dehydration at home. This clear pattern in six well matched communes, provides some indication of the potential of hygiene and sanitation training in CHC to affect health outcomes.

4.1.4 Cost effectiveness of the CHC intervention

We apply the same method of assessing cost-effectiveness in Vietnam as we did when estimating cost per beneficiary in two districts of Zimbabwe [1]. In Makoni District in two years for 68,700 beneficiaries we estimated a cost per beneficiary of US$ 0.61: this included in addition to training and running costs, support in terms of allowances and fuel and motorbikes for 14 government field workers [3]. Whilst this method of dividing the cost of operation of the project by number of beneficiaries is a fairly rough approximation, it can give some comparative data to enable assessment of cost-effectiveness in Vietnam using the same equation.

The 48 CHC in Vietnam were run by Village Health Workers, who were given a nominal incentive, but no transport or fuel allowance as they were stationed in the village. The only costs in Vietnam were for the initial training in the District, which was done in 2009. The running costs for two years was estimated in one Province at US$45,045. Taking the national average of 4.5 family members per household with 2,929 CHC member, there were **13,258** beneficiaries. Thus, cost per beneficiary can be roughly estimated at US$1.30 per annum for two years (2009–2010) per district [3].

Cost-effectiveness is determined by the number of beneficiaries and the CHC approach is a methodology which can work at scale. The Zimbabwe programme was almost 5 times larger than the Vietnam pilot project and was therefore a third of the cost per beneficiary. Generally pilot projects are not expected to be cost-effective as they tend to be small scale with large start-up costs which make them more costly per person. However, as with the pilot Community Health Club project in Vietnam, this rough calculation may provide some indication of the cost-saving that could be achieved at scale.

4.1.5 Perceptions of stakeholders of the community response

Perception of project success can be ascertained from the stakeholders and for this reason we conducted a structured interview with health officials in each province in Vietnam [16] and asked them to rate the 'popularity' of Community Health Clubs from 1 to 10.

Community Response in Phu Tho, was rated at 7 out of 10, with officials saying, 'the *CHCs are very popular because people do it voluntarily, they vote for the committee and they organise it all themselves...more focus on the practical and more participation. They do not rely on the facilitator, so it is a two-way teamwork and promotes a good spirit*.'

In Son La officials gave a score of 8 out of 10 and reported: '*We are very satisfied with the changes and expect that it can be replicated to other districts. With experience it has improved knowledge and skills, not only for district but also for provincial staff. Before we had to deal with health promotion but not in a professional way, no materials, so after CHC training we know how to do it.'*

The highest score was given by officials in Ha Tinh with 9/10, who said that community '*have better relationships with each other, and exchange information, do village clean ups, have better coordination and help improve knowledge and awareness.'* One official declared that the CHC Model is '*low cost- high impact*'.

4.2 Results from Zimbabwe

The impact on behaviour change found in Makoni [1] are now summarized. Clinical data is now provided to assess if there was an impact on health in CHC areas in Zimbabwe. By 1999 there were 42 Health Centres throughout the 20 communal wards of Makoni, of which 12 had resident Environment Health Technicians (EHTs). A communal ward consisted of five or six scattered villages and between 1,000–2,000 households of mostly subsistence farmers.

Whilst the Health Centres cater only to the local population of up to 3,000 people (usually within a 10 km radius), the district hospitals are referral centres for all the surrounding health centres, often over 50 kms away. District hospitals, therefore, did not reflect the same pattern of decrease, presumably because many patients are likely to be referred by Health Centres from areas where there may be no Community Health Clubs. Most Health Centres, on the other hand, situated within a CHC catchment area, did register some downward trend, not only in diarrhoea, but also in skin and eye diseases, ARIs, schistosomiasis and some malaria during the intervention period [15]. Bilharzia was almost eliminated from 1,310 to only one case; Acute Respiratory Diseases decreased from 2,136 to 159 and skin diseases fell from 685 to 41 reported cases.

For the purpose of this paper, we examine only diarrhoea reported cases for comparative analysis with Vietnam. We took the data collected in 8 Health Centres, between 1995 and 2003, which was two years after the end of the project in 2001 [16]. Most notable is the pattern that *in all wards* reported cases of diarrhoea start to fall in the same year that CHCs start in each ward even though the start-up year may be different in each Health Centre, as shown by the shaded areas in **Table 3**. Furthermore, cases in all 8 wards *continue to decline* until 2001 when there is a *rise or a spike* in all but two wards: the two oldest wards of Ruombwe remains low (38 cases) and never climb back to its original level of 404 as in 1995 and Mutanda maintains the fall but starts to rise the following year 2003, when the highly effective EHT left the area. Tikwiri by contrast, without an EHT after the project ended in 2001, climbed straight back to previous levels of diarrhoea in two years (437) with 124 more cases than in 1995 (**Table 3** below). The effect of the charisma of different EHTs is a variable which should be correlated more closely with behaviour change.

This lack of sustainable reduction of diarrhoea maybe attributed to the circumstances in Zimbabwe where in 2001, political change and economic inflation started to affect the country. However, if these circumstances caused the decrease in reported cases, it stands to reason that all wards would have been equally affected. The question to be asked is 'Why is it that one ward, the one which was the most diarrhoea-affected of all wards in 1995, continued to decrease in reported cases across all diseases over nine years, despite the economy and other constraints shared by all other wards?' Our explanation for this is that only in Ruombwe ward was there a dedicated EHT and active CHCs for nine years, and only in this ward was the coverage of CHC members of all households sufficiently high (80%) with 18 CHCs and 1,777 members out of 2224 households in

Health Centres	1995	1996	1997	1998	1999	2000	2001	2002	2003	1995 less 2003
Ruombwe	404	301	244	198	166	81	65	26	38	−366
Nyamidzi	325	338	162	181	79	56	50	117	125	−200
Tikwiri	303	248	266	210	191	210	56	348	427	+124
Mutanda	180	231	71	85	119	127	122	82	135	−45
Dumbamwe	144	141	119	138	92	103	66	118	143	+1
Sangano	105	163	256	200	259	293	101	221	149	−44
Inyati Mine	144	170	259	189	106	63	34	82	75	−69
Chiduku	182	148	182	204	346	89	74	94	76	−106
Total all CHC	**1787**	**1740**	**1559**	**1405**	**1358**	**1022**	**568**	**1088**	**1168**	

Shaded area indicates the span of the CHC in each of the wards. Underlining represents a decrease from previous year.

Table 3.
*Number of reported cases of Diarrhoea in 8 health Centres in Makoni District, Zimbabwe 1995–2003 [17] LINK Excel.Sheet.12 "Book1" "Sheet1!R17C2:R26C11" \a \f 4 \h * MERGEFORMATX.*

the ward participating in the programme, all of which were accessing one Health Centre (**Table 2** *above*). Furthermore, Ruombwe being the first ever CHC project received high visibility externally [15]. This finding reinforces the need for CHC activity to continue for many years to ensure that a sufficient number of people in the area are converted to good hygiene and that this standard is taken as a norm in all households. This take more than a couple of years which is the normal length of a WASH project.

In wards which had been going for five years there was a higher number of CHCs and *(See* **Table 2***)*, the downward trend of reported cases remains low. In wards where CHC had been active for one or two years (Inyati and Chiduku) downward trend was reversed the moment the project officially ended in 2001.

The total number of diarrhoea cases from all wards decrease from 1,787 to 568 between 1995 and 2000 which were the years of intervention. Although the number of cases mounts again to 1,168 two years after the end of the project, the same level is not regained in six out of eight wards by 2003.

To understand which variables affects these differences we would have needed more contextual information from that period: it could be the effectiveness of the EHT, the local leadership, the proximity of the ward to urban areas and the impact of rising HIV/AIDS infections which at the time were 30% of the population. Our sense is that the *length* of the intervention, which also affects the *spread* of CHC members is probably the most important variable, but more contextual information is needed to interpret this data.

4.2.1 Intermediate outcomes of hygiene behaviour change in Makoni District

The most significant intermediate outcomes of hygiene behaviour change were found in 10 proxy indicators showing a mean improvement of 24% ($p < 0.001$) as follows:

- Use of individual cups was 98% in CHC intervention, 66% in control
- Use of individual plates was 97% in CHC and 64% in control

- Use of pot racks was 94% in CHC, 82% in control
- Having a nutrition garden was 90% in CHC, 80% in control
- Using a rubbish pit was 93% in CHC, 82% in control
- Management of rubbish pit was 55% in CHC, 29% in control
- No open defecation was 88% in CHC, 29% in control
- Latrine built in last year was 36% in CHC, 4% in control
- Handwashing facility owned was 45% in CHC, 20% in control
- Handwash facility with water was 35% in CHC, 20% in control.

5. Discussion

This paper describes for the first time, how a seemingly 'African' approach [13] is in fact transferrable to a South East Asian context, into a very different society, but one which faces the same challenges of poverty and ill health associated with WASH related disease as Zimbabwe. The Community Health Club Approach is a method of community mobilisation and is considered culturally well aligned with traditional communal life in Africa, providing a much-needed means for the empowerment of women and their advancement through increased knowledge of basic causes and prevention of disease. From its first field trial in Zimbabwe [1], the methodology spread to at least 15 countries in Africa to our knowledge, easily replicated by one of the authors in Uganda [18], and Rwanda [17] in East Africa, in Cape Town and Kwa Zulu Natal [16] in South Africa and in Sierra Leone [19] and Guinea Bissau [20] in West Africa, and by others to Haiti in the Caribbean [21]. Monitoring data from all these projects have demonstrated measurable changes in health knowledge, hygiene and sanitation behaviour change, and even in some places an impact on health but more peer reviewed research is needed to ascertain the extent of this impact is the efficacy of CHCs to improve health is to be believed.

5.1 Comparison of values and norms

The South African concept of 'Ubuntu' on which the CHC model is based, is perhaps a universal value for 'common unity' shared with Confucian and Buddhist teaching, common in Vietnam, which recognises that the strength of the individual is contingent on an effectively integrated community with shared norms and values. In Northern Provinces of Vietnam where this pilot project took place, the values of group conformity and consensus have been developed through many years of national communism, which have discouraged individualism, and very 'western' need for self-expression which has been the hallmark of liberal democracy [22]. Instead CHC members in Vietnam readily comply with the recommended practices advocated in the Community Health Club, and there is little resistance to change. It was apparent from the numbers who joined the CHC and completed the training, that the norms cultivated by the Community Health Club resonated strongly with the existing village culture of mass organisations, who readily endorsed the activities and were part of the existing village structures under the wing of the Women's Union, which is found in all villages throughout Vietnam.

5.2 Comparison of facilities

Villages in Vietnam had the advantage of a village hall, the 'Culture House', where CHC meetings could be routinely held despite the weather, meaning that CHC activities were not dependent on the seasons unlike in Africa, where training had to be timed to avoid the wet season when attendance was affected by daily downpours of rain [18]. As meetings could be held at night, they did not take away from more pressing demands of earning a living, and provided a welcome social occasion, an outlet for the creativity and musical talent of many members, who loved to sing, deliver poems and drama for the entertainment of the whole village. With electricity and a public announcement system, the Culture Houses provided a ready means to disseminate health messages over the entire village. This sophistication would be a welcome enhancement for CHCs in Zimbabwe, where CHC meet under a tree.

5.3 Comparison of human resources

Unlike many countries in Africa, where finding facilitators within the community to run the CHC is often a challenge, every village in Vietnam already has a well-trained Village Health Worker (VHW) who usually has a basic training in primary health. In addition instead of local volunteers, VHWs in Vietnam often have a motorbike and are supported by government with a small stipend to ensure that they can sustain such community commitment. As such Vietnam is in the same league as Rwanda, the only country in Africa to adopt the CHC model into a national Community Based Environmental Health Promotion Programme, where CHCs have been started in every village in the country, under the existing staff of the Ministry of Health, who supervise Village Health Workers to facilitate health club sessions. The CHC training in Zimbabwe was done by Environmental Health Technicians stationed at each of the Health Centers, in the Makoni Pilot project, with community-based facilitators in the village. Although the National Water Policy [23] and the National Sanitation Policy [24] both call for CHCs in every village, implementation of such programmes is being done by NGOs, most of which have been trained by Africa AHEAD (Zimbabwe AHEAD, as it was from 1999 to 2015) and is not done by District Health Department.

5.4 Comparison of community mobilisation

The mobilisation of the community was as easy in Vietnam as it was in Zimbabwe. The Vietnamese manual [25] was adapted from the Zimbabwean manual [8] both written by the main author. It was translated into the vernacular and a toolkit of culturally appropriate visual aids on which this training depends enabled local Ministry of Health officials to conduct the training through existing government structures. The CHC approach holds special promise in the Vietnamese context as the socialist political system ensures a strong public sector with a vibrant network of mass organisations at community level. In addition, the National Target Programme gives overall coordination in the WASH Sector. Zimbabwe (despite having been the original birthplace of the CHC approach in 1995), still has no data base of the thousands of CHCs which have been started in most districts by over 30 NGOs in the past twenty years. Nor do District Health Departments know which CHC are still active. This is a great pity as much could be done to control cholera and Covid 19 epidemics if this was properly coordinated centrally. The obvious next step would be for CHCs to be mapped and registered in a national programme such as the Community Based Environmental Health Promotion Programme which has been so outstanding in Rwanda, so that the National Coordinating Unit which should control WASH development, can in fact coordinate NGOs and prevent the wasteful duplication which is the feature of the chaotic CHC implementation in Zimbabwe.

5.5 Adaptation of the African style CHC to SE Asian context

The hallmark of CHC programmes in Africa has been the use of a 'membership card' held by each CHC member which records their attendance of sessions and which is required to be fully completed in order that the member be awarded a certificate. It has been theorised that this is an essential part of the 'magic' of the CHC which attracts and holds a larger number of members [23] than with most other mobilisation strategies such as CLTS or PHAST. However, the authorities in Vietnam did not print or distribute membership cards; nor were certificates awarded for completion of the training to CHC members. The facilitation style in Vietnam was autocratic and didactic with top-down directives for hygiene behaviour and compliance enforced by mandatory directives from village leadership. Whilst African CHC tend to be above 80% women, in Vietnam there was more gender balance with as many men as women attending sessions. However, this perceived advantage meant that it was usually men directing proceedings, with little opportunity for gender equity. With a higher level of literacy in Vietnam, the sessions were more like conventional top-down adult education. The sessions were often done without the use of visual aids, which in many places were not printed in time for most of the training. Therefore, the participatory activities which enable women to find their voice were not done, resulting in women remaining largely passive in the meetings. This is unlike the vibrant meeting in Africa which are notable for the full participation of all women as well as men. It is surmised that in Vietnam, with stricter discipline instilled by years of communism, people are perhaps more accustomed to focus for longer periods of time as instructed, without the attraction of participatory activities and visual aids as is the case in African CHC.

5.6 Time needed to effect such change

High levels of hygiene behaviour were achieved in Vietnam which easily matches some of the best projects in Africa [2]. An interesting addition to the literature is the analysis of how long it took the majority of the CHC members to adopt total sanitation. The data collected in Vietnam shows that with weekly training in a CHC it took *at least four weeks* before the behaviour starts to shift towards zero open defecation, but that within 20 sessions all of the members had either build some sort of latrine (49%) whilst the rest were practicing cat sanitation. This is a relatively fast uptake of sanitation and supports the CHC Theory of Change [17] which advocates for at least six months of regular training in a CHC to ensure high levels of uptake of recommended practices.

In Zimbabwe the data from health centers shows that for *health gains* it needs years, not just months of CHC group pressure, to ensure non risk-hygiene behaviour is maintained and is spread to a critical mass of the population, to ensure gains in prevention of diarrhoea is maintained. Only in Ruombwe ward, the only area with over 80% spread, and nine years of CHC activity, did the number of reported cases diminish and remain low after the end of external project support. There has long been debate as to how much time is needed to achieve hygiene behaviour change. The CHC model has been one of the most thorough of training approaches arguing for 20–24 weekly sessions [2], whilst PHAST used up to six sessions [9] and CLTS expects to achieve ODF status within two face-to-face sessions with the community [10]. This research therefore supports the call by leading WASH NGOs [26], who are now joined by some esteemed academics [27, 28], calling for more long-term investment in hygiene behaviour change which is shown to be necessary if any effect on diarrhoea is to be seen through WASH interventions.

5.7 Reduction of disease

In Vietnam the reduction of diarrhoea, dysentery and food poisoning as a direct result of this pilot project was evident in Health Center records, which provides preliminary indication of some effect of the CHC on health. The fact that in the control non-CHC communes DD & DP actually *increased*, while it decreases significantly in all CHC communes gives a preliminary indication of some impact. Project monitoring reports further convey a strong pattern of sanitation and hygiene behaviour change is still believed to be efficacious in the prevention of diarrhoea [29].

5.8 Cost-effectiveness of the CHC model in Vietnam

The CHC methodology can calculate cost-effectiveness because the exact number of beneficiaries and their attendance of health sessions is known. Costs in the first year of a programme are usually higher as training materials need to be printed, but once facilitators are equipped with toolkit and transport, cost per beneficiary should decrease.

It could have been more efficient if Village Health Workers had more than one CHC to run each, as the Zimbabwean facilitators were full time, coordinating five or more health clubs per week. Also, much expenditure went on the printing billboards and posters in Vietnam which is not needed for CHC. The amount of US$ 1.30 for health promotion per person per year is still low and comparable with most CHC projects in Zimbabwe and well under the target in 'Classic CHC' Programmes of less than US$5 per beneficiary per annum for hygiene behaviour change (not including water or sanitation subsidy). With number of cases saved through safe hygiene, there is little doubt that Community Health Clubs are almost always 'low cost - high impact'.

5.9 The methodological debate

We are receiving mixed messages in recent literature on the effectiveness of WASH to reduce diarrhoea and the jury is still out as to exactly which methodology is able to change people's habits in the long term to ensure non risk hygiene and sanitation behaviour. Whilst the Burden of Disease attributable to WASH has apparently been reduced from 4.2% to 1.5% in the last 30 years [3], some recent trials has led to experienced practitioners in the public health sector to question whether WASH interventions are in fact impacting on diarrhoea [30]. Our limited research indicates that comprehensive WASH programmes such as was done in Zimbabwe and Vietnam does lead to reduction in diarrhoal disease.

6. Conclusion

Whilst epidemiologists and trialists struggle with high end statistical data, to inform the Environmental Health Departments of Ministries of Health on the efficacy of community interventions designed to prevent diarrhoea, the *curative* wing of Ministry of Health continues to rely simply and systematically on the number of reported cases at Health Centres to indicate trends in the burden of disease. These trends over time may be more reliable than snapshot interventions of clustered-randomised control trials which seldom have enough time to understand the dynamics of community response. Whilst the routine data we present here has obvious limitations in that it may fail to represent the *full* disease burden, with the crisis of reliability in the WASH literature in the past few years, we may find that watching the pattern of reported cases in the catchment area of an intervention over time may be the nearest we can get to assessing impact on health by such interventions as a Community Health Club programme.

Acknowledgements

In Vietnam, the main author was funded as a consultant by DANIDA 2009-2010 in collaboration with the Ministry of Health and acknowledges the input of local consultants and officials.

In Zimbabwe, the pilot project in Makoni District from 1999 to 2001 was funded by DANIDA in collaboration with the Ministry of Health, and we acknowledge the efforts of Environmental Health Department which was the main implementor of this programme.

Thanks also to Zimbabwe AHEAD (now Africa AHEAD) for quality of training and support to Makoni District.

Conflict of interest

The corresponding authors is the original architect of the CHC Methodology and therefore has obvious bias.

Author details

Juliet Waterkeyn[1]*, Victor K. Nyamandi[2] and Nguyen Huy Nga[3]

1 Africa AHEAD Association, Cape Town, South Africa

2 Food Safety and Port Health Services, Ministry of Health and Child Care, Harare, Zimbabwe

3 Faculty of Public Health and Nursing, Quang Trung University, Quy Nhon City, Vietnam

*Address all correspondence to: juliet@aficaahead.com

References

[1] Waterkeyn J. and Cairncross S. Creating demand for sanitation and hygiene through Community Health Clubs: a cost-effective intervention in two districts of Zimbabwe. Social Science & Medicine. Vol 61, p.1958-1970. 2005.

[2] Waterkeyn J. Hygiene behaviour change through the Community Health Club Approach: a cost-effective strategy to achieve the Millennium Development Goals for improved sanitation in Africa. Germany. Lambert Publishing. p. 144-167.

[3] Waterkeyn J, Nguyen HN. Low cost-high Impact: Hygiene Behaviour Change in Vietnam in Community Health Clubs, University of North Carolina Water Institute Conference. Available from: https://www.africaahead.org/documentation/publications/conference-papers/.2011. Accessed: 2021.03.05

[4] Africa AHEAD. Countries. [Internet] 2021. https://www.africaahead.org/countries/ [Accessed: 2021.03.08]

[5] Waterkeyn J, Matimati R, Muringaniza A, Chingono A, Ntakarutimana A, Katabarwa J, Bigirimana Z, Pantoglou J, Waterkeyn A, Cairncross S. Comparative Assessment of Hygiene Behaviour Change and Cost-effectiveness of Community Health Clubs in Rwanda and Zimbabwe. in Umar B, Rozman U, Turk SS. Healthcare Access: Regional Overviews. 2019. IntechOpen. http://doi:10.5772/intechopen.89995

[6] Government of Rwanda. Road Map for Community Based Environmental Health Promotion Programme. 2010. Revised 2020.Available from https://africaahead.org/wp-content/uploads/2015/03/2015.4.-CBEHPP-Workshop-report_AA.pdf [Accessed 2021.0308]

[7] Rosenfeld J, Berggen R, Frerichs L. A Review of the Community Health Club Literature Describing Water, Sanitation, and Hygiene Outcomes. 2021. Int.J.Environ. Res. Public Health. 18, 1880. https://doi.org/10.3390/ijerph18041880

[8] Waterkeyn J. The Community Health Club Approach: A Manual for Workshop Participants. 2009. Africa AHEAD. ISBN 978-0-620-40422-8. Zimbabwe.

[9] Srinavasan L. Tools for Community Participation. A Manual for Training Trainers in Participatory Techniques. 1990. PROWESS/United Nations Development Programme Technical Series Involving Women in Water and Sanitation. New York.

[10] Kar K. Subsidy or self-respect? Participatory Total Community Sanitation in Bangladesh. 2003. IDS Working Paper 184. Brighton UK: Institute of Development Studies.

[11] Curtis V, Kanki B. et al. Evidence of behaviour change following a hygiene promotion programme in Burkino Faso. 2001. Bulletin of the World Health Organisation. (79): 518-527

[12] Ministry of Agriculture and Rural Development. Completion Report for the RWSS National Target Program 2006-2010 and Major Contents of RWSS NTP 2011-2015

[13] Waterkeyn J, Waterkeyn A. *Creating a culture of health: hygiene behaviour change in Community Health Clubs through knowledge and positive peer pressure.* 2013. *Journal of Water, Sanitation and Hygiene for Development. Vol 3 No 2. 144-155.* Available from: https://doi.org/10.2166/washdev.2013.109

[14] Water Supply and Sanitation in Zimbabwe. Amcow Country Status

Overview. 2011. Available from https://www.wsp.org/sites/wsp/files/publications/CSO-Zimbabwe.pdf. [Accessed 2021.03.08]

[15] Waterkeyn J. Decreasing communicable diseases through improved hygiene in Community Health Clubs, In Maximizing the Benefits from Water and Environmental Sanitation, Proceedings of the 31st WEDC Conference, Kampala, Uganda, 31October – 4 November 2005. Loughborough University, UK. P.138-145. Available from https://wedc-knowledge.lboro.ac.uk/resources/conference/31/WaterkeynJ2.pdf [Accessed 2021.08 03]

[16] Rosenfeld J, Waterkeyn J. Using Cell Phones to Monitor and Evaluate Behaviour Change Through Community Health Clubs in South Africa Proceedings of WEDC International Conference, Addis Ababa, Ethiopia, 2009 water, sanitation and hygiene: sustainable development and multisectoral approaches. Available from https://repository.lboro.ac.uk/articles/conference_contribution/Using_cell_phones_to_monitor_and_evaluate_behaviour_change_through_community_health_clubs_in_South_Africa/9585668/1. [Accessed 2021.03.08]

[17] Waterkeyn J, Waterkeyn A, Uwingabire F, Pantoglou J, Ntakarutimana A, Mbirire M, Katabarwa J, Bigirimana Z, Cairncross S, Carter R. 2020. The value of monitoring data in a process evaluation of hygiene behaviour change in Community Health Clubs to explain findings from a cluster-randomised controlled trial in Rwanda. BMC Public Health 20, 98. https://doi.org/10.1186/s12889-019-7991-7

[18] Waterkeyn J, Okot P, Kwame V. Rapid Sanitation Uptake in the Internally Displaced People Camps of Northern Uganda through Community Health Clubs. 2005. Kampala. 31st WEDC Conference. Available from https://wedc-knowledge.lboro.ac.uk/resources/conference/31/WaterkeynJ.pdf. [Accessed 2021.08.03]

[19] Azurduy L, Stakem M, Wright L. Assessment of the Community Health club Approach. Koinadugu District, Sierra Leone. 2007. CARE International, Atlanta, USA. Available at https://africaahead.org/wp-content/uploads/2015/08/Capstone-report-on-CHCs.pdf. [Accessed 2021.03.08]

[20] Boone P, Elbourne D, Fazzio I, Fernandes S, Frost C, Jayanty C, King R, Mann V, Piaggio G, dos Santos A, Walker P. Effects of community heath interventions on under 5 mortality in rural Guinea Bissau (EPICS): a cluster-randomised controlled trial. 2016. Lancet Glob Health. 4: e328-35. DOI: 10.1016/s2214-109X(16)30048-1

[21] Brooks J, Adams A, Bendjemil S , Rosenfeld J. Putting heads and hands together to change knowledge and behaviours: Community Health Clubs in Port au Prince, Haiti. 2015. Waterlines 2015, 34, 379-396, doi:10.2166/washdev.2013.109.

[22] Harris D, Kooy M, Quang NP. Scaling up Rural Sanitation in Vietnam: Political Economy Constraints and Opportunities. 2011. Working paper 341. Overseas Development Institute. London. Available at https://www.researchgate.net/publication/268051069 [Accessed 2021.0308]

[23] National Water Policy. 2012. (Internet) p.26. Available from: http://ncuwash.org/newfour/wp-content/uploads/2017/08/National-Water-Policy.pdf [Accessed.2021.03.08]

[24] Government of Zimbabwe. National Sanitation and Hygiene Strategy. 2017. p.2. (Internet) Available from: http://newfour.ncuwash.org/wp-content/uploads/2017/08/

National-Sanitation-and-Hygiene-Policy-Draft-2017.pdf. [Accessed 2021. 03.08.]

[25] Government of Vietnam. Ministry of Health. Introduction to the Community Health Club Approach: Participatory Community Training Sessions for Village Health Workers. Vietnam. 2011. Ed. J.Waterkeyn. Available from: https://www.africaahead.org/wp-content/uploads/2021/03/2009-11-11-Trainers-Manual_Final.pdf. [Accessed 2021.03.08]

[26] WaterAid. Revitalising Community Led Total Sanitation: A process guide. 2009. Available from file:///C:/Users/Juliet/Downloads/community%20led%20total%20sanitation%20process%20guide.pdf [Accessed 2021.03.08]

[27] Carter RC. Can and should sanitation and hygiene programmes be expected to achieve health impacts? 2017. Waterlines, Vol. 36, No. 1: 92-103. http://doi: 10.3362/1756-3488.2017.005

[28] Schmidt WP. The elusive effect of water and sanitation on the global burden of disease. 2014. Trop Med. & Int. Health; 19.5. 522-527. https://doi:10.1111/tmi.12286

[29] Pruss-Ustun A, Bartram J, Clasen T, Colford LM, Cumming O, Curtis V, Bonjour S, Dangour A, De France J, Fewtrell l, Freeman MC, Gordan B, Hunter P, Johnston RB, Mathers C, Mausezah D, Medlicott.K, Neira M, Stocks M, Wolf J, Cairncross S. Burden of disease from inadequate water, sanitation and hygiene in low- and middle-income settings: a retrospective analysis of data from 145 countries. 2014. Trop Med & Int. Health. 19.8. 894-905. http://doi:10.1111/tmi.12329

[30] Cumming O, Arnold BF, Ban R, Clasen T, Esteves Mill J, Freeman MC, Gordon B, Guiteras R, Howard G, Hunter PR, Johnston RB, Pickering AJ, Prendergast AJ, Prüss-Ustün A, Rosenboom JW, Spears D, Sundberg S, Wolf J, Null C, Luby SP, Humphrey JH and Colford JM. 2019. The implications of three major new trials for the effect of water, sanitation and hygiene on childhood diarrhea and stunting: a consensus statement. BMC Medicine 17:173: http://doi.org/10.1186/s12916-019-1410-x

Chapter 10

New Approaches for Improved Service Delivery in Rural Settings

Isaac Oluwafemi Dipeolu

Abstract

The health status of the people in rural areas is faced with challenges primarily due to availability, acceptability, financial accessibility to healthcare services. These include traditional and cultural beliefs, behavioural norms that explain community viewpoints of social roles and various community members' functions. Rural and remote areas are medically underserved, access to healthcare services is difficult sometimes. Distance covered to access the nearest available health facility by some rural dwellers is discouraging. Thus, moving critically ill or injured persons is hampered because of long-distance or poor transportation means. In the end, many prefer to use traditional medicine than travel that long distance for medical treatment. Recently, healthcare delivery systems have focused on innovative approaches to improve health outcomes, control costs, and foster achieving the Sustainable Development Goals (SDGs). One of these innovations is mHealth (Short Messaging Service) [SMS] texts, which have peculiar attributes, making it particularly suitable for health care in rural and hard-to-reach areas in Low and Middle-Income Countries (LMICs). Moreover, text-messaging interventions are uniquely suited for underserved populations. This chapter highlights some interventions on the uses and benefits of SMS text applications in healthcare service delivery.

Keywords: mHealth, reminders, text message, rural areas, health care

1. Introduction

The term "rural area" or "rurality" is difficult to define as there is no standard definition of a rural area. There is no standard universal definition of rural area or rurality. Countries or individuals define rural areas, characterised by the main activities such as farming, type, and size [1, 2]. A rural area is considered "a place with agricultural orientation; the houses are farmhouses, barns, sheds and other structures of similar purposes" [3]. He noted that population is the main characteristic differentiating rural from urban areas, especially in developing countries. This definition and description of the rural area may seem adequate; however, this measure might not adequately capture what rural areas means to different people in different countries [3]. There are various categories of rural areas, depending on their ease of access from urban centres. These range from rural-urban fringe to remote rural areas [4]. Rural areas change over time, and these changes are triggered by three factors, namely:

IntechOpen

i. Economic factors—tourism income, farming profitability, primary sector jobs

ii. Environmental factors—land use, pollution, conservation

iii. Social factors—population change and migration, leisure time, retirement population [4].

It has been found that most rural areas are heterogeneous. Thus, defining rural areas based only on people and or one economic activity (commonly agriculture) is not enough to classify areas or regions as rural [2, 5]. Due to the difficulties in getting a unified standard definition of rural areas, census commissions or agencies at the national levels, development partners/organisations and academics in various disciplines turn to and adopt selected approaches in their definitions. However, these definitions also have their limitations [2]. Researchers and international organisations developed typologies and indicators to understand better rural areas [2, 5]. In 2018, about half (49.7%) of the population in Nigeria lived in rural areas [6]. Udo and colleagues noted that each compound houses a man, his immediate family, and some relatives in the rural areas. Some compounds make up the village, usually inhabited by people claiming a common ancestor, often the village's founder. Villages are rural areas, and they share similar characteristics along the line of various ethnic groups in Nigeria [6].

Studies on rural areas and rural residents' health is not new [7]. Freeman & Lumsden [8] reported an outbreak of typhoid in rural Virginia, USA, and some early researchers called out the need to approach health in rural areas differently. This is because rural and remote areas have scarce resources, inadequate supply of physicians and health workers, limited access to service, and an inadequate healthcare delivery system [9–16]. Knowing that rurality reflects a range of demographic, culture, social, economic, and health systems, it may be appropriate to measure these characteristics rather than using a geographic definition of rurality only [7].

2. Rural people's health status

In most developing countries, there are cultural differences between rural communities and urban centres. Even in the rural areas, there are significant cultural differences from community to community, and these reflect in the social roles and functions they are engaged in [17, 18]. So, health is a low priority, which often means that medical services and hospitals are the last resort [18, 19]. This is due to different norms, long traditions and religious practices, culture and beliefs the rural dwellers hold on to and previous experiences with healthcare workers [20–22]. One other important factor is accessibility to rural and remote communities. This is due to the physical structure and topography, with mountains, deserts and jungles of these areas, consequently creating difficulties for transportation and often complicated by varying natural disasters. Hence, no means of transportation and evacuation of critically ill or injured patients is impossible in some rural areas [18, 23].

Globally, rural people's health status is worse than urban areas [18]. Although much progress was made in the Health for All target by 2000 and the Millennium Development Goals (MDGs), some of these goals have not been attained. This is evident in the rural and remote areas where most of the world's population live [18]. In some African countries, infant mortality rates in rural and remote areas are usually higher than those obtained in urban centres [24, 25]. Children in rural and remote areas are more likely to suffer from one health challenge or the other compared with their counterparts in the urban centres [18, 26, 27].

The health status of the people in rural areas worldwide is faced with many challenges primarily due to availability, acceptability, financial accessibility to healthcare services. These include poverty resulting in low health status and high disease burden; one of the main factors responsible for rural-urban drift, traditional and cultural beliefs, behavioural norms that explain community viewpoints of social roles and various community members' functions [18]. Topography most time affects accessibility to rural and remote communities, making it difficult for transportation and sometimes complicated by varying harsh climatic conditions. As a result, moving critically ill or injured persons is hampered because of poor or no transportation means in rural and remote areas.

2.1 Limited funding and other resource constraints

Another factor affecting health services in rural and remote areas is limited funding and other resource constraints. It is a known fact that rural and remote areas are medically underserved, access to healthcare services is difficult sometimes. Some health facilities are understaffed, and in some instances, the health facilities do not have essential equipment or consumables. Distance covered to access the nearest available facility by some rural dwellers is discouraging. Many people living in rural areas have to travel or walk some kilometres from their homes to get to the nearest healthcare facilities. In the end, many prefer to use traditional medicine than travel that long distance for medical treatment.

2.2 Healthcare workers' attitude to patients

The attitude of healthcare providers is another factor influencing the health status of rural community members. There have been concerns about the attitudes of healthcare workers towards their patients in health facilities. Healthcare workers, especially nurses, sometimes do not treat patients or clients well, use abusive words on patients, and be rude and harsh. In some other instances, healthcare workers were accused of giving preferential treatment to patients they knew [28]. Studies show trends in the unprofessional behaviours and attitudes of healthcare workers towards their patients. A study in Nigeria found healthcare workers showing discriminatory attitudes and engaging in unethical behaviour towards patients with HIV/AIDS [29, 30]. In a related study, some pregnant women in South Africa expressed their hesitations in delivering in the hospital due to previous experiences of being shouted at, beaten or neglected by nurses [31, 32].

Another study revealed that healthcare workers in some hospitals also exhibited these unprofessional behaviours and attitudes by using education level as a yardstick for high-quality services [33–35]. Patients with little or no education considered "villagers or rural dwellers" were treated with impatience and disrespect, given less information, and accorded less attention [33–35].

2.3 Healthcare access in rural communities

Rural areas in developing countries, especially in Africa, are plagued with persistent social inequality, poverty, unemployment, a heavy burden of disease, and healthcare service provision's inequitable quality [36]. Inequitable quality of healthcare service bothers on accessibility, affordability, and acceptability. Accessibility and affordability of healthcare services are crucial to good health, yet rural residents face various access barriers. Access is defined as "the timely use of personal health services to achieve the best possible health outcomes" [37]. That means the rural residents should access primary care, dental care, behavioural health, emergency care, and public health services conveniently and confidently. Rural residents face serious difficulties in accessing healthcare services which are usually found in urban centres. This is a true and common feature across rural communities in most African countries. For some people who live in rural areas, the nearest health facilities are some kilometres away from their villages or townships, as the case may be. For instance, 56% of South Africa rural communities live 5 km from a health facility; and 75% of South Africa's poor people live in rural areas [36, 38].

If access to primary healthcare is a fundamental human right, primary healthcare must be brought to rural communities. Asabere reported that the main goal of primary healthcare in most developing countries, including Nigeria, was to make healthcare available, accessible and affordable to all citizens by the year 2000 [39]. This goal has not been achieved yet in most countries, and it seems it will not be soon unless there is a change. For example, despite citing some healthcare centres in rural and urban centres, about two-thirds of the Nigerian population are still medically underserved for many reasons, some of which have been highlighted. Suttle reported that accessing, delivering, or providing healthcare services in rural areas presents unique challenges [40]. Some rural dwellers may travel between two to 3 h to get to the closest health facilities.

Despite the huge gap between developed and developing countries, the main point is that rural health is the same worldwide [41]. The major rural health challenges are availability, accessibility, affordability, and inadequate health workers [15, 42]. Even in countries where most of the population lives in rural areas, the resources are concentrated in the cities [15, 43, 44]. With the concentration of poverty, low health status, and high disease burden in rural areas, there is a need to re-strategize the healthcare delivery systems. Attention must be paid to improving people's health in rural and remote areas if the rural-urban drift (a common trend now) is reversed remarkably [18].

3. New approaches to improving health services delivery in the rural areas

With the concentration of poverty, low health status and high burden of diseases in rural areas, there is a need to focus specifically on improving people's health in rural and remote areas, particularly if the urban drift is to be reversed. A paradigm shift in the healthcare delivery system focuses on finding new and innovative approaches and organisational frameworks to improve health outcomes, control costs, and improve population health. Lunze, Higgins-Steele, Simen-Kapeu, Vesel, Kim and Dickson [45] pointed out that "innovative approaches have the potential to accelerate progress and to lead to better health outcomes", especially in medically underserved areas. In addition, to achieve the Sustainable Development Goals (SDGs), designing and implementing innovative approaches in the health systems is germane. For instance, immunisation is one of the best global health investments, and it is of great import in achieving 14 of the 17 SDGs. As one of the most far-reaching health interventions, it closely reflects the ethos of the SDGs, "leaving no one behind". Other proven interventions that reduce the burden of diseases and mortality are well established; these interventions are not implemented on a large scale in most Low-and-middle-income countries (LMICs) [45–47].

Improvements in technology and new approaches to organising healthcare delivery are occurring quickly. Information and Communication Technologies (ICTs) are now integrated into existing facilities to stimulate development and enhance service delivery [48]. For example, ICT is integrated into service delivery to manage conditions, monitor progress, improve patients' health, and use reminders for clinic appointments and service uptake, disaster management, and emergency. It is also used in seeking feedback from patients in developed and developing nations [49]. Information and Communication Technologies improve service delivery in various ways, such as increasing accessibility to basic needs and increasing efficiency by increasing connectivity and knowledge sharing [50]. The inclusion of different forms of ICTs into health workers daily routines and their patients is common worldwide [51]. The health status of the masses in developing countries is very poor and providing healthcare services to people living in rural and remote areas is a challenge [52]. This is due to inadequate planning for the populace, predominantly rural areas, rising poverty levels, cultural beliefs, inadequate human resources for health in most rural areas, and increased population size [52].

About half of most countries live in rural areas with a high disease burden and are always left behind during planning and budgetary allocation. Nyasulu and Chawinga pointed out that 11% of the world's population is projected to be in Africa, with a global disease burden estimated to be 22% [48]. To take care of this population, additional 1.5 million health workers must fill the existing human resource for health gap. Information and communication technologies have a growing influence on all areas of human life, and the health care sector can leverage this [53]. They can transform health services delivery [54].

4. Delivery of healthcare services via technologies

Technology drives the world today, and new technologies are making a significant impact on healthcare delivery. Transformation in healthcare will be driven by future technological innovation. While development in new drugs and treatments, new machines and devices, smartphones, new social media platforms for healthcare, etc., will drive innovation, human factors will remain one of the stable limitations of these innovations [55]. Personal electronics used for communication and social networking are ubiquitous, spreading into mobile healthcare (mHealth) [56]. In Mobile Health News, Jeffrey Shuren, director of the US Food and Drug Administration's Center for Devices and Radiologic Health, was quoted thus, "the use of mobile medical apps on smartphones and tablets is revolutionising health care delivery" [57]. Thus, we can leverage this to improve healthcare access and delivery in rural areas. Mobile Medical Applications (MMAs) tools can be useful in managing or preventing some health conditions. With smartphones everywhere and their revolution in our day-to-day activities, the thousands of MMAs currently available can take some of the strain off the healthcare system [57].

Kabachinski also noted that, as the number of all cadre of health workers continues to shrink, the sick and elderly Americans continue to increase. mHealth and other innovations can readily be deployed to mitigate these frightening developments [56]. Today, it is remarkable to see how mobile devices and applications are incorporated into healthcare systems to deliver effective and improved services. Almost all health workers have smartphones, and their ownership is expected to increase yearly. Many health workers with multiple mobile devices use them at the point of care [58]. Mobile technology is making a significant impact on human life today, and its application in healthcare systems is on the increase. Some of the apps in the mobile devices have been applied in various areas of health services delivery ranging from enquiry/consultation, clinic appointment reminders, adherence, diagnosis to treatment. Specifically, apps malaria diagnosis, check blood pressure and blood sugar levels are common today, thus providing quick feedback to patients. Unlike before, the waiting time for clinic consultation or appointment is always long, and the results of some tests or investigations take longer to be ready. Learning through the mobile app is on the increase in the healthcare community. Apart from its primary use, today's mobile devices have apps that allow patients to complain to doctors, refill prescriptions, or find the nearest healthcare facility. Efforts are being made to leverage mobile technology for improved communication in healthcare systems [56].

In developing countries, healthcare services and product uptake face barriers, particularly in rural areas. Therefore, emphasis should be on the adoption of cost-effective and cost-efficient and user-friendly technology for sustainability. Mobile devices such as mobile phones fall into this category and have been used effectively in various health programmes or interventions. These include improvement in service delivery and uptake, disease surveillance, prevention, diagnosis, management and behaviour modification [59, 60]. Some patients used their mobile phones to remind themselves to take medication or attend their clinic appointments; some patients and health workers accessed websites and used social media to gather health information [61, 62]. Schwebel and Larimer presented a summary of a systematic review on the impact of reminders messages on the targeted health outcomes [63].

5. Prospect of mHealth and mobile phone text messages in public health interventions in rural areas

There is an increased mobile phone usage with Short Messaging Service (SMS) applications in interventions to deliver health care services. With high success rates in previous intervention in developed countries, Short Messaging Service (SMS) texts have peculiar attributes, making it particularly suitable for health care in rural and hard-to-reach areas in Low and Middle-Income Countries (LMICs). Moreover, text-messaging interventions are uniquely suited for underserved populations. This section highlights some interventions on the uses and benefits of SMS text applications in healthcare service delivery. These interventions are categorised into three major areas, namely

1. SMS used to enhance the efficiency of healthcare service delivery

2. SMS used to improve diagnosis, treatment and rehabilitation of illness

3. SMS used in public health programmes

5.1 SMS used to enhance the efficiency of healthcare service delivery

Mobile text messaging communication has proven to be an effective way to foster desired behaviour change in patients and improve the way care is delivered. A review shows many ways SMS enhances healthcare service delivery efficiency; some of these are highlighted below.

5.1.1 Appointment reminders

Atun, Sittampalam and Mohan reported that missed appointments in England led to substantial costs for many health systems and the National Health System (NHS) [64]. These costs are due to direct costs involved in arranging the appointment and the opportunity cost of missed appointments. For instance, in 2019, about 307 million were sessions scheduled with doctors, nurses, therapists and other practise staff every year, and 5%—one in twenty, 15.4 million—are missed without enough notice to invite other patients [65]. Most of the doctors pointed out that patients missed clinic appointments due to forgetfulness [64]. Almost all the respondents stressed that patients who missed clinic appointments wasted NHS resources. Most doctors also stated that these behaviours from patients have negative impacts on running the NHS efficiently. Most doctors, therefore, noted that they would consider de-list patients who missed clinic appointments repeatedly. However, most doctors opined that charging patients for missed appointments might reduce the challenge [64, 66].

According to the report, the estimated cost of a GP appointment is £18, while that for a nurse is £7 [64]. Thus, in England, the annual direct cost of missed appointments to the NHS is £180 million for GP appointments and £34 million for practice nurse appointments [64, 66]. Hence, in England, missed appointments cost the NHS £789 million a year. To reduce the extent of the problem, the Department of Health (DOH) in England issued a Missed Appointment Guidance, which identifies ways GP surgeries can improve attendance rates for hospital and GP appointments [67]. To address this problem, some pilot trials, which use mobile phone SMS to remind patients to attend NHS appointments, were launched in England in 2003. Some of these pilots reported success or benefits [64, 67], while others identified organisational factors influencing the uptake and adoption of the reminder messages. Poor healthcare service uptake influenced by ineffective administrative staff stuck to the business-as-usual idea could be enhanced when clinicians sign up patients to the innovations on health-related mobile apps [68].

Reminder SMS is now used in imaging diagnostics [69], paediatrics, sexually transmitted infections, maternal health, antenatal clinics, child, adolescent and mental health, and dental services [64]. Reminder SMS was used for mothers of infants in rural areas on appointment keeping of routine immunisation in Nigeria [54]. The intervention using reminder SMS enhanced infant immunisation timely uptake, completion and service delivery.

5.1.2 Improving communication between healthcare workers

Short Messaging Service has been identified as a useful communication tool between surgeons with enhanced coordination of patient care, improved efficiency of administrative activities, greater accuracy of messages, and even increased responsiveness to urgent cases. Communication problems between health care professionals were observed to be one of the factors that lead to errors within healthcare systems, which adversely affect patients' well-being [64, 70]. According to Atun and colleagues, it was noted then that much of the clinical information used by doctors come from peers, personal notes on patients or diagnostic tests [64]. Doctors prefer to seek the opinion of experts rather than consult guidelines, manuals or computer-aided decision systems. SMS is now used to enhance communication among healthcare workers [64, 67, 71].

5.1.3 Managing queues

It has been observed that long waiting times and queuing when accessing health care services led to customer dissatisfaction. Hence, efficient waiting times and queue management are critical to improving service quality and user satisfaction [64, 72–75]. One of the hospitals in England, for instance, has reduced patients waiting time for drug refill and collection of dispensed drugs. Patients receive a text message to inform them when their prescription is ready for collection [76]. This has reduced long waiting times in the hospital and provided much the flexibility to return any time during the day to collect their medication [64].

5.1.4 Contacting blood donors

Customised SMS is used to invite older adolescents and young adults for blood donation. The providers also use the opportunity to develop a database on blood groups of individuals so that donors can be contacted in emergencies, particularly blood of rare groups is needed [77, 78]. In addition, in India, evidence shows that when a blood centre issued a text message-based request to potential donors for blood to help a young patient with leukaemia was made, 150 calls were received offering donations within an hour [79].

5.1.5 Enhancing access of disabled people to services

Narasimhan and colleagues reported that people with disabilities, such as the deaf and hard of hearing (DHH) or mute, could benefit from SMS-based applications to contact emergency services [80]. Yousaf, Mehmood, Saba, Rehman, Rashid, Altaf, and Shuguang modelled and evaluated a mobile phone application that utilises speech-to-text and text-to-sign language to visualise the sign language using an avatar and convert the sign language to text [81]. This enables DHH individuals and hearing people communicate. Text messaging services to contact emergency and health services for the deaf and hard of hearing have been launched in some countries, such as Poland. Finding from this intervention show that without this solution, a deaf person would, in many cases, not be able to call for help [82].

5.2 SMS used to improve diagnosis, treatment and rehabilitation of illness

5.2.1 Improving adherence to health advice and medication

Adherence is the extent to which a patient's actions are consistent with the advice given by his or her doctor or nurse. According to Kalogianni [83] and Demoz, Berha, Alebachew Woldu, Yifter, Shibeshi and Engidawork, 50% of patients with chronic diseases do *not* use their *medications as* recommended, particularly problematic for long-term conditions which require daily medication [84]. Adverse health outcomes are always the consequences for patients and lead to significant expenses to the health systems. Non-adherence to treatment/medication often result to relapse in patients' health condition leads to hospital admission. This interruption of treatment for infections may result in the emergence of resistant strains. Reminder SMS would be useful to remind patients of the need to use their medication at the right time. The same reminder SMS would be useful in encouraging and reminding patients of the benefits of treatment regimens completion for a wide range of conditions, including acne, asthma [85], diabetes [86, 87], tuberculosis, and AIDS [88, 89] and teenagers on contraceptive [90]. A study was conducted among a cohort of 32 young adult asthma patients. They used SMS text messages written in 'txtspk' from a fictitious friend 'Max' (e.g., "yo dude, it is Max reminding U2 take ur inhaler"). A stream of celebrity gossip and horoscope messages accompanied the SMS and was reported to be successful. Findings showed that participants described the service as acceptable and said they had developed a rapport with Max's fictitious character [91].

A double-blind, randomised clinical trial in Spain, which involved 26 primary healthcare centres, analysed the effect of printed information followed by two SMS text messages (on lifestyle or a reminder to take the medication) on adherence and lifestyle changes in patients with hypertension. Although there was no difference in the rate of non-adherence in both groups, the experimental group could control blood pressure and bodyweight reduction better [92]. Another study from Spain involved the administration of hepatitis A and B vaccines to patients, patients in the intervention group received reminder SMS for follow-up vaccination. Those in the control group did not receive any reminders. Results showed that the vaccination completion rate was higher in the intervention group than the control group, and this difference was statistically significant [93].

5.2.2 Monitoring of illness and medical interventions

In 2005, the World Health Organisation noted that effective monitoring of medical conditions, especially chronic illness, improves health outcomes and reduces health care costs [94]. SMS applications are being used in various settings to monitor acute and chronic conditions and monitor the effectiveness of health interventions. For instance, a rheumatologist experimented with a patient reporting system that uses SMS. Patients who received corticosteroid injections for joints of soft tissue inflammation are to report whether injections were beneficial in alleviating pain or improving movement. This allowed remote monitoring and reduced the need for follow-up clinic appointments, thus reducing treatment costs [95]. Reminder SMS was also used in South Africa in monitoring people living with HIV and who receive anti-retroviral drugs. Affected persons can use the app in reporting side effects directly to health workers [96]. In Italy, cancer patients used SMS applications, which enabled them to report their symptoms systematically from home to doctors. Thus, reducing the need for hospital admission for monitoring [64]. Moreover, SMS has enabled improved self-monitoring by diabetic patients and more regular reporting to clinicians in England, France and Thailand [64].

The monitoring of patients in the intensive care unit has been improved through an innovative application. The nurses will send alerts to clinicians through SMS when specific changes are noticed in the patient's physiological status. Through this application, the clinician received a quick update about critical patients' conditions compared with pagers [97]. Furthermore, the feasibility and impact of using SMS to improve asthma self-care by reminding patients of their medication, recording symptoms, measuring peak flow rate and completing an SMS-based asthma diary to send to clinicians were tested in Denmark. Findings from the study showed that patients could effectively use the SMS-based asthma diary and gave them excitement. This gave them more control over their condition [98].

A randomised control trial evaluated the impact of the use of SMS on asthma symptom profile monitoring. The intervention was requested to send the peak flow results to their clinicians daily through SMS and a matched control group who were only counselled to monitor theirs. Findings show that the symptom profiling in the intervention group was better than that in the control group. It was also noted that the patients found the intervention suitable [64].

5.2.3 Provision of psychological support

The literature indicates that some health conditions, such as bulimia, can be better managed and improved if healthcare providers maintain continuous support through mobile apps. For patients on hospital admissions who have restricted interaction with the outside world, for instance, immuno-suppressed patients or those who had an infection and required isolation, psychological supports and interaction with other patients and relatives could have a therapeutic effect. Text messages may be a useful option in such instances.

Several interventions have been used to encourage young people to access counsellors to seek support on a range of issues, such as bulimia [99, 100], chronic illness, managing stress during end-of-year exams, and receiving advice on health or relationship problems [64]. A randomised controlled trial was conducted using SMS in supporting and prompting young diabetes patients to keep clinic appointments. A customised reminders SMS in a system called 'Sweet Talk' uses progressive goal setting to stimulate health behaviour, help patients set self-management goals, and improve glycemic control. Findings show significant improvement in diabetes control (as measured by metabolic control and self-efficacy) in the intervention group who used "Sweet Talk", as compared with those who received standard care [101–103]. Finding from another study, which explored the acceptability and feasibility of SMS based psychological support among patients with bulimia nervosa, show that SMS intervention is appropriate for aftercare after hospital discharge [104].

5.2.4 Communicating results of diagnostic tests

In recent times, it has been found that traditional approaches used to communicate diagnostic results are time-consuming and inefficient as these often require the patients to return to the provider unit in person to receive the results. Text messaging interventions have been used in developed countries to communicate results of in-vitro diagnostic tests (such as blood or microbiology tests) [105–108] and radiological imaging for breast cancer screening [109], sexually transmitted infection screening [110, 111]. In developing countries, where healthcare services access barriers exist, reminder SMS was used more effectively in sending results to clinics in rural areas [112]. Text messaging has also been used to accelerate communication to employers of occupational health examination results on foreign workers [105, 106].

5.3 SMS used in public health programmes

5.3.1 Contact tracing and partner notification for communicable diseases

An increase in the incidence and prevalence of sexually transmitted infections (STIs) is a significant public health challenge worldwide. Partner notification (partner management or contact tracing) is an essential public health strategy in controlling STIs because sexual partners of those with STIs are likely to be infected. If asymptomatic, they might not seek care [113, 114]. Text messages applications are being used to notify partners of individuals with STIs [115] and strengthen control efforts for major global public health problems such as tuberculosis, HIV, and SARS [116–118]. StarHub and the Singapore Tourism Board launched a text alert service named "SARS Contact Tracing SMS" to trace persons in case of future SARS outbreaks in Singapore [119].

Tomnay, Pitts and Fairley reported that clients attending a STIs clinic found calls or SMS to mobile telephones as acceptable and efficient means to contact tracing. Recent sexual partners could be traced, details of a website that had information on the STIs to which he or she can potentially be exposed are provided [120]. On the other hand, an SMS can be sent from the clinic to the client and forwarded to their partner(s)—thereby maintaining the anonymity of the partner [120]. Newell further described how text messaging was used to reach the client's partner, who was diagnosed with an infection after the initial visit to the STIs clinic. Even though the partner was unaware of why his girlfriend participated in a STIs clinic, the text message he received from her contained the diagnosis code used to initiate appropriate treatment. Therefore, SMS may be adjunct to contact slips for contact tracing in genito-urinary clinics [121].

5.3.2 Communicating health information to the public

Short Messaging Service is beneficial for rapid communication of health information to the general public for public health emergencies during an outbreak of infectious diseases like COVID-19, Ebola, Lassa fever, and avian influenza. It can also be used for rapid communication when a group of people or patients are accidentally exposed to an infectious agent. It has been a valuable tool in rapidly reaching people to recall harmful food products or pharmaceuticals [122–124].

Short Messaging Service has also been used in public awareness campaigns in India to inform and educate the public on WHO tuberculosis control strategy; in Kenya, Nigeria and Mali, to educate the public on HIV and malaria control programmes [116]. It has been used in Iraq to support polio immunisation campaigns targeting about 5 million children [125]. During the SARS epidemic in Hong Kong, one of the mobile telecommunication operators sent SMS to the citizens, educating every one of safety measures that helped reduce the risk of exposure to the virus [126].

Programmed bulk SMS can also be used for a specific population effectively. After the floods in India, most people in Mumbai were exposed to floodwaters. Through sent text messages, everyone in the area was advised to take 200 mg of doxycycline to prevent leptospirosis infection [127]. In the UK, health promotion advice and information was provided through NHS Direct Interactive text messages to people with long-term conditions like diabetes and asthma [128]. Shortly after, other UK health organisations adopted text messages to address the health challenges of people living in rural areas [116]; health educate students [118, 129, 130]. This interactive text message was used to provide confidential health information to pupils [131], provide teenagers and young people with information on sexual health, anti-smoking education, mental health, pollen count to asthmatics or hay fever sufferers and alerts on high levels of smog and air pollution to high-risk groups [116].

5.3.3 Use of SMS in smoking cessation programmes

Short Message Service has been used in Australia, New Zealand, Spain, and the UK to provide health education, anti-smoking campaigns, and assist behavioural change in people trying to quit smoking [132, 133].

Findings from a randomised control trial on SMS effectiveness in smoking cessation programmes in New Zealand found that the proportion of participants who stopped smoking in the intervention group who received reminder SMS support was significantly higher than the control group [134]. Findings from the follow-up study show similar results [135]. Findings from a cohort study assessing smoking cessation among college students in the US showed higher cessation rates among the group that used Web and text-messaging programmes than those in minimal-contact or self-help smoking-cessation interventions [136]. In conclusion, studies reviewed from the literature demonstrate wide use of SMS-based applications with benefits in health outcomes. These studies also show that SMS-based healthcare applications are acceptable to patients: thus, it can be concluded that SMS can develop new service delivery models.

6. Potential challenges of reminder SMS

No innovation comes without one challenge or the other. The same applies to using reminder SMS or messages in health programmes or interventions. A frequently cited challenge in its use in healthcare treatment pertains to patient confidentiality, especially regarding diseases that run in some families (such as mental illness, genetic diseases), predisposing the bearers to discrimination if made publicly known [63, 137]. Although the confidentiality of patients poses some risks, some steps can be taken to mitigate the concern. These steps include sending generic and coded reminders informing patients to open messages in a private place and delete messages after reading them [63].

One major obstacle with sending reminder SMS is for individuals not reading the messages they have received. Recipients of reminders SMS may sometimes become annoyed at receiving multiple messages over time.

7. Future directions

Reminder messages show great potential for use across the broad spectrum of healthcare services. They are effective as appointment and drug/medical compliance reminders. Additionally, SMS reminders effectively prompted other health behaviours, including self-medical examinations, socialisation, and goal-directed behaviours. It is currently unclear the most effective dose of reminder messages (i.e., timing, frequency, and the total number of messages) and under what conditions the dosage should be changed over time [63]. Dosage varies between individuals and is impacted by the perceived importance of the reminder (e.g., if something is crucial to one's health or for changing behaviour) [63]. Further research on these areas can help inform future implementations of reminder messages in healthcare service delivery.

8. Conclusion

Accessibility and affordability are the major issues about rural health around the world. In the countries where most of the population lives in rural areas, the resources are concentrated in the cities. Rural areas worldwide are faced with transport and communication difficulties, and they all face the challenge of shortages of doctors and other health professionals in rural and remote areas. Many rural people are caught in a downward spiral of poverty—ill-health—low productivity, particularly in developing countries.

Reminder messages have tremendous and untapped potential in transforming health systems in low- and middle-income countries (LMICs) predicated on the growing availability and use of mobile phones among communities members, families and health care service providers. They are relatively inexpensive, easily customised, sent directly to individuals, and a part of many daily lives. These attributes further explain why many studies utilise SMS as a reminder to help improve healthcare services. Several studies reviewed on reminder messages to improve health outcomes in developed countries show promising results. Adopting and integrating this innovation into existing health delivery systems will have robust health outcomes in rural communities. It presents a convenient and cost-effective method to support healthcare interventions. Reminder SMS can function as a reminder for periodic (e.g., daily medication adherence) and distal, one-time (e.g., to complete a follow-up vaccination 2 months after initial vaccination) behaviours.

DOI: http://dx.doi.org/10.5772/intechopen.101705

Author details

Isaac Oluwafemi Dipeolu
Faculty of Public Health, Department of Health Promotion and Education, University of Ibadan, Ibadan, Nigeria

*Address all correspondence to: oludipeolu@yahoo.com

References

[1] Food and Agriculture Organization of the United Nations [FAO]. Guidelines on defining rural areas and compiling indicators for development policy. Publication prepared in the framework of the Global Strategy to improve Agricultural and Rural Statistics. 2018. Available from: http://www.fao.org/3/ca6392en/ca6392en.pdf

[2] Madu IA. The structure and pattern of rurality in Nigeria. GeoJournal. 2010;**75**(2):175-184

[3] Egbe EJ. Rural and community development in Nigeria: An assessment. Nigerian Chapter of Arabian Journal of Business and Management Review. 2014;**62**(1101):1-14

[4] British Broadcasting Corporation (BBC). What is a rural area?—Characteristics of rural areas—GCSE [Online]. 2021. Available from: https://www.bbc.co.uk/bitesize/guides/zpmq4j6/revision/1 [Accessed: 2 February 2021]

[5] Wineman A, Alia DY, Anderson CL. Definitions of "rural" and "urban" and understandings of economic transformation: Evidence from Tanzania. Journal of Rural Studies. 2020;**79**:254-268

[6] Udo RK, Kirk-Greene AHM, Falola TO, Ade-Ajayi JF. Nigeria. Encyclopedia Britannica. 2021. Available from: https://www.britannica.com/place/Nigeria [Accessed: 5 April 2021]

[7] Bennett KJ, Borders TF, Holmes GM, Kozhimannil KB, Ziller E. What is rural? Challenges and implications of definitions that inadequately encompass rural people and places. Health Affairs. 2019;**38**(12):1985-1992

[8] Freeman AW, Lumsden LL. Typhoid fever in rural Virginia a preliminary report. American Journal of Public Health. 1912;**2**(4):240-252. DOI: 10.2105/ajph.2.4.240

[9] Knopf SA. The modern aspect of the tuberculosis problem in rural communities and the duty of the health officers. American Journal of Public Health. 1914;**4**(12):1127-1135. DOI: 10.2105/ajph.4.12.1127-a

[10] Ruediger GF. A program of public health for towns, villages and rural communities. American Journal of Public Health. 1917;**7**(3):235-239

[11] Mustard HS, Mountin JW. Measurements of efficiency and adequacy of rural health service. American Journal of Public Health and the Nations Health. 1929;**19**(8):887-892

[12] Mountin JW, Pennell EH, Brockett GS. Location and movement of physicians, 1923 and 1938: Changes in urban and rural totals for established physicians. In: Public Health Reports (1896-1970). London, EC1Y 1SP: Sage Publications, Inc., 1945. pp. 173-185

[13] Ebuehi OM, Campbell PC. Attraction and retention of qualified health workers to rural areas in Nigeria: A case study of four LGAs in Ogun State, Nigeria. Rural and Remote Health. 2011;**11**(1):41

[14] Eley DS, Laurence C, Cloninger CR, Walters L. Who attracts whom to rural general practice?: Variation in temperament and character profiles of GP registrars across different vocational training pathways. Rural and Remote Health. 2015;**15**(4):82

[15] Strasser R, Kam SM, Regalado SM. Rural health care access and policy in developing countries. Annual Review of Public Health. 2016;**37**:395-412

[16] Webster CS, McKillop A, Bennett W, Bagg W. A qualitative and semiquantitative exploration of the experience of a rural and regional clinical placement programme. Medical Science Educator. 2020;**30**(2):783-789

[17] Pew Research Center. What Unites and Divides Urban, Suburban and Rural Communities [Online]. 2018. Available from: https://webcache.googleusercontent.com/search?q=cache:RT9hFZC6xWoJ:https://www.pewresearch.org/social-trends/2018/05/22/what-unites-and-divides-urban-suburban-and-rural-communities/+&cd=15&hl=en&ct=clnk&gl=ng [Accessed: February 2021]

[18] Strasser R. Rural health around the world: Challenges and solutions. Family Practice. 2003;**20**(4):457-463

[19] National Academies of Sciences, Engineering, and Medicine; Health and Medicine Division; Board on Health Care Services; Committee on Health Care Utilization and Adults with Disabilities. Factors that affect healthcare utilization. In: Health-Care Utilization as a Proxy in Disability Determination. Washington (DC): National Academies Press (US); 2018

[20] Ejike CN. The Influence of Culture on the Use of Healthcare Services by Refugees in Southcentral Kentucky: A Mixed Study [Dissertations]. Paper 116. 2017. Available from: http://digitalcommons.wku.edu/diss/116

[21] Arousell J, Carlbom A. Culture and religious beliefs in relation to reproductive health. Best Practice & Research Clinical Obstetrics & Gynaecology. 2016;**32**:77-87

[22] Rumun AJ. Influence of religious beliefs on healthcare practice. International Journal of Education and Research. 2014;**2**(4):37-48

[23] Brovarone EE, Cotella G. Improving rural accessibility: A multilayer approach. Sustainability. 2020;**12**(7):2876

[24] Akinyemi JO, Chisumpa VH, Odimegwu CO. Household structure, maternal characteristics and childhood mortality in rural sub-Saharan Africa. Rural and Remote Health. 2016;**16**(2):117

[25] Van de Poel E, O'donnell O, Van Doorslaer E. What explains the rural-urban gap in infant mortality: Household or community characteristics? Demography. 2009;**46**(4):827-850

[26] Teckle P, Hannaford P, Sutton M. Is the health of people living in rural areas different from those in cities? Evidence from routine data linked with the Scottish Health Survey. BMC Health Services Research. 2012;**12**(1):1-16

[27] Clark SJ, Savitz LA, Randolph RK. Rural children's health. Western Journal of Medicine. 2001;**174**(2):142

[28] Dapaah JM. Attitudes and Behaviours of Health Workers and the Use of HIV/AIDS Health Care Services. Nursing Research and Practice. 2016; **2016**:5172497. DOI: 10.1155/2016/5172497

[29] Amoran OE. HIV related stigmatising attitude and practice among health care workers in Northern Nigeria. Journal of Infectious Diseases and Immunity. 2011;**3**(13):226-232

[30] Reis C, Heisler M, Amowitz LL, Moreland RS, Mafeni JO, Anyamele C, et al. Discriminatory attitudes and practices by health workers toward patients with HIV/AIDS in Nigeria. PLoS Medicine. 2005;**2**(8):e246

[31] Kruger LM, Schoombee C. The other side of caring: Abuse in a South African maternity ward. Journal of Reproductive and Infant Psychology. 2010;**28**(1):84-101

[32] Jewkes R, Abrahams N, Mvo Z. Why do nurses abuse patients? Reflections from South African obstetric services. Social Science & Medicine. 1998;**47**(11):1781-1795

[33] Andersen HM. "Villagers": Differential treatment in a Ghanaian hospital. Social Science & Medicine. 2004;**59**(10):2003-2012

[34] Umar N, Quaife M, Exley J, Shuaibu A, Hill Z, Marchant T. Toward improving respectful maternity care: A discrete choice experiment with rural women in northeast Nigeria. BMJ Global Health. 2020;**5**(3):e002135

[35] Afulani PA, Kelly AM, Buback L, Asunka J, Kirumbi L, Lyndon A. Providers' perceptions of disrespect and abuse during childbirth: A mixed-methods study in Kenya. Health Policy and Planning. 2020;**35**(5):577-586

[36] de Villiers K. Bridging the health inequality gap: An examination of South Africa's social innovation in health landscape. Infectious Diseases of Poverty. 2021;**10**(19):1-7. DOI: 10.1186/s40249-021-00804-9

[37] Rural Health Information Hub. Healthcare Access in Rural Communities [Online]. 2019. Available from: https://www.ruralhealthinfo.org/topics/healthcare-access [Accessed: 2 February 2021]

[38] Axsel C. Strategic Location Modeling for Mobile Clinics in Rural Areas in South Africa [Unpublished Bachelor's Degree Project]. South Africa: University of Pretoria; 2015

[39] Asabere NY. mMES: A mobile medical expert system for health institutions in Ghana. International Journal of Science and Technology. 2012;**2**(6):333-344. ISSN 2224-3577

[40] Suttle A. Using technology to improve rural health care. Harvard Business Review. October 18, 2017:1-5

[41] Strasser R, Neusy AJ. Context counts: Training health workers in and for rural and remote areas. Bulletin of the World Health Organization. 2010;**88**:777-782

[42] Dassah E, Aldersey H, McColl MA, Davison C. Factors affecting access to primary health care services for persons with disabilities in rural areas: A "best-fit" framework synthesis. Global Health Research and Policy. 2018;**3**(1):1-13

[43] Adogu PO, Egenti BN, Ubajaka C, Onwasigwe C, Nnebue CC. Utilization of maternal health services in urban and rural communities of Anambra State, Nigeria. Nigerian Journal of Medicine. 2014;**23**:61-69

[44] Scheil-Adlung X. Global evidence on inequities in rural health protection: New data on rural deficits in health coverage for 174 countries. ESS Doc. 47. Geneva: Int. Labour Organ; 2015. Available from: http://www.social-protection.org/gimi/gess/RessourcePDF.action?ressource.ressou

[45] Lunze K, Higgins-Steele A, Simen-Kapeu A, Vesel L, Kim J, Dickson K. Innovative approaches for improving maternal and newborn health-a landscape analysis. BMC Pregnancy and Childbirth. 2015;**15**(1):1-19

[46] Besnier E, Thomson K, Stonkute D, Mohammad T, Akhter N, Todd A, et al. Which public health interventions are effective in reducing morbidity, mortality and health inequalities from infectious diseases amongst children in low-income and middle-income countries (LMICs): Protocol for an umbrella review. BMJ Open. 2019;**9**(12):e032981

[47] Stover J, Hardee K, Ganatra B, García-Moreno C, Horton S. Interventions to improve reproductive health. In: Black RE, Laxminarayan R, Temmerman M, et al., editors. Reproductive, Maternal, Newborn, and Child Health: Disease Control Priorities. 3rd ed. Vol. 2. Washington (DC): The International Bank for Reconstruction and Development/The World Bank; 2016. Chapter 6. pp. 95-114. DOI: 10.1596/978-1-4648-0348-2_ch6

[48] Nyasulu C, Chawinga WD. The role of information and communication technologies in the delivery of health services in rural communities: Experiences from Malawi. South African Journal of Information Management. 2018;**20**(1):a888. DOI: 10.4102/sajim.v20i1.888

[49] Ramachandran D, Canny J, Das PD, Cutrell E. Mobilizing health workers in rural India. In: Proceedings of the ACM Special Interest Group on Computer-Human Interaction (SIGCHI) Conference on Human Factors in Computing Systems; ACM, Atlanta, GA; April 10-15. New York, NY, United States: Association for Computing Machinery (ACM); 2010. pp. 1889-1898

[50] Ruxwana NL, Herselman ME, Conraide DP. ICT Application as e-Health Solutions in Rural Healthcare in the Eastern Cape Province of South Africa. Health Information Management Journal. 2010;**39**(1):1833-3575

[51] World Health Organization (WHO). Strategy 2004-2007. e-Health for healthcare delivery. [Online]. 2004. Available from: http://www.who.int/eht/en/eHealth_HCD.pdf [Accessed 2 February 2021]

[52] Shekar M, Otto K. ICTs for health in Africa [Online]. 2014. Available from: http://siteresources.worldbank.org/extinformationandcommunicationandtechnologies/Resources/282822-1346223280837/Health.pdf [Accessed: February 2021]

[53] Nair P. ICT based health governance practices: The Indian experience. Journal of Health Management. 2014;**16**(1):25-40. DOI: 10.1177/0972063413518678

[54] Oladepo O, Dipeolu IO, Oladunni O. Outcome of reminder text messages intervention on completion of routine immunization in rural areas, Nigeria. Health Promotion International. 2021;**36**(3):765-773

[55] Thimbleby H. Technology and the future of healthcare. Journal of Public Health Research. 2013;**2**(3):e28

[56] Kabachinski J. Mobile medical apps changing healthcare technology. Biomedical Instrumentation & Technology. 2011;**45**(6):482-486

[57] Mobile Health News. Wireless Health: State of The Industry 2009 Year End Report. 2010

[58] Ventola CL. Mobile devices and apps for health care professionals: Uses and benefits. Pharmacy and Therapeutics. 2014;**39**(5):356-364

[59] Carrillo MA, Kroeger A, Sanchez RC, Monsalve SD, Runge-Ranzinger S. The use of mobile phones for the prevention and control of arboviral diseases: A scoping review. BMC Public Health. 2021;**21**(1):1-16

[60] Grantz KH, Meredith HR, Cummings DA, Metcalf CJE, Grenfell BT, Giles JR, et al. The use of mobile phone data to inform analysis of COVID-19 pandemic epidemiology. Nature Communications. 2020;**11**(1):1-8

[61] Balogun MR, Boateng GO, Adams YJ, Ransome-Kuti B, Sekoni A, Adams EA. Using mobile phones to promote maternal and child health: Knowledge and attitudes of primary health care providers in southwest Nigeria. Journal of Global Health Reports. 2020;**4**:e2020060. DOI: 10.29392/001c.13507

[62] Watkins JOTA, Goudge J, Gómez-Olivé FX, Griffiths F. Mobile phone use among patients and health workers to enhance primary healthcare: A qualitative study in rural South Africa. Social Science & Medicine. 2018;**198**:139-147

[63] Schwebel FJ, Larimer ME. Using text message reminders in health care

services: A narrative literature review. Internet Interventions. 2018;**13**:82-104. DOI: 10.1016/j.invent.2018.06.002

[64] Atun RA, Sittampalam SR, Mohan A. Uses and Benefits of SMS in Healthcare Delivery. Discussion Paper V 21.1. London: Centre for Health Management, Tanaka Business School, Imperial College; 2005

[65] National Health System (NHS). Missed GP appointments costing NHS millions. England: National Health System; 2020

[66] Curtis L, Netten A. Unit Costs of Health and Social Care 2005. Canterbury: Personal Social Services Research Unit, University of Kent; 2005

[67] NHS Connecting for Health. A Guide to the National Programme for Information Technology. Delivering Better Care. London: Department of Health; 2005. p. 3. Available from: www.connectingforhealth.nhs.uk/resources/brochures/npfit_brochure_apr_05_final.pdf

[68] Vodafone Text Message Pilot Evaluation. Homerton University Hospital NHS Foundation Trust; 2004

[69] Hospitals embrace SMS technology. 2004. Available from: http://www.textually.org/textually/archives/2004/08/004930.htm

[70] Zinn C. 14000 preventable deaths in Australian hospitals. BMJ. 1995;**310**:1487

[71] Sherry E, Colloridi B, Warnke PH. Short message service (SMS): A useful communication tool for surgeons. ANZ Journal of Surgery. 2002;**72**(5):369

[72] Davis MM, Heineke J. Understanding the roles of the customer and the operation for better queue management. International Journal of Operations & Production Management. 1994;**14**(5):21-34

[73] Pierce RA II, Rogers EM, Sharp MH, Musulin M. Outpatient pharmacy redesign to improve work flow, waiting time, and patient satisfaction. American Journal of Hospital Pharmacy. 1990;**47**(2):351-356

[74] Jones P, Dent M. Improving service: Managing response time in hospitality operations. International Journal of Operations & Production Management. 1994;**14**(5):52-58

[75] Lin AC, Jang R, Lobas N, Heaton P, Ivey M, Nam B. Identification of factors leading to excessive waiting times in an ambulatory pharmacy. Hospital Pharmacy. 1999;**34**(6):707-713

[76] Medicine text alert to offer patients greater choice. 1998. Available from: http://www.uhb.nhs.uk/news/press_releases/05_04.htm#2

[77] The Times of India. 2013. Now, blood is available just an SMS away. Available from: http://timesofindia.indiatimes.com/city/mysuru/Now-blood-is-available-just-an-SMS-away/articleshow/17879908.cms

[78] PRNewswire. AT & T Wireless Grant Helps Blood Center Use Technology to Reach Blood Donors. 2004. Available from: http://www.prnewswire.com/news-releases/att-wireless-grant-helps-blood-center-use-technology-to-reach-blood-donors-72220192.html

[79] Cell Phone mobilize support in medical emergencies. 2005. Available from: https://textually.org/textually/archives/2005/08/009518.htm/ [Accessed: December 2020]

[80] Narasimhan N, Leblois A, Bharthur D, Haridas L, Lal P, Looms, et al. Making mobile phones and services accessible for persons with disabilities. A joint report of ITU—The International Telecommunication Union

and G3ict—The global initiative for inclusive ICTs. 2012

[81] Yousaf K, Mehmood Z, Saba T, Rehman A, Rashid M, Altaf M, et al. A novel technique for speech recognition and visualization based mobile application to support two-way communication between deaf-mute and normal peoples. Wireless Communications and Mobile Computing. 2018;(7):1-12

[82] Observatory for Public Sector Innovation. Mobile application "Deaf Help"—Deaf assistance in emergency situations. 2018. Available from: https://oecd-opsi.org/innovations/mobile-application-deaf-help-deaf-assistance-in-emergency-situations/

[83] Kalogianni A. Factors affect in patient adherence to medication regimen. Health Science Journal. 2011;**5**(3):157

[84] Demoz GT, Berha AB, Alebachew Woldu M, Yifter H, Shibeshi W, Engidawork E. Drug therapy problems, medication adherence and treatment satisfaction among diabetic patients on follow-up care at Tikur Anbessa Specialized Hospital, Addis Ababa, Ethiopia. PLoS One. 2019;**14**(10): e0222985

[85] Yun TJ, Arriaga RI. A text message a day keeps the pulmonologist away. Proceedings of the SIGCHI Conference on Human Factors in Computing Systems; Paris, France; April 27–May 02, 2013. Also available at Association for Computing Machinery. 2013. pp. 1769-1778. DOI: 10.1145/2470654.2466233. Available from: http://www.cc.gatech.edu/~arriaga/YunArriagaCHI13.pdf

[86] Ferrer-Roca O, Cárdenas A, Diaz-Cardama A, Pulido P. Mobile phone text messaging in the management of diabetes. Journal of Telemedicine and Telecare. 2004;**10**:282-286

[87] McMahon GT, Gomes HE, Hohne SH, Hu TM-J, Levine BA, Conlin PR. Web-based care management in patients with poorly controlled diabetes mellitus. Diabetes Care. 2005;**28**(7):1624-1629

[88] Harris JL, Furberg R, Martin N, et al. Implementing an SMS-based intervention for persons living with human immunodeficiency virus. Journal of Public Health Management & Practice. 2013;**19**(2):E9-E16

[89] Lewis MA, Uhrig JD, Bann CM, et al. Tailored text messaging intervention for HIV adherence: A proof-of-concept study. Health Psychology. 2013;**32**(3): 248-253. DOI: 10.1037/a0028109. Epub 2012 Apr 30.

[90] Johns Hopkins Medicine. Text messages can help boost teen birth control compliance. ScienceDaily, May 19. 2015. Available from: www.sciencedaily.com/releases/2015/05/150519083307.htm

[91] Neville R, Greene A, McLeod J, Tracy A, Surie J. Mobile phone text messaging can help young people manage asthma. BMJ. 2002;**325**:600

[92] Marquez Contreras E, de la Figuera von Wichmann M, Gil Guillen V, Ylla-Catala A, Figueras M, Balana M, et al. Effectiveness of an intervention to provide information to patients with hypertension as short text messages of reminders sent to their mobile phone (HTA-Alert). Atencion Primaria. 2004;**34**(8):399-407

[93] Vilella A, Bayas J, Diaz M, Guinovart C, Diez C, Simó D, et al. The role of mobile phones in improving vaccination rates in travelers. Preventive Medicine. 2004;**38**:503-509

[94] World Health Organisation. Preventing chronic diseases: A vital investment. World Health Organization.

2005. Available from: http://www.who.int/chp/chronic_disease_report/en/

[95] Pal B. The doctor will text you now: Is there a role for the mobile telephone in health care? BMJ: British Medical Journal. 2003;**326**(7389):607

[96] Pérez GM, Hwang B, Bygrave H, Venables E. Designing text-messaging (SMS) in HIV programs: Ethics-framed recommendations from the field. Pan African Medical Journal. 2015;**21**:201

[97] Chen HT, Ma WC, Liou DM. Design and implementation of a real-time clinical alerting system for intensive care unit. In: Proceedings of the American Medical Informatics Association Symposium. Bethesda MD, USA: American Medical Informatics Association; 2002. pp. 131-135

[98] Anhøj J, Møldrup C. Feasibility of collecting diary data from asthma patients through mobile phones and SMS (short message service): Response rate analysis and focus group evaluation from a pilot study. Journal of Medical Internet Research. 2004;**6**(4):e42. DOI: 10.2196/jmir.6.4.e42. Available from: http://www.jmir.org/2004/4/e42/

[99] Hazelwood A. Using text messaging in the treatment of eating disorders. Nursing Times. 2008;**104**(40):28-29

[100] Walsh R. Texting can be bulimia aid. The New Zealand Herald. 2004. Available from: http://www.nzherald.co.nz/nz/news/article.cfm?c_id=1&objectid=3566605

[101] Franklin V, Greene S. Sweet talk: A text messaging support system. Journal of Diabetes Nursing. 2007;**11**(1):22-26

[102] Franklin VL, Waller A, Pagliari C, Greene SA. A randomized controlled trial of Sweet Talk, a text-messaging system to support young people with diabetes. Diabetic Medicine. 2006;**23**(12):1332-1338

[103] Franklin V, Waller A, Pagliari C, Greene S. "Sweet Talk": Text messaging support for intensive insulin therapy for young people with diabetes. Diabetes Technology & Therapeutics. 2003;**5**(6):991-996

[104] Bauer S, Percevic R, Okon E, Meermann R, Kordy H. Use of text messaging in the aftercare of patients with bulimia nervosa. European Eating Disorders Review. 2003;**11**:279-290

[105] Gurol-Urganci I, de Jongh T, Vodopivec-Jamsek V, Car J, Atun R. Mobile phone messaging for communicating results of medical investigations. Cochrane Database of Systematic Reviews. 2012;**13**(6):CD007456. DOI: 10.1002/14651858.CD007456.pub2

[106] Atun RA, Sittampalam S. A review of the characteristics and benefits of SMS in delivering healthcare. In: Atun RA et al., editors. The Role of Mobile Phones in Increasing Accessibility and Efficiency in Healthcare. London: Vodafone Group PLC; 2006

[107] Lim EJ, Haar J, Morgan J. Can text messaging results reduce time to treatment of *Chlamydia trachomatis*? Sexually Transmitted Infections. 2008;**84**(7):563-564

[108] Menon-Johansson AS, McNaught F, Mandalia S, Sullivan AK. Texting decreases the time to treatment for genital *Chlamydia trachomatis* infection. Sexually Transmitted Infections. 2006;**82**(1):49-51

[109] Lamont M. Text messaging and breaking bad news. British Medical Journal. 2005;**330**:1217

[110] Lovitt CJ. Patient choice? British Medical Journal. 2005;**330**:1217. DOI: 10.1136/bmj.330.7501.1217

[111] Bradbeer C, Mears A. STI services in the United Kingdom: How shall we

cope? Sexually Transmitted Infections. 2003;**79**(6):435-438

[112] Wright B. Rural Doctors Advance Care With Wireless: A South African pilot project lets a developer test under extreme conditions. New York, NY: M Business, CMP Media LLC; 2001

[113] World Health Organisation. Sexually transmitted infections (STIs). Fact sheet No. 110. 2015

[114] Centers for Disease Control and Prevention (CDC). Trends in Reportable Sexually Transmitted Diseases in the United States, 2004: National Surveillance Data for Chlamydia, Gonorrhea, and Syphillis. Atlanta, USA: Centers for Disease Control and Prevention; 2005

[115] Swendeman D, RotheramBorus MJ. Innovation in sexually transmitted disease and HIV prevention: Internet and mobile phone delivery vehicles for global diffusion. Current Opinion in Psychiatry. (London, United Kingdom: Wolters Kluwer Health, Inc.,) 2010;**23**(2):139-144. DOI: 10.1097/YCO.0b013e328336656a

[116] Déglise C, Suggs LS, Odermatt P. Short message service (SMS) applications for disease prevention in developing countries. Journal of Medical Internet Research. 2012;**14**(1):e3. DOI: 10.2196/jmir.1823. Available from: http://www.jmir.org/2012/1/e3/

[117] Nsubuga P, White ME, Thacker SB, et al. Public health surveillance: A tool for targeting and monitoring interventions. In: Jamison DT, Breman JG, Measham AR, et al., editors. Disease Control Priorities in Developing Countries. 2nd ed. Washington (DC): World Bank; 2006. Chapter 53. Available from: http://www.ncbi.nlm.nih.gov/books/NBK11770/

[118] Vital Wave Consulting. mHealth for Development: The Opportunity of Mobile Technology for Healthcare in the Developing World. Washington, D.C. and Berkshire, UK: UN Foundation-Vodafone Foundation Partnership; 2009

[119] SARS contact tracing SMS program. 2003. Available from: https://textually.org/textually/archives/2003/05/000689.htm

[120] Tomnay JE, Pitts MK, Fairley CK. New technology and partner notification--why aren't we using them? International Journal of STD & AIDS. 2005;**16**(1):19-22

[121] Newell A. A mobile phone text message and *Trichomonas vaginalis*. Sexually Transmitted Infections. 2001;**77**(3):225

[122] Revere D, Calhoun R, Baseman J, Oberle M. Exploring bi-directional and SMS messaging for communications between Public Health Agencies and their stakeholders: A qualitative study. BMC Public Health. 2015;**15**:621. DOI: 10.1186/s12889-015-1980-2

[123] Baseman JG, Revere D, Painter I, Toyoji M, Thiede H, Duchin J. Public health communications and alert fatigue. BMC Health Services Research. 2013;**13**:295. DOI: 10.1186/1472-6963-13-295

[124] Free C, Phillips G, Felix L, Galli L, Patel V, Edwards P. The effectiveness of M-health technologies for improving health and health services: A systematic review protocol. BMC Research Notes. 2010;**3**(1):1-7

[125] Cell phones alert users of natural disasters. 2005. Available from: https://textually.org/textually/archives/2005/01/006683.htm.

[126] America's Network. The SARS files: How telcos kept Asia on its feet during the crisis. Article by Clark R. 2003. p. 18

[127] D'Silva J. Rx: Beat leptospirosis with Doxycycline. The Economic Times.

The Times of India Group. Bennett, Coleman & Co. Ltd. All rights reserved. 2005. Available from: www.economictimes.com

[128] Colledge A, Car J, Donnelly A, Majeed A. Health information for patients: Time to look beyond patient information leaflets. Journal of the Royal Society of Medicine. 2008;**101**(9): 447-453. DOI: 10.1258/jrsm.2008.080149

[129] Blackburn L, Blatnik A. Promoting sexual health with SMS texting technology. Nursing for Women's Health. 2013;**17**:465-469. DOI: 10.1111/1751-486X.12074

[130] Chen Z, Fang L, Chen L, Dai H. Comparison of an SMS text messaging and phone reminder to improve attendance at a health promotion center: A randomized controlled trial. Journal of Zhejiang University. Science. B. 2008;**9**(1):34-38. DOI: 10.1631/jzus.B071464

[131] Health Organization. mHealth: New Horizons for Health through Mobile Technologies: Second Global Survey on eHealth. 20 Avenue Appia, 1211 Geneva 27, Switzerland: World Health Organization; 2011

[132] Chamberlain C, O'Mara-Eves A, Oliver S, Caird JR, Perlen SM, Eades SJ, et al. Psychosocial interventions for supporting women to stop smoking in pregnancy. The Cochrane Database of Systematic Reviews. 2013;**10**:CD001055. DOI: 10.1002/14651858.CD001055.pub4

[133] Abroms LC, Whittaker R, Free C, Mendel Van Alstyne J, Schindler-Ruwisch JM. Developing and pretesting a text messaging program for health behaviour change: Recommended steps. Journal of Medical Internet Research mHealth and uHealth. 2015;**3**(4):e107. DOI: 10.2196/mhealth.4917

[134] Rodgers A, Corbett T, Bramley D, Riddell T, Wills M, Lin RB, et al. Do u smoke after txt? Results of a randomized trial of smoking cessation using mobile phone text messaging. Tobacco Control. 2005;**14**:255-261

[135] Bramley D, Riddell T, Whittaker R, Corbett T, Lin R, Wills M, et al. Smoking cessation using mobile phone text messaging is as effective in Maori as non-Maori. The New Zealand Medical Journal. 2005;**118**(1216):U1494

[136] Obermayer JL, Riley WT, Asif O, Jean-Mary J. College smoking-cessation using cell phone text messaging. Journal of American College Health. 2004;**53**(2):71-78. DOI: 10.3200/JACH.53.2.71-78

[137] Branson CE, Clemmey P, Mukherjee P. Text message reminders to improve outpatient therapy attendance among adolescents: A pilot study. Psychological Services. 2013;**10**(3): 298-303

Section 8

Early Cancer Diagnosis

Chapter 11

Forty Years of Arctic Primary Care Research on the Early Diagnosis of Cancer

Knut Holtedahl

Abstract

Usually, before a patient with cancer can be treated in a hospital, a general practitioner (GP) must suspect the diagnosis and refer the patient. GPs often worry that they could have done better for some of their cancer patients. Had there been an unreasonable delay of diagnosis? In the arctic, rural/urban city of Tromsø, this question became the subject of several scientific articles. Symptoms was an evident gateway to thinking about cancer in patients. In later years, there has been an explosion of good research studies about early diagnosis both in primary and secondary care. Through a northern gaze, the reader will be guided through a journey covering forty years of primary care-based research aiming at earlier diagnosis of cancer. Summing up, suggestions are given for: How to react upon signals from the body? And for the GP: 1. Explain unusual symptoms. 2. Add results from clinical findings and testing to symptoms. 3. Refer when the probability based on symptoms and findings exceed 3%. 4. Consider 'fast track' when you seriously suspect cancer. 5. Think of early diagnosis of cancer as an important, challenging and interesting part of your effort to serve the patients who consult you!

Keywords: Neoplasm, Oncology, Early diagnosis, Primary care, General practice, Family practice, Public Health

1. Introduction

Care for people with cancer: the task is universal, but conditions vary in different areas of the world. Tromsø, in the beginning of the 1970s, was a small city with a recently established university, the northernmost university in the world. The oncological department was yet to come, and surgeons and internists dealt with patients in collaboration with oncologists in the bigger, southern cities.

Then there were the general practitioners (GPs). In the homes, some of the patients were ill with cancer. Time to talk, some relief, morphine for pain, and repeated visits, this was enriching for the GP and sometimes comforting for the patient and the family. Tromsø covered a large, arctic island community, part urban and part rural, with closeness to sea and mountains, where summer brings the midnight sun and winter features northern light and pastel colours and snow. For a GP, home visits were many, always on duty nights, and sometimes also on ordinary working days to patients calling the surgery. Means of transport, on sunny days and through winter wind and snow, were private cars, but also all kinds and sizes of boats and exceptionally a seaplane or a helicopter. Occasionally, medical things were put in a rucksack in order to go skiing to the patient – a mode of home visit that was more common and over greater distances in the previous generation of GPs. Many Norwegian GPs would recognise descriptions and photos in Berger & Mohr's beautiful book about a fortunate man [1]. The book follows an English rural GP, dedicated to his practice and his patients, trying to combine empathy and lessons from life with wide-ranging theoretical learning that can help his patients. Landscapes may differ, but the GP's tasks were much the same.

In these homes, as well as in the surgeries, many questions came to mind. This article will concentrate on a question which arose naturally in this primary care context: Can cancer be diagnosed earlier? Many researchers have contributed to the present-day knowledge and understanding. Some early studies were performed in Tromsø. They may be a suitable starting point for a somewhat personal story about the modern development of early diagnosis primary care research. Altogether, in 2021, there are some answers to the question.

2. Early diagnosis of cancer, in primary care

GPs see some patients requiring urgent hospitalisation, turning out to have incurable cancer. Often, GPs will ask themselves whether they have reacted reasonably quickly to worries and symptoms presented? Could something have been done better? What about the young woman with a seemingly innocent lump on her neck, turning out to be an oral cancer? Or the man with long-standing abdominal pain who got a follow-up appointment but never returned? He died from a stomach cancer. An elderly woman got antibiotics twice after delivering bloody urine specimen to our lab. The third time, she was contacted and asked to come for an appointment, and yes, the blood came from a cervical cancer.

GPs benefit from much trust. People expect their GP to understand and react professionally, without delaying a diagnosis like cancer and the time before treatment may start. A patient seen by an oncologist or a surgeon would commonly be rapidly diagnosed. However, how would the specialist know about that patient if the GP did not refer, or only did so after the cancer had spread?

3. Why writing now?

Hopefully, senior medical students and young doctors in vocational training could learn something useful from this story. Younger GPs -including GPs working in rural areas where they often know their patients well – might become more confident in their clinical practice, and some might open to the possibility of transforming good questions into research. Contributing to the knowledge base is important for the exercise of medicine. Some of this knowledge should be produced in primary care, in order to get the whole picture of diagnostic challenges. Primary care must be an integrated part of the research community.

Finally, it would be nice if some readers think they get a better idea about when to see their GP if the thought of cancer bothers them, and about what to expect from the GP. The language here is simple enough for lay people to follow.

As this story develops, some results have been quoted and short commentaries given. For detailed methodologies and more extensive discussions, the reader may consult the articles in the literature list.

4. The leap into research: 1977-1984

In Norwegian medical schools, general practice was not taught as a specific topic until around 1970. General practice was not among the more prestigious disciplines in medicine, and GPs were not frequently authors of scientific papers.

Still, most students graduating from medical schools found work in general practice. During the 1950s and 60s, some brave British GPs like John Fry and John Howie ventured into more systematic studies. Even before them, the productive Robert Braun in Austria had made diagnostic checklists for general practice. In Norway, Bent Bentsen gathered practice registration material in his own surgery [2].

At this time, academic departments of general practice appeared in several countries, introducing relevant student teaching and new research agendas. A formal specialty of general practice was acknowledged in more and more countries.

One interesting initiative occurred in Norway: The national medical association decided to encourage this revival and financed the first professorship in general practice in Oslo. And: They gave practice compensation payment for up to six months for GPs wanting to take a research leave after presentation of a project.

This encouragement resulted in a project description and an application from Tromsø. Did some cancer patients have their diagnosis delayed by incorrect handling in primary care? A friendly librarian at the University library searched their recently acquired databases for articles combining keywords 'cancer' and 'general practice'. Articles were found, saying for instance that an early diagnosis was often important for patient prognosis [3, 4]. And there it was, the word matching many previous thoughts: DELAY. Diagnostic delay. Somebody had been interested in this, and had written about it [5, 6], a couple of them in general practice [7, 8]!

5. Delay

All GPs in Tromsø agreed to find medical journals for patients diagnosed with cancer, and one GP researcher went through all journals, taking structured notes. On request, the Norwegian Cancer registry furnished a list of all 108 patients in Tromsø municipality having been diagnosed with cancer in 1976. The following was noted from the medical journals: Age, sex, civil state, rural/urban habitat, weeks from first symptom to first consultation, weeks from first consultation to diagnosis. Also, laboratory tests and X-rays taken the last year, and an admittedly subjective but criteria-based evaluation of what seemed like reasonable actions for that type of cancer, in the situations described in the journals. Did the medical history appear sparse, adequate, penetrating? Was the clinical examination insufficient, good local/regional, or extensive? Did the researcher think there was diagnostic delay, based on the conclusion in the medical journal notes, the type of cancer and the number of weeks noted for the two intervals examined? If so, was this due to what the patient did, or to what the GP did? Given the conclusion the GP described at the end of the consultation, did the researcher think that the GP could have done a better job there and then, and thereby reduced a possible delay?

The University hospital also gave access to their archives. The same kind of anonymous structured notes were taken from their machine written journals, altogether 25 archives from primary or secondary care, for a population of 45000 inhabitants.

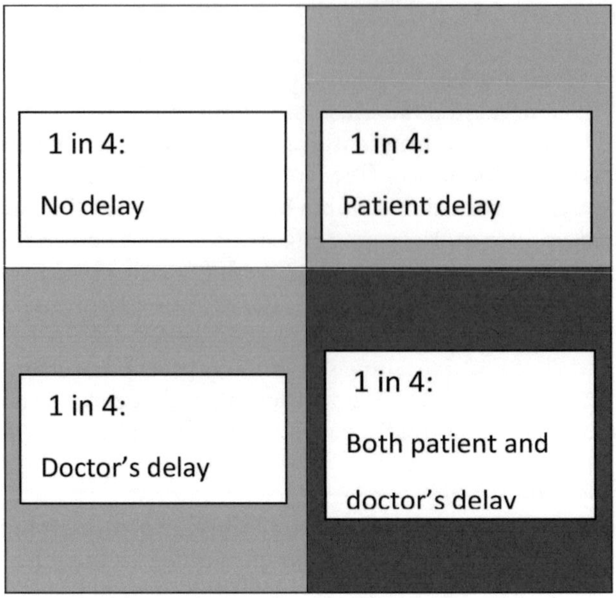

Figure 1.
Diagnostic delay of cancer in medical journal study, 108 patients in Tromsø, Norway, 1976.

5.1 Results

Three quarters of the patients could have had their diagnosis made earlier: Half of all patients saw their GP rather late in the course of the disease. In half of the cases the GP or the hospital doctor could have improved the diagnostic work-up. The overlap left one fourth of all patients with no kind of delay. Long waiting lists in primary or secondary care also played a part (**Figure 1**).

What could have been done better? For 43 of the 108 patients, one or more of these were noted: Apparently no follow-up when needed, insufficient medical history, insufficient clinical examination, lack of relevant laboratory examination or of x-ray referral, no or late referral to secondary care.

5.2 Short reflection

What was lacking, was good old GP work, with a potential of improvement through vocational training and continuous education!

6. Symptoms: seven warning signals of cancer

Symptoms patients had presented at consultation, also were recorded from the medical journals. Medical journals are not reliable sources of everything going on in a consultation, but symptoms seem to be among the well documented topics [9]. Many symptoms had been noted in medical journals from both primary and secondary care.

At that time, in most patient waiting rooms, there were posters quoting 'Seven warning signals of cancer' (**Table 1**). The posters advised patients to tell their doctor if they experienced any such symptoms. The first mention of 'the danger signals of cancer' occurred in a pamphlet developed during World War I, in a desire to

Seven 'classical' warning signals of cancer
1. Any sore which does not heal
2. Lumps anywhere in the body, especially in the breasts, and even if they are painless
3. Abnormal bleeding from body orifices
4. Changes in colour or size of warts or moles
5. Indigestion or change in bowel habits, if this is not rapidly normalised
6. Hoarseness or coughing without any apparent reason
7. Weight loss without any apparent reason
Abbreviations used in text:
1. Sore
2. Lump
3. Bleeding
4. Mole
5. Indigestion
6. Cough/hoarseness
7. Weight loss

Table 1.
Seven 'classical' warning signals of cancer.

stretch medical resources and to emphasise disease prevention. Three such signals were soon distributed to the public, and by 1929 they had been translated into 22 different languages, despite no scientific studies validating the signals. By 1951, the number of signals had increased to seven (Personal communication, Gerry de Harven, American Cancer Society). By 1982, 'danger signals' had changed names to 'warning signals', and a minor revision made the first letter in each signal form the word CAUTION. The Norwegian translation was a quite accurate translation from the American original.

6.1 Results

One or more of the seven symptoms had been presented by 68 of the 108 patients with cancer. However, 35 patients presented other symptoms, a quite varied list. Most symptoms, including those on the list, were common and it could only be assumed whether the symptom stemmed from the cancer. Still, with a known cancer location, many recorded symptoms seemed to fit with the diagnosis. Some symptoms seemed to be better known than others by the public: lumps and irregular bleeding more quickly than other symptoms led to GP consultations. Overall, non-warning symptoms did not lead to slower consultation than warning signals.

6.2 Short reflection

It was possible that the list had a mission in reminding the GPs of being vigilant. The public may be more aware of some symptoms than of others. The role of warning signals seemed to merit further studies.

7. Publish!

The Journal of the Norwegian Medical Association published this study. A first article detailed the background, method, results and conclusions, and a second article gave casuistic examples of what the GP might improve [10, 11].

By now, a regular contact at the university library had been established. What had been written previously about early cancer diagnosis, was eagerly studied. In a British article from 1966, Grey [12] described how cancer can bring patients to GPs and the possible reactions of the doctor. Whole person medicine is the GP's starting point in consultations. From there, the medical history, the clinical examination and various tests and referral possibilities is the way to go. Patient delay, GP delay, hospital delay and even government delay from insufficient financing of health services, were described with casuistic examples.

Patient delay had been discussed considering social psychological factors in two articles from the US [13, 14]. Some hospital based articles described delay in relation to specific forms of cancer [15]. Jenkins' article on delay and Macadam's article focusing on gastrointestinal cancer were contemporary investigations from general practice [16, 17].

New questions were triggered by the original study. How frequent were the warning symptoms among patients consulting in general practice? - according to GP registrations, and according to patients interviewed after their consultation? In a general population? Had newly diagnosed cancer patients consulted for warning signals more often than other GP patients? Over the next three years, these questions were studied with a basis in general practice in Tromsø.

8. Warning signals in patients who consult

Fourteen GPs from four group practices, almost all GPs in Tromsø, registered anonymously for six months consecutive patients on an A6 card immediately after the consultation, marking initials, sex and date of birth. A cross in a square, one for each symptom, identified patients who presented one or more of the seven warning signals.

8.1 Results

In 11606 patients, 649 symptoms were recorded. Three of the signals, 'lump', 'bleeding' and 'indigestion' (**Table 1**) occurred far more often than the other signals. On average, warning signals were presented in 5.4% of all consultations, more frequently in women than in men. This was expected because of the possibility of lumps in breasts. The rate of warning signals increased with age, except for 'lump' which was frequent in children and young persons, and 'bleeding', frequent in younger women.

8.2 Short reflection

At that time, Norwegian GPs saw approximately 20 patients a day. If one in twenty patients presents a warning signal of cancer, it meant that on average, one such patient would consult a GP every day. That did not mean that many of them had cancer, but it meant that GPs had to think of that possibility at least once most of our working days!

9. Warning signals in the general population

The posters in waiting rooms and in the municipal bus aimed at informing patients and the general population. The symptoms should initiate a visit at their GP's surgery. How frequent were these symptoms? Did people really go see their doctor?

Two medical students in Tromsø volunteered to do a door-to-door survey in two areas of Tromsø, one with small houses and many elderly inhabitants, and one with a more suburban mix of higher concrete buildings and rows of houses. Every other entrance or house were visited in early evenings by one or the other student. Local papers had informed about the study. The presentation procedure and questioning had been standardised. People who consented to participate, were asked whether they during the last three months had experienced any of the seven symptoms which were read to them one by one. The A6 cards from the consultation study served to record the answers.

Moreover, one of the students was engaged to sit for one day at the waiting room of each of the four group practices while the consultation study was being done. When a patient came out of a GP's office, the students would ask for a brief interview and record symptoms the patient thought they had presented to the doctor. The answers were compared to the GP's registration for the same consultation.

9.1 Results

In 299 persons from the general population, one fourth said they sometimes during the last three months had felt one of the symptoms read aloud to them. There was no difference between age groups. Half of these people had visited the GP for this reason, more so in the highest age group. These were higher proportions than what used to be found in studies about why people see a doctor [18], suggesting that the warning signals do promote visits to the GP. 'Indigestion', 'lump' and 'cough/hoarseness' were frequent. During the four interview-days in the surgeries, more patients than GPs thought that the patient had presented this kind of symptoms, 28% versus 10%.

9.2 Short reflection

The symptoms in question no doubt are present in people's mind, far more frequently than when they signify cancer. Increased consultation may become a burden for the health services; on the other hand, the symptoms have been shown to be relevant for cancer, and an increased tendency for consultation may be a good thing when cancer can cause the symptom. The GPs seem to have stricter criteria for recognising warning signals than people consulting them.

10. The first control groups: case–control study

If you investigate a group of patients, it is difficult to have a clear idea of what caused or expressed disease without a similarly constituted control group. The consultation registrations took place during six months in 1981–1982. A new retrospective study of medical journals was planned. For these six months, the Norwegian cancer registry again furnished a list of patients diagnosed with new cancer in Tromsø. For each of the 65 cancer patients, a control patient was found among the group of patients having consulted before any diagnosis of cancer had been made in

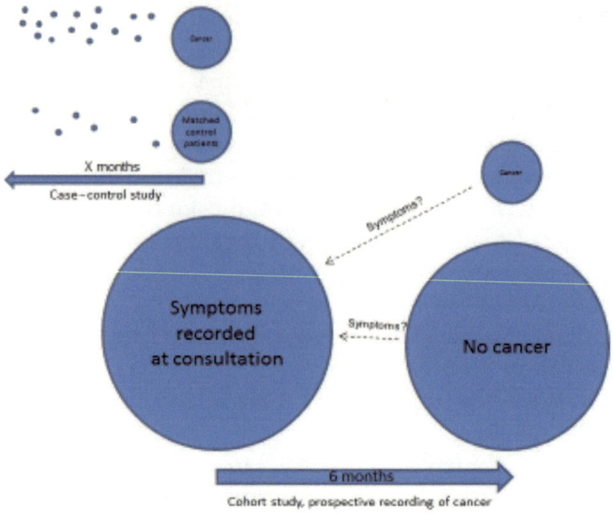

Figure 2.
Two kinds of study design: case–control study (looking back in time), and Cohort study with prospective recording of cancer (looking forward).

the cohort (**Figure 2**). Matching criteria were same sex and the closest possible date of birth. This time, criteria were made for early versus late symptoms in the cancer patients, to see the potential prognostic gain from early diagnosis.

10.1 Results

Two third of cancer patients had presented early warning signals, and about 35% of control patients had presented corresponding symptoms. The difference was statistically significant both for males and females.

10.2 Short reflection

When early warning signals are more frequent in cancer patients than in other consulting patients, a window of diagnostic opportunity exists for GPs.

Altogether five articles were now sent to the Norwegian medical journal [19], including a discussion of the content of the list of warning signals, and possibilities given by observations of the person-related data. Also, some more common diagnostic traps facing the GPs were discussed (**Table 2**).

Later, a list of Tromsø cancer patients diagnosed during the first eighteen months after the symptom registrations, was provided by the Cancer registry. Eighty of these cancer patients could be found among the recorded consulting patients. A new matching with 80 control patients based on the same criteria as in the previous study, was performed. Additionally, three GPs performed an inter-observer agreement study concerning what warning signals were found by each of them in the medical records.

10.3 Results

Warning signals were registered from the journals of 78% of cancer patients, before patient or doctor knew that the patient would get a cancer diagnosis, and in 26% of control patients. Again, this was a significant difference. Warning signals recorded only at consultation occurred in 20 cancer patients and 13 control patients. This difference did not reach statistical significance [20]. Agreement about the presence of warning signals in the journals, measured with kappa statistics, was

Traps for GPs in early diagnosis of cancer
1. GP does not follow-up positive findings
2. Two most common clinical omissions: rectal examination, and not taking seriously what a woman feels in her breast if GP cannot confirm
3. Early diagnostic hypothesis may be wrong
4. Trauma in history is too easily accepted as an explanation for present symptom
5. Comorbid benign disease is too easily taken as an explanation for present symptom
6. Not all cancers produce the most common symptom; GP may sometimes repeat negative test
7. If symptoms are diffuse, consider exploring deeper in medical history
8. If symptoms are confusing, consider hormonal explanation – and if hormonal, consider cancer

Table 2.
Traps for GPs in early diagnosis of cancer.

good both for cancer patients and control patients, with some variation between different symptoms and less good in control patients [21].

10.4 Short reflection

The greater frequency of warning signals in cancer patients, found in the retrospective medical journal study, was not evident in the prospective recording of cancer patients. However, the tendency was in the same direction. Overall, based on all the studies, a majority of cancer patients experienced a cancer-related symptom which was communicated to a doctor some time before diagnosis. Furthermore, it seemed possible to rely quite well on registrations of symptoms from medical journals.

11. Strengthening the academic basis in the north: 1984–1991

During the 1980s, the topic of early diagnosis gained visibility in vocational training – in the North, and soon nationally. A GP colleague in Oslo started a PhD thesis in the same cancer field [22] and initiated a book about different cancer topics for GPs [23]. The next couple of years, GPs attended continuing education seminars and studied books that gave better insight in clinical epidemiology [24] and statistics [25]. Based on the investigations in the north, a thesis [26] and a practical manual for GPs [27] were written. The Arctic University had a Department of Community medicine, led by a GP professor, and several GPs started teaching and research in combined academic and clinical positions.

At this time, a big step in technology also created important changes: The typewriter had previously necessitated total re-writing of manuscripts needing changes. Now, the two-diskette-slot personal computer had appeared and developed into a movable computer with a 20-megabyte hard-disk and one diskette slot, opening a new world of free writing that could easily be corrected again and again.

12. A theoretical basis: understanding how probabilities may change

It had become quite certain that the probability of diagnosing cancer in a patient presenting a warning signal, was greater than in a patient without such symptoms.

However, with the many non-cancer patients presenting similar symptoms, it was clear that the probability of cancer was still very low. In order to refer a patient, a GP should be able to convince specialists that investigations in hospital would have a reasonable chance of revealing a cancer, preferably an early-stage cancer. Working with the Tromsø data, it was calculated how many of the patients with one or more warning signals had turned out to have cancer: this proportion, known to GPs as the *positive predictive value* (PPV), was 3.7%. Perhaps not very impressive in a referral letter, but we will get back to this figure.

A chapter in a book about decision analysis showed how the 18th century Bayesian thinking allow to update the probabilities of a hypothesis when evidence is added [28]. This is the way a GP works! The patient presents a symptom. The GP already knows something about the patient: age, sex, perhaps something about heredity and profession. Then the GP starts to explore the problem: a further medical history, a focused clinical examination. Cumulated additional information may allow upgrading the probability of cancer, or in many cases, dismiss such a hypothesis without bothering the patient or the specialist or the system with unnecessary procedures. The new information may not be independent of what we already know, but the GP may then apply Bayes' axioms of conditional probability to arrive at a reasonable update of the previous probability.

Three more articles resulted: two were about diagnostic indexes allowing quantitative judgement about the relationship between symptoms and cancer [29, 30]. The third article gave examples of revising probabilities of cancer: Based on data from the 1982 study, positive predictive value (PPV) was calculated from consultation data and then revised adding new information from the medical journals [31]:

12.1 Results/examples

A 60–69 years-old male with 'indigestion' had a PPV of 2.3% for colorectal cancer. Adding information about a positive test for occult blood, PPV rose to 13.3%.

A 60–69 years-old male with 'cough/hoarseness' had a PPV of 6.4% for lung cancer. Adding the information that this man was a daily smoker, PPV increased to 8.5%. If the man was a non-smoker, PPV decreased to 3.3%. The increase is smaller than for the occult blood example. This is because it may be assumed that 'indigestion' and occult bleeding are independent of each other, while 'cough/hoarseness' and daily smoking are less independent.

12.2 Short reflection

Such indexes can be calculated on the basis of empirical data. However, they also fit well with the more approximate way a GP works when analysing a patient problem. It is a way of thinking that implies both quantitative and qualitative considerations, and which most GPs apply intuitively and approximatively.

It is nice to be able to give examples based on data collected in primary care. However, we were still only in 1990 when these articles were published. Registrations in databases like Medline were in its infancy. The scientific journal, owned by Springer Verlag, ceased to appear the year after, and the articles in "Allgemeinmedizin" are not searchable in current databases. If you want to read the articles, you may use the Arctic University web-link given in the references. Also, for this and other examples of older articles in the reference list, a university library may help.

13. Academia: on the right track, with mixed feelings of enthusiasm and professional loneliness: 1992–1999

After rich years of full-time general practice, teaching and research at the university became a full time task for this author, although still with one day a week in the group practice in general practice. The 1990s was a period of increasing activity in primary care reunions, nationally and internationally, and many doctors presented primary care-based research. In some seminars and workshops, colleagues were asked to bring a cancer case of their own to discuss in small groups. This was motivating for the participants, who soon eagerly discussed how to improve their early diagnosis of cancer. Such group work later became part of the compulsory program in vocational training for the specialty of general practice in Norway. However, not everything was easy. The Arctic university was a young university, which admitted its first medical students in 1973. For the first decades, the competition for research grants was difficult with limited earmarking for primary care and competition with the more established universities. When grants were obtained, applicants for research positions were few. It was difficult to tempt colleagues living in the more populated south of Norway to apply for positions in the beautiful, but longer-winter north.

However, international primary care publications dealing with the early diagnosis of cancer, were relatively few during the 1990s. In workshops and congresses for GPs, interest in the subject was vivid, but with some exceptions [32, 33], the interest was only modestly reflected in studies from general practice. The focus on the early diagnosis topic weakened for a while at our department. General practice is a good place to get research ideas and produce evidence about many different clinical questions [34].

14. The times they are a-changin' – fortunately: research boost and Ca-PRI - from year 2000 and onward

Soon, however, a remarkable change occurred: Some GP based researchers, especially in the UK, but also in Denmark, Sweden, Belgium, the Netherlands, Australia, published interesting studies about the early diagnosis of cancer. They often drew upon large number of patients found in GP based databases and in official registries, and focused on major types of cancer [35, 36], in addition to cancer in general [37–40]. A GP can never know what kind of cancer the next patient presents, and it is useful to be prepared to diagnose just any cancer, frequent or rare. However, the frequent ones are more frequent and merit a closer look.

At this time in the north, all the almost 4000 GPs in Norway were invited to participate in an audit-type, one-sheet questionnaire study with much of the same intent as in previous studies, but this time recording cancer prospectively after an initial symptom registration in consecutive GP patients [41] (Cohort study, **Figure 2**). About 10% of the invited GPs volunteered to take part. In these studies, cancer suspicion was examined more closely.

14.1 Results

GPs' correct cancer suspicions were found to be six times more frequent than their erroneous lack of suspicion. Patient comorbidity and multiple consultations seemed to be underestimated by GPs as factors associated with cancer.

The discussion dealt with how GPs in their diagnostic attentiveness could consider ways of thinking, interpersonal awareness and relevant information related to symptoms and other factors [42]. The study also showed how a comprehensive GP approach should include knowledge derived from clinical examination and test results. This could increase sensitivity, i.e. findings correctly identifying patients with cancer, and help correctly suspect a diagnosis of cancer, in some cases with 'low-risk-but-not-no-risk' symptoms, or even without any relevant symptom [43].

14.2 Short reflection

The study suggests how knowledgeable, empathic medical work in primary care can make a positive difference for early cancer diagnostics.

Also, Johansen [44] interviewed GPs about the essential question "How does the thought of cancer arise in a general practice consultation?"

14.3 Results

Several contexts of attention were found: Practising basic knowledge, interpersonal awareness, intuitive knowing and fear of cancer. Such fear could affect both patient and doctor. Intuitive knowing was described as a tacit feeling of alarm which could be difficult to verbalise, but nevertheless was helpful. Intuition was supposed to build on the three other elements: knowledge, awareness, fear.

14.4 Short reflection

The complex quality of diagnostic analysis is demonstrated here through a qualitative approach. The study was performed around the same time as the previous, quantitative study. The results show how different methodological approaches may create complementary knowledge.

In 2008 our department was invited to participate in the creation of a permanent workshop promoting research about cancer in primary care; The Cancer and Primary Care Research International Network (Ca-PRI) [45]. This forum has proved to be an inspiration for many researchers in primary care, generating ideas and developing new ways and new standards for producing good knowledge about all aspects of cancer, with early diagnosis and cancer care as backbones. The important role of primary care in providing research-based knowledge about cancer, has been highlighted [46]. Now, in 2021, a first nationwide formal GP research practice network is about to be established in Norway.

To-day, it would be impossible to reproduce the delay findings based on the subjective criteria from the 1970s. A more modern approach emphasises the different intervals and milestones from first symptom to start of treatment, and encourages shortening of the different intervals with patients, GPs, hospital doctors and the administrative system as stakeholders. Not only the intervals from symptom to consultation, and from consultation to diagnosis counts: the time from diagnosis to first treatment is important as well [47]. The intervals have been clarified and standardised for research purposes [48, 49], and the Ca-PRI workshop is an active hot-spot for ideas and discussions.

In the last decade, many countries have organised different kinds of 'fast track' for patients suspected to have cancer [50]. This has helped shortening the time from symptom to treatment, which is in itself a good thing, and there is hope that it could also contribute to lowering cancer mortality.

One welcome result of Ca-PRI connections was a six-country study of a new cohort of general practice patients, focusing on abdominal symptoms. Consultation data were collected in 2011, and cancer was registered prospectively after six months or more. A question to the GPs about cancer suspicion now distinguished between different reasons for such suspicion: symptoms, clinical findings, intuition.

14.5 Results

Unexpectedly, in statistical analyses intuition ranged higher than symptoms or clinical findings in the association with a subsequent new cancer [51]. The study further demonstrated that a wide range of symptoms may signal abdominal cancer, with 'rectal bleeding' reaching the highest association with cancer. PPV above 3% was found for visible bleeding in the urine or from rectum, and for weight loss that was associated with a more specific abdominal symptom [52].

An analysis of the subgroup with colorectal cancer demonstrated clinically important differences between colon and rectal cancer, and between proximal and distal colon cancer. Proximal colon cancer often has scarcity or slow debut of symptoms, slow development of anaemia and fewer positive findings on clinical examination, which may explain more urgent but less fast track referrals and less implication of the GP in the initiation of diagnosis. The challenges of the GP's work is discussed in the article [53].

14.6 Short reflection

Again, GPs' clinical competence seems to be essential for the work with early diagnosis of cancer. A process of better understanding of diagnostic approaches towards symptom poor cancer is ongoing and will need further research.

The results from these studies seem to suggest why GPs working professionally quite often may arrive at correct cancer suspicions [42]. At the same time, the subjective assessment of probability will always be influenced by ideas about similarity or representativeness or other prior notions which easily may bias conclusions [54]. It would have been too much to expect that GPs could correctly suspect all subsequent cancers. One fourth of cancer cases in the six-country study were not suspected by the GP, but with good clinical training it should be possible to lower this proportion in the future.

In the UK, the NICE guidelines [55] give GPs a rational way to deal with probabilities. Patients suspected of cancer should be referred when the positive predictive value reaches 3%. This may be a surprisingly low risk threshold, but a single symptom by itself usually has a lower PPV [56]. The seemingly low PPV of 3.7% for any warning signal in relation to cancer that was reported in 1991 [26] might well justify a referral in some cases. Later studies referred to here, seem to support this.

15. Summing up/conclusion

15.1 Avoiding patient delay

What can the layman do to react rationally to signals from the body? First, it is important to know your own body. A few common symptoms should always have an explanation, especially if your age or habits put you in a risk group for a certain cancer. Bleeding unexpectedly from a body orifice is perhaps the most important of such symptoms. Often one can understand that some innocent condition caused it, but if not, see your GP. The same way of thinking goes for a lump that is new or changing in size, for a mole growing or changing in colour, or a sore that does not heal. Cancer lodged deep in the body is more difficult, needing a certain size before signalled in the body. Cancer in an early stage is rarely painful. Pain may still be a relevant symptom, but you should know that pain is more than other symptoms caused by numerous non-cancerous conditions. Sometimes the best you can do is to observe and react to unexpected changes in the body, especially when they do not go away when you think they should.

15.2 Promoting early diagnosis in general practice

This article follows some of the stepstones leading up to present-day thinking about the early diagnosis of cancer. Some findings are in line with wise thoughts written even more than 40 years ago: Cox [57] worked in medical education and had been a professor of surgery before that. He wrote that "..beliefs about how likely different events and outcomes are derived from some facts, some habits and some hopes." Cox listed five important factors which are quoted backwards, in order to start with the most basic: Fifth, decisions are based on subjective probabilities, not objective probabilities. Fourth, probabilities are about this individual 50 year-old male with both his cough and his unique genetic, family, socio-economic mix and disease history, not only any 50 year-old male with a cough. Third, what clinicians need is a probability given that symptom, not incidence figures. Second, clinicians think in probabilities in rather course categories, such as common, possible, rare. And first, when a probability is very low, its exact quantity is not important.

His further discussion is well worth reading, too. However, his article suffers the same lack of visibility as many early papers: the journal in question has been digitalised only from 2002. Again, try a university library.

Hence, how is this to be summed up for to-day's GPs?

1. Explain unusual symptoms

   The vocational training of doctors should make them acquainted with the literature about warning signals, or alarm symptoms, as they are also called. Some symptoms like unexpected bleeding always need an explanation: Although often having a benign cause, it is important to exclude serious disease like cancer. Sometimes the distinction between symptoms and signs is blurred: In the early cancer context, anaemia is most often a sign discovered through the GP's blood tests rather than something the patient feels.

2. Add results from clinical findings and testing to symptoms

   Most patients with cancer consult when their cancer can still be treated with a curative intent. This is motivating for a GP's work. In an early stage, less than half of cancer patients present with a warning signal in the consultation, but more than half have a warning signal and/or some other cancer relevant but low-risk symptom. Adding findings from clinical examination and testing, the GP will be able to suspect cancer in about four of five cases a short time after a patient consults [43].

3. Refer when the probability based on symptoms and findings exceed 3%

   Usually, a GP needs some other information pointing in the same direction as the symptom, or replacing the symptom, to revise a PPV above the 3% NICE level. If you do your GP job and examine carefully, you may even add your intuitive suspicion, which has been shown to be of importance.

4. Consider 'fast track' when you seriously suspect cancer

   Patients with a warning signal have a greater probability to be referred to cancer patient pathways. The difficult challenge for GPs is to pursue more vague symptoms and refer relevant patients when a suspicion persists. Ordinary, comprehensive GP clinical work, attentive to details and to who the patient is, can facilitate this.

5. Last, but not least: Think of early diagnosis of cancer as an important, challenging, and interesting part of your effort to serve the patients who consult you!

Acknowledgements

Primarily, to all good GP colleagues who over the years helped with registrations. Also, to my university colleagues who gradually helped me understand scientific reasoning and method. Finally, to my co-authors over the years, to referees who gave constructive criticism to scientific manuscripts and to everybody who helped facilitate the research.

Funding

The publication charges for this article has been funded by a grant from the publication fund of UiT The Arctic University of Norway.

Conflict of interest

The author declares no conflict of interest.

Author details

Knut Holtedahl
Department of Community Medicine, UiT The Arctic University of Norway, Tromsø, Norway

*Address all correspondence to: knut.holtedahl@uit.no

References

[1] Berger J, Mohr J. A fortunate man. London: Canongate; 1967.

[2] Bentsen B. The accuracy of recording patient problems in general practice. J Medic Educ. 1976;51:311-6.

[3] Editorial: The image of cancer. Lancet. 1975;1(7919):1284.

[4] Miller DG. What is early diagnosis doing? Cancer. 1976;37(S1):426-32. doi:10.1002/1097-0142(197601)37: 1+<426::Aid-cncr2820370704> 3.0.Co;2-p

[5] Pack G, Gallo J. The culpability for delay in the treatment of cancer. American Journal of Cancer. 1938;33:443-62.

[6] Leach J, Robbins G. Delay in the diagnosis of cancer. JAMA. 1947;135:5-8.

[7] McWhinney I. The early diagnosis of cancer. Five years' experience in general practice. J R Coll Gen Pract. 1962;5:404-14.

[8] Starey CJ. The diagnosis and treatment of cancer in a general practice. J Coll Gen Pract. 1966;12(1):32-42.

[9] Feinstein AR, Pritchett JA, Schimpff CR. The epidemiology of cancer therapy. IV. The extraction of data from medical records. Ann Intern Med. 1969;123:571-90.

[10] Holtedahl KA. [Diagnosis of cancer in general practice. I. Can diagnosis be made earlier?]. Tidsskrift for den Norske laegeforening : tidsskrift for praktisk medicin, ny raekke. 1980;100(19-21):1219-23. English summary. . Available from: https://hdl.handle.net/10037/12542.

[11] Holtedahl KA. [Diagnosis of cancer in general practice. II. What can the general practitioner improve? Case reports as a teaching aid]. Tidsskrift for den Norske laegeforening : tidsskrift for praktisk medicin, ny raekke. 1980;100(19-21):1224-6. Available from: https://hdl.handle.net/10037/12539.

[12] Gray DJP. The role of the general practitioner in the early detection of malignant disease. Transactions Hunterian Soc (London). 1966;25:121-75.

[13] Cobb B, Clark RL, Jr., Mc GC, Howe CD. Patient-responsible delay of treatment in cancer; a social psychological study. Cancer. 1954;7(5):920-6. doi:10.1002/1097-0142(195409)7:5<920::aid-cncr2820070516>3.0.co;2-r

[14] Hackett TP, Cassem NH, Raker JW. Patient delay in cancer. The New England journal of medicine. 1973;289(1):14-20. doi:10.1056/NEJM197307052890104

[15] Howson JY. Observations on the delay period in the diagnosis of pelvic cancer. Med Clin North Am. 1948;32:1573-81. doi:10.1016/s0025-7125(16)35623-1

[16] Jenkins S. Diagnostic delay in neoplastic disease. J R Coll Gen Pract. 1978;28(197):724-8.

[17] Macadam DB. A study in general practice of the symptoms and delay patterns in the diagnosis of gastrointestinal cancer. J R Coll Gen Pract. 1979;29(209):723-9.

[18] White KL, Williams TF, Greenberg BG. The ecology of medical care. The New England journal of medicine. 1961;265:885-92. doi:10.1056/NEJM196111022651805

[19] Holtedahl KA. [Cancer diagnosis in general practice III-VII. The general

practitioner's recording of cancer warning signals in their patients. IV. Recording of interviews on cancer warning signals. Patients in general practice and in the general population. V. Patients with and without cancer. Who consults the physician for the 7 warning cancer signals? VI. The content of the warning signals. Is persistent pain relevant as a warning signal? VII. Alarm bell symptoms, alarm bell data and pitfalls. Some useful reminders for the general practitioner's work in cancer diagnosis]. English summary. Tidsskrift for den Norske laegeforening. 1984;104(12):799-812. Available from: https://hdl.handle.net/10037/12543 ; https://hdl.handle.net/10037/12544 ; https://hdl.handle.net/10037/12545 ; https://hdl.handle.net/10037/12547 ; https://hdl.handle.net/10037/12548.

[20] Holtedahl KA. The value of warning signals of cancer in general practice. Scand J Prim Health Care. 1987;5(3):140-3. doi:10.3109/02813438709013994

[21] Holtedahl KA. Inter-observer variation on registration of signals of cancer. Scand J Prim Health Care. 1987;5(3):133-9. doi:10.3109/02813438709013993

[22] Nylenna M. Diagnosing cancer in general practice: from suspicion to certainty. Br Med J (Clin Res Ed). 1986;293(6542):314-7. doi:10.1136/bmj.293.6542.314

[23] Nylenna M, Gundersen S, Johannessen JV, (eds). Kreft i almenpraksis [Cancer in General Practice]. Oslo: Landsforeningen mot kreft, Universitetsforlaget; 1985. In Norwegian.

[24] Sackett Dl, Haynes R, Tugwell P. Clinical epidemiology. A basic science for clinical medicine. . First edition. (Second edition 1991) ed. Boston: Little, Brown and Company; 1985.

[25] Bland M. An introduction to medical statistics. Oxford: Oxford University Press; 1987.

[26] Holtedahl KA. Diagnosis of cancer in general practice. A study of delay problems and warning signals of cancer, with implications for public cancer information and for cancer diagnostic strategies in general practice (Thesis) University of Tromsø, Norway: ISM skriftserie nr. 16, 1991. : http://hdl.handle.net/10037/2325

[27] Holtedahl KA. Early diagnosis of cancer in general practice. A manual. Berlin: Springer Verlag; 1990.

[28] Chapter 4. The use of diagnostic information to revise probabilities. In: Weinstein MC, Fineberg, H.V, editor. Clinical decision analysis. Philadelphia: W.B. Saunders Company; 1980.

[29] Holtedahl KA. A method of calculating diagnostic indexes for possible cancer symptoms in general practice. Allgemeinmedizin. 1990;19:74-9. Available from: http://hdl.handle.net/10037/12484.

[30] Holtedahl KA. More diagnostic indexes from general practice for some important forms of cancer. Allgemeinmedizin. 1990;19:80-5. Available from: https://munin.uit.no/handle/10037/12487.

[31] Holtedahl KA. Probability revision in general practice: the cases of occult blood in stool in patients with indigestion, and daily smoking in patients who cough. Allgemeinmedizin. 1990;19:35-8. Available from: http://hdl.handle.net/10037/12453.

[32] Mansson J, Bjorkelund C, Hultborn R. Symptom pattern and diagnostic work-up of malignancy at first symptom presentation as related to level of care. A retrospective study from the primary health care centre area of Kungsbacka, Sweden. Neoplasma. 1999;46(2):93-9.

[33] Buntinx F, Wauters W. The diagnostic value of macroscopic haematuria in diagnosing urological cancers: a meta-analysis. Family Practice. 1997;14:63-8.

[34] Holtedahl K. Research and practice combined--ideas for a life in general practice. Fam Pract. 2008;25(2):132-6. doi:10.1093/fampra/cmn002

[35] Bruyninckx R, Buntinx F, Aertgeerts B, Van Casteren V. The diagnostic value of macroscopic haematuria for the diagnosis of urological cancer in general practice. Br J Gen Pract. 2003;53(486):31-5.

[36] Hamilton W, Round A, Sharp D, Peters TJ. Clinical features of colorectal cancer before diagnosis: a population-based case-control study. Br J Cancer. 2005;93(4):399-405. doi:10.1038/sj.bjc.6602714

[37] Hamilton W. The CAPER studies: five case-control studies aimed at identifying and quantifying the risk of cancer in symptomatic primary care patients. Br J Cancer. 2009;101:S80-S6.

[38] Jones R, Latinovic R, Charlton J, Gulliford MC. Alarm symptoms in early diagnosis of cancer in primary care: cohort study using General Practice Research Database. BMJ. 2007;334:1040-4. doi:10.1136/bmi.39171.637106.AE

[39] Lyratzopoulos G, Neal RD, Barbiere JM, Rubin GP, Abel GA. Variation in number of general practitioner consultations before hospital referral for cancer: findings from the 2010 National Cancer Patient Experience Survey in England. Lancet Oncol. 2012;13(4):353-65. doi:10.1016/S1470-2045(12)70041-4

[40] Rubin G, Vedsted P, Emery J. Improving cancer outcomes: better access to diagnostics in primary care could be critical. Br J Gen Pract. 2011;61(586):317-8. doi:10.3399/bjgp11X572283

[41] Ingebrigtsen SG, Scheel BI, Hart B, Thorsen T, Holtedahl K. Frequency of 'warning signs of cancer' in Norwegian general practice, with prospective recording of subsequent cancer. Fam Pract. 2013;30(2):153-60. doi:10.1093/fampra/cms065

[42] Scheel BI, Ingebrigtsen SG, Thorsen T, Holtedahl K. Cancer suspicion in general practice: the role of symptoms and patient characteristics, and their association with subsequent cancer. Br J Gen Pract. 2013;63(614):e627-35. doi:10.3399/bjgp13X671614

[43] Scheel BI, Holtedahl K. Symptoms, signs, and tests: The general practitioner's comprehensive approach towards a cancer diagnosis. Scand J Prim Health Care. 2015;33(3):170-7. doi:10.3109/02813432.2015.1067512

[44] Johansen ML, Holtedahl KA, Rudebeck CE. How does the thought of cancer arise in a general practice consultation? Interviews with GPs. Scand J Prim Health Care. 2012;30(3):135-40. doi:10.3109/02813432.2012.688701

[45] The Cancer and Primary Care Research International Network (Ca-PRI) [Internet]. [cited 13 June 2021]. Available from: https://www.ed.ac.uk/usher/cancer-primary-care-research-international-network.

[46] Rubin G, Berendsen A, Crawford SM, Dommett R, Earle C, Emery J, et al. The expanding role of primary care in cancer control. The Lancet Oncology. 2015;16(12):1231-72. doi:http://dx.doi.org/10.1016/S1470-2045(15)00205-3

[47] Hanna TP, King WD, Thibodeau S, Jalink M, Paulin GA, Harvey-Jones E, et al. Mortality due to cancer treatment delay: systematic review and meta-analysis. BMJ. 2020;371:m4087. doi:10.1136/bmj.m4087

[48] Olesen F, Hansen RP, Vedsted P. Delay in diagnosis: the experience in Denmark. Br J Cancer. 2009;101 Suppl 2:S5-8. doi:10.1038/sj.bjc.6605383

[49] Weller D, Vedsted P, Rubin G, Walter FM, Emery J, Scott S, et al. The Aarhus statement: improving design and reporting of studies on early cancer diagnosis. Br J Cancer. 2012;106(7):1262-7. doi:10.1038/bjc.2012.68

[50] Holtedahl K. Challenges in early diagnosis of cancer: the fast track. (Editorial). Scand J Prim Health Care. 2020;38(3):251-2. doi:10.1080/02813432.2020.1794415

[51] Holtedahl K, Vedsted P, Borgquist L, Donker GA, Buntinx F, Weller D, et al. Abdominal symptoms in general practice: Frequency, cancer suspicions raised, and actions taken by GPs in six European countries. Cohort study with prospective registration of cancer. Heliyon. 2017;3(6):e00328. doi:10.1016/j.heliyon.2017.e00328

[52] Holtedahl K, Hjertholm P, Borgquist L, Donker GA, Buntinx F, Weller D, et al. Abdominal symptoms and cancer in the abdomen: prospective cohort study in European primary care. Br J Gen Pract. 2018;68(670):e301-e10. doi:10.3399/bjgp18X695777

[53] Holtedahl K, Borgquist L, Donker GA, Buntinx F, Weller D, Campbell C, et al. Symptoms and signs of colorectal cancer, with differences between proximal and distal colon cancer. A prospective cohort study of diagnostic accuracy in primary care. BMC Family Practice. 2021. DOI: 10.1186/s12875-021-01452-6

[54] Tversky A, Kahneman D. Judgment under Uncertainty: Heuristics and Biases. Science. 1974;185(4157):1124-31. doi:10.1126/science.185.4157.1124

[55] Suspected Cancer: Recognition and Referral (NICE guideline 12). London 2015. Available from: https://www.ncbi.nlm.nih.gov/pubmed/26180880.

[56] Shapley M, Mansell G, Jordan JL, Jordan KP. Positive predictive values of >/=5% in primary care for cancer: systematic review. Br J Gen Pract. 2010;60(578):e366-77. doi:10.3399/bjgp10X515412

[57] Cox KR. The GP and the cancer patient. What does a GP do about the person who might have cancer? Australian Family Physician. 1978;7(June):757-68.

Section 9

Zoonotic and Veterinary Diseases and Food Safety Concerns

Chapter 12

Fascioliasis: A Foodborne Disease of Veterinary and Zoonotic Importance

Tolulope Ebenezer Atalabi and Omotosho Taiye Lawal

Abstract

Fascioliasis is a food-borne neglected disease caused by digenetic trematodes in the genus *Fasciola*. There is a significant increase in the global prevalence of human fascioliasis with a strong correlation with a high infection rate among ruminant definitive hosts. *Fasciola* is a liver fluke with complex life cycle. Fascioliasis is endemic in every continent of the world with the exception of Antarctica. Discharge of the metabolites of liver flukes into the circulatory system of hosts has pathological consequences. Fascioliasis has been diagnosed by parasitological, immunological, and molecular means, and it is being reliably treated chemotherapeutically. The emerging drug-resistant strains of liver flukes have led to the need for vaccine development. Most vaccine candidates were first isolated as native proteins from adult worms. Several of the early antigens, including cathepsin L proteases, Glutathione S-transferase (GST), and fatty acid binding protein (FABP), significantly reduced worm burden, egg output, and liver pathology in cattle and sheep. Climate change, emerging drug resistance, and the development of new parasite strains through hybridization are the current challenges that could potentially alter the epidemiology of fascioliasis soon. Therefore, researchers need to produce promising vaccines that offer maximum protection to farm animals and humans.

Keywords: fascioliasis, veterinary, zoonosis, epidemiology, diagnosis, pathology, control, vaccines, Nigeria

1. Introduction

Fascioliasis is an ancient food-borne neglected zoonotic disease of medical importance caused by some species of macroscopic and leaf-like digenetic trematodes in the genus *Fasciola* [1]. The disease came into public health limelight in 1379 when Jehan De Brie, a French scientist, described the first ever known parasite, *Fasciola hepatica* [2]. In 1874, Professor James McConnell, a pathologist and resident physician in Calcutta, discovered *Clonorchis sinensis,* a Chinese human liver fluke, when he carried out autopsy on the corpse of a 20-year old carpenter [3]. Currently, suspected hybrid species of *F. hepatica* and *F. gigantica* are being investigated to ascertain their true taxonomic status [4].

Since every continent is infested with these trematodes, 180 million people are at risk, while an estimated 2.4 million people living in more than 70 countries of the world are suffering from the scourge of fascioliasis [1, 5]. Meanwhile, it has been estimated that *F. hepatica* infects over 300 million cattle and 250 million sheep globally and in consonance with *F. gigantica* causes economic loss estimated at USD 3billion annually [6].

Recently, there has been a significant increase in the global prevalence of human fascioliasis [1, 7] with a strong correlation with a high infection rate among ruminant definitive hosts [8].

A broad range of cosmopolitan freshwater snails in the family Limnaeidae are responsible for the transmission of fascioliasis. For instance, *Austropeplea tomentosa, Hinkleyia caperata, Stagnicola corvus, Galba truncatula, Radix rubiginosa,* and *Pseudosuccinea columella*, which are endemic (but not limited) to Australia, North America, Europe, Africa, Asia, and South America, respectively, have been reported previously [9]. Fascioliasis due to *F. gigantica* is predominantly endemic in the lower altitudes of tropical and subtropical parts of the world. Consequently, more cases of the disease are reported in larger part of sub-Saharan Africa (SSA) where suitable snail intermediate hosts naturally inhabit [10–12].

2. Life cycle

Liver flukes have a complex life cycle with a wide range of mammalian definitive hosts [9]. Humans are accidental definitive host of *Fasciola* species [13]. The infective form of this parasite is the metacercariae which, upon infecting man, temporarily settle down in the peritoneal cavity for about 24 hours after burrowing through the wall of the small intestine. Various species of liver flukes have affinity for intrahepatic or extrahepatic biliary tree [14]. At hepatic stage, which is assumed to last for about 6–7 weeks in *F. hepatica* [15], metacercariae invade the parenchyma mechanically through the liver capsule and eventually find their way into the biliary duct; this is the biliary stage. They settle down there, attain maturity, and lay eggs after sexual reproduction [5, 15]. In humans, metacercariae attain maturity within 3–4 months [5].

The number of eggs extruded by each adult worm per day varies from one definitive host to the other. Report has shown that as much as 25,000 eggs, 12,000 eggs, and 2,150 eggs could be extruded in sheep, cow, and black rats, respectively [16, 17]. Elsewhere, it has been reported that an individual liver fluke could extrude about 40,000 eggs per day [9]. These unembryonated eggs are transported in the bile medium to the small intestine, where they mix up with feces [18]. In ruminant definitive hosts, they are passed out in the pasture and undergo a period of embryonation under suitable ambient temperature and humidity.

Since freshwater body is crucial to the development of the larval stages of liver flukes [18], hatching takes place in response to external stimuli of light, temperature, and humidity [9, 19, 20]. The emerging free-swimming ciliated miracidia are genetically configured to locate a suitable Limnaeid snail intermediate host via thin films of water [21], in less than 24 hours through positive chemotactic and phototactic movements [9]. By means of their piercing stylets and proteolytic enzymes, they mechanically invade their snail hosts' body wall and tissues [20, 22] and develop into sporocysts. The sporocysts further metamorphose into mother rediae, which develop into the daughter rediae. The metamorphosis in the snail host culminates in the emergence of cercariae, which are capable of passively infecting suitable vertebrate hosts and humans who drink infested water [18, 23–25]. Relative humidity above 65%, annual rainfall >100 mm, and ambient temperature of between 25 and 30°C have been reported as the factors that are suitable for the growth and shedding of cercariae [26, 27].

Finally, the cercariae locate the wet leaves of herbaceous plants by negative geotactic movement, encyst, and metamorphose into metacercariae. When ingested by suitable ruminant definitive hosts during grazing, the cyst is digested by the hosts' enzyme and the metacercariae migrate to the duodenum where they re-encyst [18, 28]. **Figure 1** below shows a summary of the life cycle of liver flukes.

3. Epidemiology of fascioliasis

3.1 The distribution of fascioliasis

Fascioliasis is endemic in every continent of the world with the exception of Antarctica (**Figure 1**). The disease is being reported from Africa, Asia, the Caribbean, Europe, parts of Latin America, Middle East, and Oceania [29]. High transmission rate of human fascioliasis has been reported from the Andean highlands of Bolivia, Peru, the Nile valley, the Caspean sea basin, East Asia, and South East Asia [30].

In sub-Saharan Africa (SSA), fascioliasis has been reported in West Africa [12, 31], East Africa [32], and South African countries [33, 34]. However, it has also been reported in Egypt (outside SSA), North Africa [35, 36].

The distribution of fascioliasis in Nigeria covers every geo-political zone. There have been reports from North West [37, 38], North Central [39, 40], North East [41, 42], South West [43, 44], South South [45, 46] and South East [47, 48].

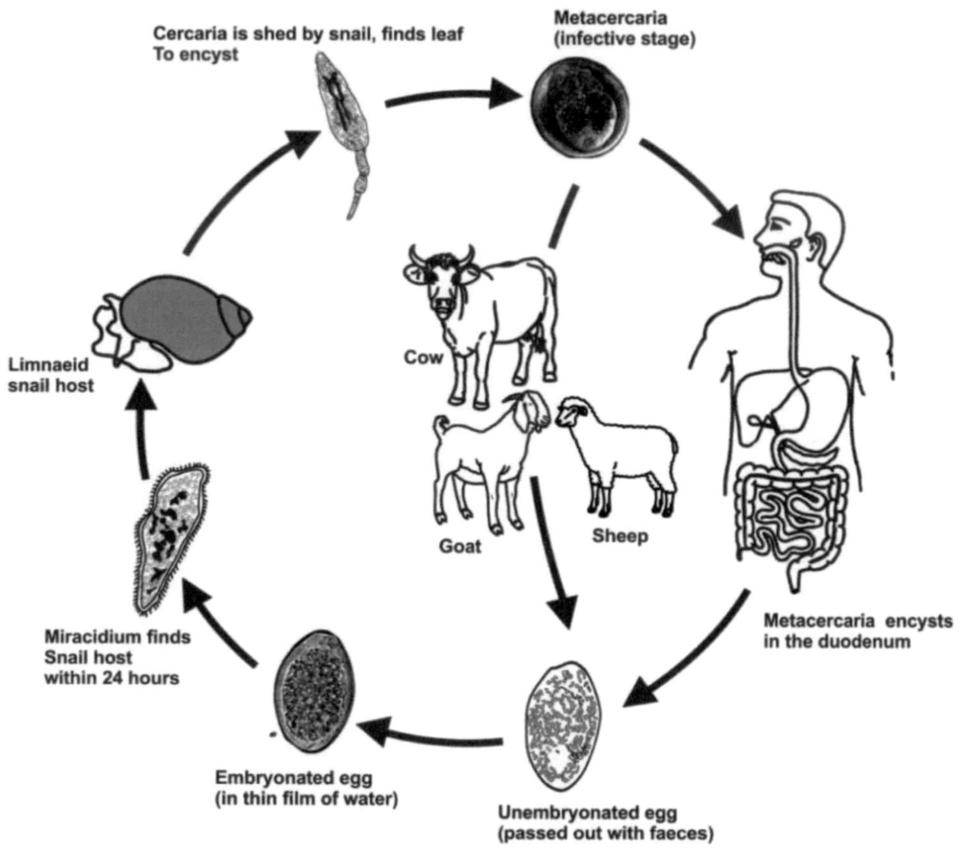

Figure 1.
Life cycle of liver flukes.

3.2 The ecology and transmission pattern of fascioliasis

In 1939, Eugene Pavlovsky, a Russian Academician propounded the theory of disease focality, which suggests that some disease-causing organisms (pathogens) naturally occur in specific ecosystems [49, 50]. This implies that the population of the pathogens is an integral part of that natural landscape [51]. Characteristically, pathogens are transmitted in such settings irrespective of the presence of humans. Consequently, humans become accidental definitive hosts when their ecological niche overlaps with suitable hosts from such landscapes and they become infected after establishing contact [52]. Researchers have found out that the epidemiology of fascioliasis has a strong link with the ecology of the settings where the disease is transmitted [30].

Pavlovsky's theory explains why fascioliasis is categorized as a focal infectious disease [29]. It could be transmitted independent of human presence. Drawing analogy from Pavlovsky's theory, there are three important elements that play key roles in the transmission pattern of fascioliasis. These are the snail intermediate hosts, ruminant vertebrate hosts, and humans who are the accidental hosts (see **Figure 2** below).

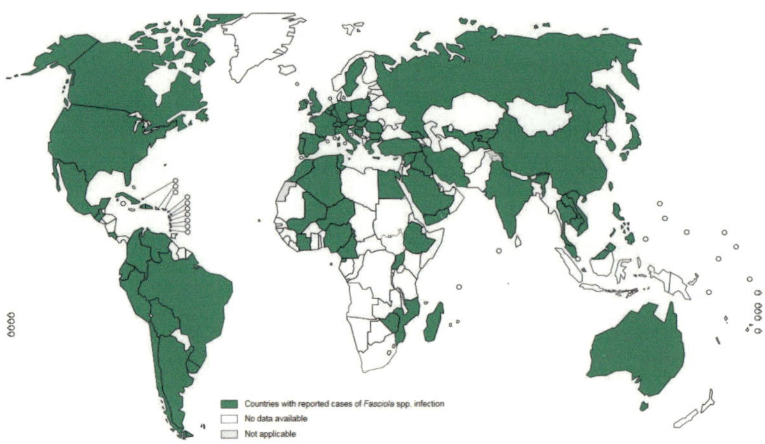

Figure 2.
Global distribution of fascioliasis. Source: Reprinted from [53].

The transmission patterns of fascioliasis vary in different epidemiological settings [30]. In the last 20 years, some researchers proposed that the patterns of the disease can be classified as fascioliasis due to influx of immigrants, human endemic/non-human (animal) endemic areas, native or isolated cases, and the three human degrees of endemicity. The fourth classification is further grouped as hypoendemic [prevalence rate < 1% while Arithmetic Mean Intensity of Infection (AMII) < 50 eggs/gram of feces], mesoendemic [prevalence rate of 1–10% while AMII 50–300 eggs/gram of feces], and hyper-endemic [prevalence rate > 10% while AMII >300 eggs/gram of feces]. In mesoendemic settings, school-age children (SAC) [5–15 years] may have higher prevalence rates while in hyper-endemic settings, SAC usually record higher prevalence rates [54, 55].

3.3 The effects of climate change on fascioliasis transmission

The role of climate in the ecology of disease-causing organisms cannot be overemphasized. In fact, climate is regarded as a basic concept of ecology. Climate triggers environmental changes [56], which in turn affect the ecosystems where parasites are transmitted, reproduced, and complete their life cycles. Because life cycles, transmission rates, and pattern *vis a vis* the biology of their intermediate hosts are weather-sensitive, climate change has the capacity to significantly increase the prevalence and intensity of infection with liver flukes [57]. Besides, it could widen the geographical distribution [58] as well as determine the survival and transmission of the infective stage (metacercariae) [56, 59].

3.4 The risk factors of fascioliasis

Factors that predispose humans and animals to infectious diseases are referred to as risk factors. At different times and locations, many researchers have carried out spatial regression analysis of environmental variables to determine the risk factors of fascioliasis in humans and domestic ruminants. Consequently, significant associations have been described between fascioliasis and streams, wetlands, pastures [60], raising more than five sheep, dog ownership, familiarity with aquatic plants, drinking alfalfa juice, dizzy spells, history of jaundice, peripheral eosinophilia, presence of *Ascaris lumbricoides* eggs in feces [61], seasonal precipitation, temperature, elevation, and several land covers [62].

Meanwhile, gender, age, epidemiological settings (rural, urban, or rural-urban), feeding habit, familial, and social factors have been reported as the major risk factors of fascioliasis among humans [55].

3.4.1 Gender

In areas that are hyper-endemic for human fascioliasis (e.g., Egypt and Bolivia), females have reportedly recorded higher prevalence and intensity rates [55, 63, 64].

3.4.2 Age

All age groups have been found to be at risk of infection with fascioliasis but school-age children (5–15 years) have the highest prevalence and intensity [30, 64].

3.4.3 Epidemiological settings (rural, urban, or rural-urban)

People from low-middle income countries are more likely to suffer from fascioliasis. However, inhabitants from developed countries could be infected when they feed on imported infested plants that elude quarantine measures [30]. During field trips, urban inhabitants could be at a high risk of infection due to fascioliasis [55].

3.4.4 Human feeding habits

Source of food and water consumed is an important epidemiological factor of human fascioliasis. Uncontrolled markets of vegetables (like carrot, cucumber, cabbage, onions, tomatoes, spinach, etc.) coupled with drinking infested water or beverages/juice made from local plants could predispose humans to infection since liver flukes have affinity for all plants. Reports have also shown that consumption of raw liver plays a vital role in infection transmission [55, 65].

3.5 The prevalence and intensity of fascioliasis in Nigeria

Information on the prevalence of fascioliasis in Nigeria is more available compared to the intensity of infection: researchers seem to report the former more than the latter. *Fasciola gigantica* has a higher geographical coverage than *F. hepatica* and other helminthes of veterinary importance [38].

In a recent cross-sectional study conducted in North Central Nigeria where 686 fecal samples were collected from cattle in 11 villages, 110 were found to test positive for the eggs of *F. gigantica*, implying a prevalence of 16% (95% CI: 13–19%) [31]. However, a decade long study (2005–2014) of the prevalence of bovine fascioliasis in the States in that geopolitical zone shows a prevalence of 32.34% (95% CI: 30.28–34.46%) [40].

Meanwhile, a study carried out in South-South Nigeria revealed a fascioliasis prevalence (due to *F. gigantica* and *F. hepatica*) of 44.8 and 36% in cattle and goats, respectively. Intensity of infection showed that for every cattle infected, 8–10 liver flukes were recovered. Conversely, 4–5 flukes were recovered from the liver of every goat infected [45]. A similar study carried out elsewhere in the same zone reported a low prevalence of 5.34% from a total number of 712 randomly sampled cattle [46].

Nevertheless, in the North-East, a fascioliasis (without distinction) prevalence of 28.2% was reported where 262 gall bladders of White Fulani cattle were examined [42]. In a recent longitudinal study carried out in another part of North-East, Nigeria, where 7640 samples of feces and gall bladders were collected from slaughtered cattle, sheep, and goats in seven local government areas, 3092 were positive for the eggs and adults of *F. gigantica* and *F. hepatica*, giving a prevalence of 40.5% [41].

Moreover, a cross-sectional study on bovine fascioliasis in southwestern Nigeria where 905 samples of feces were screened for the eggs and adult of both species shows the predominance of *F. gigantica* (84.38%) over *F. hepatica* (1.56%) with an overall prevalence of 7.07% [44]. Conversely, the report of a longitudinal study conducted between 1994 and 2004 in another part of the zone revealed a prevalence of 2.31% after a total of 1,640,095 cattle were screened [66].

Furthermore, a cross-sectional survey carried out in North-West Nigeria reported a prevalence of 27.68% after fecal and bile samples were examined from 224 cattle [37]. Another cross-sectional survey of slaughtered cattle, sheep, and goats carried out in similar zone reported a prevalence of 29.6% for *F. hepatica* [67].

Finally, a longitudinal study carried out in South-East 8 years ago reported a prevalence of 17.2% after fecal and liver samples from 367 slaughtered sheep were examined for the presence of *F. gigantica* [47]. Interestingly, in a more recent study carried out 2 years ago in the same geo-political zone, a prevalence of 16.4% was reported for *F. hepatica* after the liver of 128 slaughtered cattle were examined [48].

The pattern of the prevalence rate of fascioliasis in Nigeria has proven the focal nature of the disease irrespective of the class of ruminant animals examined.

4. Pathology of fascioliasis

Oriental forms of liver flukes cause cholangiocarcinoma, a type of liver cancer that is peculiar to areas where *Opisthorchis felineus, O. viverrini*, and *Clonorchis sinensis* are endemic [68]. Bile ducts and gall bladders become enlarged when liver flukes establish themselves in these locations in large numbers. Discharge of the metabolites of liver flukes into the circulatory system of hosts has reportedly led to anemia, increased level of serum enzyme concentration, and dysfunction of the thyroid and adrenal glands [69].

5. Diagnosis of fascioliasis

The parasitological means of examining fecal samples for the presence of liver flukes' eggs is the use of microscope [68]. Eggs become visible after 8–10 weeks post infection. This, however, varies from one host species to another. The limitation of this method is that the sensitivity of the Fecal Egg Count (FEC) may be undermined by factors like the age of the host, quantity of water in each fecal sample, and how representative the number of aliquots is per fecal sample examined [70]. Furthermore, a report has shown that in definitive hosts suffering from the acute phase of the disease, adverse effects of fascioliasis become evident much earlier before the pre-patent period [71]. Consequently, at necropsy, quantitative fecal examination and finding the hepatic fluke load will grossly downplay the severity of the disease [69, 72].

Quite a number of relatively cheap antibody detection indirect enzyme-linked immunosorbent assays (ELISA) with high sensitivity and specificity have been developed. Most of these techniques are based on excretory-secretory products and cathepsin L proteases [70, 73].

Increase in parasite-specific IgG (which becomes detectable after 4 weeks post infection) is peculiar to infection with fascioliasis [74]. The limitation of this technique is that after many months of successful treatment, antibodies could remain in serum, giving a false impression that the infection status is positive [70].

Excellent specificity and sensitivity has been reported for a serodiagnostic technique developed in 2011 for human fascioliasis. SeroFluke, as it is called, is a lateral flow test which has fared better compared with ELISA test (MM3-SERO) [70, 75].

Nonetheless, report has shown the superiority of antigen detection to that of antibody in the diagnosis of human fascioliasis. Coproantigens (antigens in fecal samples) are preferred to antigenemia (the presence of antigens in blood) because in the latter, circulating antigens disappear soon in the serum of patients. Besides, most of them appear in form of immune complex which are not freely detectable [76].

Less than a decade ago, a nested-PCR was developed to boost the sensitivity and specificity of current diagnostic techniques with the view that the fascioliasis could be detected in the feces of sheep 2 weeks post infection. This method entails the amplification of a 423 bp fragment of the Cytochrome C Oxidase 1 gene [70, 77]. Interestingly, similar result was achieved a year later in lesser time by amplifying a 292 bp fragment of ITS2 gene [70, 78]. Because molecular diagnosis using PCR is not readily available everywhere and as well undermined by irreproducibility of published methods, loop-mediated isothermal amplification (LAMP) has been introduced as an alternative. LAMP has proven to be more specific and sensitive by detecting fascioliasis 1 week post infection in sheep within a much shorter time—about 2½ times faster than PCR [70, 79].

6. Control of fascioliasis in Nigeria

6.1 Chemotherapeutic control

Chemotherapeutic approach has been in practice in fascioliasis control for 20 years. Based on its effectiveness, it has been predicted that the *status quo* shall be maintained in the future [80, 81]. Epidemiological and meteorological data-based treatment with drugs of choice is important for the control of fascioliasis [82]. Such drug categories include: "halogenated phenol (niclofolan, bithionol, hexachlorophene, and nitroxynil); salicylanides (rafoxanide, oxyclozanide, and closantel), benzimidazoles (triclabendazole and albendazole); sulphonamides (clorsulon), and phenoxyalkanes (diamphenethides)" [82, 83]. These drugs differ in their effectiveness against adults and immature liver flukes. However, Triclabendazole (TCZ) has been the preferred drug for treating fascioliasis since 1983 as a result of its high efficacy against the adult and all larval stages of liver flukes [82, 84–86].

The single dose of 10 mg/kg body weight is effective against the adult in the bile ducts and on immature flukes migrating through the liver [80, 85]. However, TCZ resistance has been reported in animals [87, 88] and in humans [89]. Reports have shown that drug resistance could frustrate fascioliasis control programmes [18]. Besides, TCZ is not commercially available because it is solely distributed by Novartis Pharma. Inc. (Basel, Switzerland). Consequently, it is not recommended for mass administration of medicines (MAM) [80, 90]. The unavailability of the drug, specifically to treat fascioliasis, has been reported to result in outbreaks of the disease more than a decade ago [91].

Periodic antihelmintic use at 12–13 week intervals is effective against both mature and immature flukes. By this strategic control measure, intensity of infection with liver flukes significantly reduces over time. In the tropics where incidence of fascioliasis occurs all year round, annual treatment of up to four times is recommended [82, 92].

In Nigeria, some parts have reported seasonal trends in fascioliasis while some Southern parts of the country have reported an all-year-round occurrence [93]. A recent 46- year meta-analysis of the prevalence and distribution of helminthes of veterinary and zoonotic importance in Nigeria has identified failure of control programmes in the area of strategic deworming, snail host control, and adequate sanitation as the reason for the highest pooled prevalence in southwestern Nigeria [38]. Some authorities recommend that cattle be dewormed regularly [94], while others recommend treatment upon onset of clinical fascioliasis. Meanwhile, two or three annual treatments have been proposed: at the start of the rainy season, mid rainy season, and at the start of the dry season [95]. Currently, the anthelminthic drugs in use in Nigeria include: albendazole, nitroxynil, clorsulon and levamisole. However, a report has shown that the drug of choice against fascioliasis (triclabendazole) is not available for use in Nigeria [82].

6.2 Vaccination against fascioliasis

The emerging drug-resistant strains of liver flukes have led to the need for vaccine development. Despite the immense effort of researchers in this regard, no commercial vaccine is available yet [96]. Cysteine proteases produced by every stage in the life cycle of the liver flukes are common virulence mediators [97], which mediate biological functions like excystment, tissue invasion, and immune evasion [98].

Adult fluke cathepsin L and newly excysted juvenile (NEJ) cathepsin B are the prominent proteolytic enzymes of their respective excretory secretory (ES) materials [97]. Cathepsin L5 and cathepsin B synthesized by *F. hepatica* as well as cathepsin L1 synthesized by *F. gigantica* are promising targets for vaccines against fascioliasis [99–101].

Recombinant protein expression is critical to the assessment of cysteine protein vaccine potential [97]. The yeast expression system has been a useful tool for the functional expression of cathepsin L1 and L2 [102], cathepsin L5, and cathepsin B [101].

A larger part of these vaccine candidates was first isolated as native proteins from adult worm ES products. Several of these early antigens, including cathepsin L proteases, glutathione S-transferase (GST), and fatty acid binding protein (FABP) significantly reduced worm burden, egg output, and liver pathology in cattle and sheep [96, 103].

7. Conclusion

Fascioliasis has been established as an important foodborne disease of veterinary and zoonotic importance. Climate change, emerging drug resistance, and the development of new parasite strains through hybridization are the current challenges that could potentially alter the epidemiology of the disease in the nearest future [70]. To this end, researchers need to step up their effort to produce promising vaccines that offer maximum protection to farm animals and humans and as well contribute immensely to global elimination of the disease by reducing its prevalence and intensity. Government of countries in the tropics and subtropics should endeavor to provide more funds for researchers.

Acknowledgements

The authors sincerely appreciate the effort of Mr. Osuntuyi Mabayoje Pius who did the art work on the Life Cycle of liver flukes. We extend our gratitude to the World Health Organization for granting us the permission to use the map of the world showing the global distribution of fascioliasis under the request ID 312094.

Conflicts of interest

The authors do not have any conflicts of interest to declare.

Author details

Tolulope Ebenezer Atalabi[1*] and Omotosho Taiye Lawal[2]

1 Department of Biological Sciences, Faculty of Life Sciences, Federal University Dutsin-Ma, Dutsin-Ma, Katsina State, Nigeria

2 Department of Microbiology, Faculty of Life Sciences, Federal University Dutsin-Ma, Dutsin-Ma, Katsina State, Nigeria

*Address all correspondence to: ebenezer2k2@gmail.com

References

[1] World Health Organization. Foodborne trematode infections: Fascioliasis [Internet]. 2019a. Available from: https://www.who.int/foodborne_trematode_infections/fascioliasis/en/ [Accessed: 04 November 2019]

[2] Hugh-Jones ME, Hubbert WT, Hagstad HV. Chronology of Events in Zoonoses: Recognition, Control, and Prevention. Iowa: Iowa State University Press; 1995. p. 11

[3] Wikivisually. Ascaridida [Internet]. 2019. Available from: https://wikivisually.com/wiki/Ascaridida [Accessed: 04 November 2019]

[4] Centre for Disease Control. Fasciola [Internet]. 2018a. Available from: https://www.cdc.gov/parasites / fasciola/biology.html [Accessed: 04 November 2019]

[5] World Health Organization. Neglected tropical diseases: Fascioliasis-infection with the "Neglected" neglected worms [Internet]. 2019b. Available from: https://www.who.int/neglected_ diseases /integrated_media /integrated_media_fascioliasis/en/ [Accessed: 04 November 2019]

[6] Mas-Coma S, Bargues MD, Valero MA. Fascioliasis and other plant-borne trematode zoonoses. International Journal for Parasitology. 2005;**35**:1255-1278

[7] Diyana JNA, Lokman IH, Fazila SHN, Latiffah H, Ibitoye EB, Hazfalinda HN, et al. A retrospective study on bovine fascioliasis in veterinary regional laboratories in Peninsular Malaysia. Journal of Parasitology Research. 2019;**2019**:7903682. DOI: 10.1155/2019/7903682

[8] Ashrafi K, Bargues MD, O'Neill S, Mas-Coma S. Fascioliasis: A worldwide parasitic disease of importance in travel medicine. Travel Medicine and Infectious Disease. 2014;**12**:636-649

[9] Vázquez AA, Alda P, Lounnas M, Sabourin E, Alba A, Pointier J-P, et al. Lymnaeid snails hosts of *Fasciola hepatica* and *Fasciola gigantica* (Trematoda: Digenea): A worldwide review. Centre for Agriculture and Bioscience International. 2018;**13**(62):1-15

[10] Taylor MA, Coop RL, Wall RL. Veterinary Parasitology. 3rd ed. London: John Wiley and Sons Ltd; 2007. p. 874

[11] Abunna F, Asfaw L, Megersa B, Regassa A. Bovine fasciolosis: Coprological, abattoir survey and its economic impact due to liver condemnation at Soddo municipal abattoir, Southern Ethiopia. Tropical Animal Health and Production. 2010;**42**:289-292. DOI: 10.1007/s11250-009-9419-3

[12] Kelly RF, Mazer S, Hartley C, Hamma SM, Ngwa VN, Nkongho EF, et al. Assessing the performance of a *Fasciola gigantica* serum antibody ELISA to estimate prevalence in cattle in Cameroon. BMC Veterinary Research. 2019;**15**:8

[13] World Health Organization. Zoonosis and veterinary public health: Trematodosis [Internet]. 2019c. Available from: https://www.who.int/zoonoses/diseases/trematodosis/en/ [Accessed: 16 November 2019]

[14] Moazeni M, Ahmadi A. Controversial aspects of the life cycle of *Fasciola hepatica*. Experimental Parasitology. 2016;**169**:81-89. DOI: 10.1016/j.exppara.2016.07.010

[15] Ishikawa T, Meier-Stephenson V, Heitman SJ. Biliary obstruction caused by the liver fluke, *Fasciola hepatica*.

CMAJ. 2016;**188**(7):524-526. DOI: 10.1503 /cmaj.150696

[16] Boray JC. Experimental fascioliasis in Australia. Advances in Parasitology. 1969;**8**:95-210

[17] Valero MA, Panova M, Comes AM, Fons R, Mas-Coma S. Patterns in size and shedding of *Fasciola hepatica* eggs by naturally and experimentally infected murid rodents. The Journal of Parasitology. 2002;**88**(2):308-313

[18] Nyindo M, Lukambagire A-H. Fascioliasis: An ongoing zoonotic trematode infection. BioMed Research International. 2015;**2015**:786195. DOI: 10.1155/2015/786195

[19] Andrews SJ. The life cycle of *Fasciola hepatica*. In: Dalton JP, editor. Fasciolosis. 3rd ed. Wallingford: CABI Publishing; 1999. p. 30

[20] Zhang X-X, Cwiklinski K, Hu R-S, Zheng W-B, Sheng Z-A, Zhang F-K, et al. Complex and dynamic transcriptional changes allow the helminth *Fasciola gigantica* to adjust to its intermediate snail and definitive mammalian hosts. BMC Genomics. 2019;**20**:729. DOI: 10.1186/s12864-019-6103-5

[21] Sustainable Control of Parasites (SCOPS). Internal parasites: Liver fluke [Internet]. 2019. Available from: https://www.scops.org.uk/internal-parasites/liver-fluke/lifecycle/ [Accessed: 18 November 2019]

[22] Graczyk TK, Fried B. Development of *Fasciola hepatica* in the intermediate host. In: Dalton JP, editor. Fasciolosis. CABI Publishing; 1999. pp. 31-46

[23] Rondelaud D, Belfaiza M, Vignoles P, Moncef M, Dreyfuss G. Redial generations of *Fasciola hepatica*: A review. Journal of Helminthology. 2009;**83**:245-254

[24] Valero MA, Perez-Crespo I, Periago MV, Khoubbane M, Mas-Coma S. Fluke egg characteristics for the diagnosis of human and animal fascioliasis by *Fasciola hepatica* and *F. gigantica*. Acta Tropica. 2009;**111**(2):150-159

[25] Carrique-Mas JJ, Bryant JE. A review of foodborne bacterial and parasitic zoonoses in Vietnam. EcoHealth. 2013;**10**(4):465-489

[26] Rahman MH, Begum N, Alim A. Factors for the development of Furcocercus and other cercariae in snails and their release. Bangladesh Veterinarian. 1997;**14**:29

[27] Dodangeh S, Daryani A, Sharif M, Gholami S, Kialashaki E, Moosazadeh M, et al. Freshwater snails as the intermediate host of trematodes in Iran: A systematic review. Epidemiol Health. 2019;**41**:e2019001. DOI: 10.4178/epih.e2019001

[28] Hotez PJ, Savioli L, Fenwick A. Neglected tropical diseases of the middle east and north africa: Review of their prevalence, distribution, and opportunities for control. PLoS Neglected Tropical Diseases. 2012;**6**(2):e1475

[29] Centre for Disease Control. *Fasciola*: Epidemiology and risk factors [Internet]. 2018b. Available from: https://www.cdc.gov/ parasites/fasciola/epi.html [Accessed: 19 November 2019]

[30] World Health Organization. Food-borne trematode infections: Fascioliasis epidemiology [Internet]. 2019d. Available from: https://www.who.int/foodborne_trematode_infections/fascioliasis/fascioliasis_epidemiology/en/ [Accessed: 19 November 2019]

[31] Elelu N, Ambali A, Coles GC, Eisler MC. Cross-sectional study of *Fasciola gigantica* and other trematode infections of cattle in Edu

local government area, Kwara state, North-Central Nigeria. Parasites & Vectors. 2016;**9**:470. DOI: 10.1186/s13071-016-1737-5

[32] Dida GO, Gelder FB, Anyona DN, Matano A-S, Abuom PO, Adoka SO, et al. Distribution and abundance of schistosomiasis and fascioliasis host snails along the Mara River in Kenya and Tanzania. Infection Ecology & Epidemiology. 2014;**4**:24281. DOI: 10.3402/iee.v4.24281

[33] Mochankana ME, Robertson ID. A retrospective study of the prevalence of bovine fasciolosis at major abattoirs in Botswana. Onderstepoort Journal of Veterinary Research. 2016;**83**(1):a1015. DOI: 10.4102/ojvr.v83i1.1015

[34] Nyirenda SS, Sakala M, Moonde L, Kayesa E, Fandamu P, Banda F, et al. Prevalence of bovine fascioliasis and economic impact associated with liver condemnation in abattoirs in Mongu district of Zambia. BMC Veterinary Research. 2019;**15**:33. DOI: 10.1186/s12917-019-1777-0

[35] Keiser J, Sayed H, El-Ghanam M, Sabry H, Anani S, El-Wakeel A, et al. Efficacy and safety of Artemether in the treatment of chronic fascioliasis in Egypt: Exploratory phase-2 trials. PLoS Neglected Tropical Diseases. 2011;**5**(9):e1285. DOI: 10.1371/journal.pntd.0001285

[36] Elshraway NT, Mahmoud WG. Prevalence of fascioliasis (liver flukes) infection in cattle and buffaloes slaughtered at the municipal abattoir of El-Kharga, Egypt. Veterinary World. 2017;**10**(8):914-917. DOI: 10.14202/vetworld.2017.914-917

[37] Magaji AA, Ibrahim K, Salihu MD, Saulawa MA, Mohammed AA, Musawa AI. Prevalence of fascioliasis in cattle slaughtered in Sokoto Metropolitan Abattoir, Sokoto, Nigeria. Advances in Epidemiology. 2014;**2014**:247258. DOI: 10.1155/2014/247258

[38] Karshima SN, Maikai B, Kwaga JKP. Helminths of veterinary and zoonotic importance in Nigerian ruminants: A 46-year meta-analysis (1970-2016) of their prevalence and distribution. Infectious Diseases of Poverty. 2018;**7**:52. DOI: 10.1186/s40249-018-0438-z

[39] Ekong PS, Juryit R, Dika NM, Nguku P, Musenero M. Prevalence and risk factors for zoonotic helminth infection among humans and animals - Jos, Nigeria, 2005-2009. The Pan African Medical Journal. 2012;**12**:6

[40] Yatswako S, Alhaji NB. Survey of bovine fasciolosis burdens in trade cattle slaughtered at abattoirs in north-Central Nigeria: The associated predisposing factors and economic implication. Parasite Epidemiology and Control. 2017;**2**:30-39

[41] Isah UM. Studies on the prevalence of fascioliasis among ruminant animals in northern Bauchi state, North-Eastern Nigeria. Parasite Epidemiology and Control. 2019;**3**:e00090

[42] Shinggu PA, Olufemi OT, Nwuku JA, Baba-Onoja EBT, Iyawa PD. Liver Flukes Egg Infection and Associated Risk Factors in White Fulani Cattle Slaughtered in Wukari, Southern Taraba State, Nigeria. Advances in Preventive Medicine. 2019;**2019**:2671620. 5p. DOI: 10.1155/2019/2671620

[43] Ibironke AA, Fasina FO. Socio-economic implications of bovine liver rejection in a major abattoir in South-Western Nigeria. Revista de Ciências Agrárias. 2010;**33**:2

[44] Afolabi OJ, Olususi FC. The prevalence of Fascioliasis among slaughtered cattle in Akure, Nigeria. Molecular Pathogens. 2016;**7**(1):1-5. DOI: 10.5376/mp.2016.07.0001

[45] Abraham JT, Jude IB. Fascioliasis in cattle and goat slaughtered at Calabar abattoirs. Journal of Biology, Agriculture and Healthcare. 2014;**4**(18):34-40

[46] Eze NC, Briggs AA. Prevalence of Fascioliasis and histopathology of the liver in cattle slaughtered in Port Harcourt Abbatoir, Rivers state Nigeria. World News of Natural Sciences. 2018;**16**:105-116

[47] Njoku-Tony RF, Okoli GC. Prevalence of fascioliasis among slaughter sheep in selected abattoirs in Imo State, Nigeria. American Journal of Science. 2011;**7**(2):361-366

[48] Anyaegbunam LC, Ajana U. *Fasciola hepatica* infestation in slaughtered cow liver in Eke Uli market abattoir, Ihiala local government area of Anambra State, Nigeria. Tropical Journal of Applied Natural Sciences. 2017;**2**(1):21-24

[49] Malkhazova SM, Mironova VA, Kotova TV, Shartova NV, Orlov DS. Natural-focal diseases: Mapping experience in Russia. International Journal of Health Geographics. 2014;**13**:21. DOI: 10.1186/1476-072X-13-21

[50] Pavlovsky EN. Fundamentals of the theory of natural focality of transmissible human diseases. Zhurnal Obshcheĭ Biologii. 1946;**7**(1):3-33

[51] Korenberg EI. Natural focality of infections: Current problems and prospects of research. The Biological Bulletin. 2010;**37**(7):665-676. DOI: 10.1134/S1062359010070010

[52] Reisen WK. Landscape epidemiology of vector-borne diseases. Annual Review of Entomology. 2010;**55**:461-483. DOI: 10.1146/annurev-ento-112408-085419

[53] World Health Organization. Food-borne trematode infections [Internet]. 2019e. Available from: https://www.who.int/foodborne_trematode_ infections/en/ [Accessed: 19 November 2019]

[54] Mas-Coma S, Esteban JG, Bargues MD. Epidemiology of human fascioliasis: A review and proposed new classification. Bulletin of the World Health Organization. 1999;**77**:340-346

[55] Mas-Coma S, Bargues MD, Valero MA. Human fascioliasis infection sources, their diversity, incidence factors, analytical methods and prevention measures. Parasitology. 2018:1-35. DOI: 10.1017/S0031182018000914

[56] Mas-Coma S, Valero MA, Bargues MD. Climate change effects on trematodiases, with emphasis on zoonotic fascioliasis and schistosomiasis. Veterinary Parasitology. 2009;**163**:264-280

[57] Houghton JT, Jenkins GJ, Ephraums JJ, editors. Scientific Assessment of Climate Change. Report of Working Group I of the Intergovernmental Panel of Climate Change (IPCC). Cambridge: Cambridge University Press; 1990. p. 357

[58] Lafferty KD, Porter JW, Ford SE. Are diseases increasing in the ocean? Annual Review of Ecology, Evolution, and Systematics. 2004;**35**:31-54

[59] Cattadori IM, Haydon DT, Hudson PJ. Parasites and climate synchronize red grouse populations. Nature. 2005;**433**:737-741

[60] Olsen A, Frankena K, Bødker R, Toft N, Thamsborg SM, Enemark HL, et al. Prevalence, risk factors and spatial analysis of liver fluke infections in Danish cattle herds. Parasites & Vectors. 2015;**8**:160. DOI: 10.1186/s13071-015-0773-x

[61] Marcos LA, Maco V, Samalvides F, Terashima A, Espinoza JR, Gotuzzo E.

Risk factors for Fasciola hepatica infection in children: A case-control study. Transactions of the Royal Society of Tropical Medicine and Hygiene. 2006;**100**(2):158-166. DOI: 10.1016/j.trstmh.2005.05.016

[62] Rahman AKMA, Islam SKS, Talukder MH, Hassan MK, Dhand NK, Ward MP. Fascioliasis risk factors and space-time clusters in domestic ruminants in Bangladesh. Parasites & Vectors. 2017;**10**:228. DOI: 10.1186/s13071-017-2168-7

[63] Esteban JG, Flores A, Angles R, Mas-Coma S. High endemicity of human fascioliasis between Lake Titicaca and La Paz valley, Bolivia. Transactions of the Royal Society of Tropical Medicine and Hygiene. 1999;**93**:151-156

[64] Esteban JG, Gonzalez C, Curtale F, Muñoz-Antoli C, Valero MA, Bargues MD, et al. Hyperendemic fascioliasis associated with schistosomiasis in villages in the Nile Delta of Egypt. The American Journal of Tropical Medicine and Hygiene. 2003;**69**:429-437

[65] Zumaquero-Rios JL, Sarracent-Perez J, Rojas-Garcia R, Rojas-Rivero L, Martinez-Tovilla Y, Valero MA, et al. Fascioliasis and intestinal parasitoses affecting schoolchildren in Atlixco, Puebla State, Mexico: Epidemiology and treatment with nitazoxanide. PLoS Neglected Tropical Diseases. 2013;7(11):e2553

[66] Oladele-Bukola MO, Odetokun IA. Prevalence of bovine fasciolosis at the Ibadan Municipal Abattoir, Nigeria. African Journal of Food Agriculture Nutrition and Development. 2014;**14**(4):9055-9070

[67] Kiran S, Asma'US T. Prevalence of fascioliasis among animals slaughtered at Sokoto state Abattoir. International Journal of Malaria and Tropical Diseases. 2017;**1**(11):059-062

[68] World Health Organization. The management of bloody diarrhoea in young children (unpublished document). Bulletin of the World Health Organization. 1995;**73**(3):397-401

[69] Sharma RL, Godara R, Thilagar MB. Epizootiology, pathogenesis and immunoprophylactic trends to control tropical bubaline fasciolosis: An overview. Journal of Parasitic Diseases. 2011;**35**(1):1-9. DOI: 10.1007/s12639-011-0025-8

[70] Beesley NJ, Caminade C, Charlier J, Flynn J, Hodgkinson JE, Martinez-Moreno A, et al. Fasciola and fasciolosis in ruminants in Europe: Identifying research needs. Transboundary and Emerging Diseases. 2018;**65**(Suppl 1):199-216. DOI: 10.1111/tbed.12682

[71] Dixit AK, Pooja D, Sharma RL. Immunodiagnostic/protective role of Cathepsin L cysteine proteinases secreted by Fasciola sp.—A review. Veterinary Parasitology. 2008;**154**:177-184

[72] Garg R, Yadav CL, Kumar RR, Banerjee PS, Vatsya S, Godara R. The epidemiology of fasciolosis in ruminants in different geo-climatic regions of North India. Tropical Animal Health and Production. 2009;**41**:1695-1700

[73] Jezek J, El Ridi R, Salah M, Wagih A, Aziz HW, Tallima H, et al. *Fasciola gigantica* cathepsin L proteinase-based synthetic peptide for immunodiagnosis and prevention of sheep fasciolosis. Biopolymers. 2008;**90**(3):349-357

[74] Martınez-Perez JM, Robles-Perez D, Rojo-Vazquez FA, Martınez-Valladares M. Immunological features of LPS from *Ochrobactrum intermedium* on sheep experimentally infected with *Fasciola hepatica*. Research in Veterinary Science. 2014;**97**:329-332

[75] Martınez-Sernandez V, Muino L, Perteguer MJ, Garate T, Mezo M, Gonzalez-Warleta M, et al. Development and evaluation of a new lateral flow immunoassay for serodiagnosis of human fasciolosis. PLoS Neglected Tropical Diseases. 2011;**5**:e1376

[76] Sarkari B, Khabisi SA. Immunodiagnosis of human fascioliasis: An update of concepts and performances of the serological assays. Journal of Clinical and Diagnostic Research. 2017;**11**(6):OE05-OE10. DOI: 10.7860/JCDR/2017/26066.10086

[77] Martınez-Perez JM, Robles-Perez D, Rojo-Vazquez FA, Martınez-Valladares M. Comparison of three different techniques to diagnose *Fasciola hepatica* infection in experimentally and naturally infected sheep. Veterinary Parasitology. 2012;**190**:80-86

[78] Robles-Perez D, Martınez-Perez JM, Rojo-Vazquez FA, Martınez-Valladares M. The diagnosis of fasciolosis in feces of sheep by means of a PCR and its application in the detection of anthelmintic resistance in sheep flocks naturally infected. Veterinary Parasitology. 2013;**197**:277-282

[79] Martınez-Valladares M, Rojo-Vazquez FA. Loop-mediated isothermal amplification (LAMP) assay for the diagnosis of fasciolosis in sheep and its application under field conditions. Parasites & Vectors. 2016;**9**:73-77

[80] Soliman MFM. Epidemiological review of human and animal fascioliasis in Egypt. Journal of Infection in Developing Countries. 2008;**2**(3):182-189

[81] Fairweather I. Reducing the future threat from (liver) fluke: Realistic prospect or quixotic fantasy? Veterinary Parasitology. 2011;**180**(1-2):133-143. DOI: 10.1016/j.vetpar.2011.05.034

[82] Elelu N, Eisler MC. A review of bovine fasciolosis and other trematode infections in Nigeria. Journal of Helminthology. 2018;**92**(2):128-141. DOI: 10.1017/S0022149X17000402

[83] Fairweather I, Boray JC. Fasciolicides: Efficacy, actions, resistance and its management. The Veterinary Journal. 1999;**158**:81-112

[84] Boray J, Crowfoot P, Strong M, Allison J, Schellenbaum M, Von Orelli M, et al. Treatment of immature and mature *Fasciola hepatica* infections in sheep with triclabendazole. The Veterinary Record. 1983;**113**:315-317

[85] World Health Organization. Report of the WHO Informal Meeting on use of triclabendazole in fascioliasis control [Internet]. 2007. Available from: http://www.who.int/neglected_diseases/preventive chemotherapy/WHO_CDS_NTD_PCT_2007.1.pdf [Accessed: 18 December 2019]

[86] Mas-Coma S, Bargues MD, Valero MA. Diagnosis of human fascioliasis by stool and blood techniques: Update for the present global scenario. Parasitology. 2014;**141**:1918-1946

[87] Olaechea F, Lovera V, Larroza M, Raffo V, Cabrera R. Resistance of *Fasciola hepatica* against triclabendazole in cattle in Patagonia (Argentina). Veterinary Parasitology. 2011;**178**(3-4):364-366

[88] Ortiz P, Scarcella S, Cerna C, Rosales C, Cabrera M, Guzman M, et al. Resistance of *Fasciola hepatica* against Triclabendazole in cattle in Cajamarca (Peru): A clinical trial and an *in vivo* efficacy test in sheep. Veterinary Parasitology. 2013;**195**(1-2):118-121. DOI: 10.1016/j.vetpar.2013.01.001

[89] Winkelhagen AJS, Mank T, de Vries PJ, Soetekouw R. Apparent

Triclabendazole-resistant human *Fasciola hepatica* infection, the Netherlands. Emerging Infectious Diseases. 2012;**18**(6):1028-1029

[90] Keiser J, Utzinger J. Emerging foodborne trematodiasis. Emerging Infectious Diseases. 2005;**11**(10):1507-1514

[91] Parkinson M, O'Neill SM, Dalton JP. Endemic human fasciolosis in the Bolivian Altiplano. Epidemiology and Infection. 2007;**135**(4):669-674

[92] Torgerson P, Claxton J. Epidemiology and control. In: Dalton JP, editor. Fasciolosis. 1st ed. Wallingford: CABI Publishing; 1999. pp. 113-149

[93] Gboeloh LB. Seasonal prevalence of *Fasciola gigantica* in slaghter cattle in major abattoirs in port-Harcourt. Advances in Agriculture, Sciences and Engineering Research. 2012;**2**:336-340

[94] Aliyu AA, Ajogi IA, Ajanusi OJ, Reuben RC. Epidemiological studies of *Fasciola gigantica* in cattle in Zaria, Nigeria using coprology and serology. Journal of Public Health. 2014;**6**:85-91

[95] Damwesh SD, Ardo MB. Detection of *Fasciola gigantic* antibodies using Pourquier ELISA kit. Sokoto Journal of Veterinary Sciences. 2013;**11**:43-48

[96] Molina-Hernández V, Mulcahy G, Pérez J, Martínez-Moreno Á, Donnelly S, O'Neill SM, et al. Fasciola hepatica vaccine: We may not be there yet but we're on the right road. Veterinary Parasitology. 2015;**208**(1-2):101-111. DOI: 10.1016/j.vetpar.2015.01.004

[97] Jayaraj R, Piedrafita D, Dynon K, Gramsc R, Spithill TW, Smooker PM. Liver fluke vaccines: Vaccination against fasciolosis by a multivalent vaccine of recombinant stage-specific antigens. Procedia in Vaccinology. 2010;**2**(1):82-85. DOI: 10.1016/j.provac.2010.03.015

[98] Sajid M, McKerrow JH. Cysteine proteases of parasitic organisms. Molecular and Biochemical Parasitology. 2002;**120**(1):1-21

[99] Grams R, Vichasri-Grams S, Sobhon P, Upatham ES, Viyanant V. Molecular cloning and characterization of cathepsin L encoding genes from *Fasciola gigantica*. Parasitology International. 2001;**50**(2):105-114

[100] Irving JA, Spithill TW, Pike RN, Whisstock JC, Smooker PM. The evolution of enzyme specificity in Fasciola spp. Journal of Molecular Evolution. 2003;**57**(1):1-15

[101] Beckham SA, Law RHP, Smooker PM, Quinsey NS, Caffrey CR, McKerrow JH, et al. Production and processing of a recombinant Fasciola hepatica cathepsin B-like enzyme (FhcatB1) reveals potential processing mechanisms in the parasite. Biological Chemistry. 2006;**387**:1053-1061. DOI: 10.1515/BC.2006.130

[102] Dowd AJ, Smith AM, McGonigle S, Dalton JP. Purification and characterisation of a second cathepsin L proteinase secreted by the parasitic trematode *Fasciola hepatica*. European Journal of Biochemistry. 1994;**223**(1):91-98

[103] Toet H, Piedrafita DM, Spithill TW. Liver fluke vaccines in ruminants: Strategies, progress and future opportunities. International Journal for Parasitology. 2014;**44**(12):915-927. DOI: 10.1016/j.ijpara.2014.07.011

Chapter 13

Impact of Covid-19 on Agricultural System and Food Prices: The Case of India

Pradyot Ranjan Jena, Rajesh Kalli and Purna Chandra Tanti

Abstract

The present study focused on evaluating the impact of Covid-19 lockdown on the agriculture system in India. A telephonic interview was conducted with farmers among various states between April to May 2020. A total of 494 farmers participated in the survey identifying the challenges they faced during the lockdown. First, the study has outlined the knowledge and perception of respondents on the Covid-19 virus and second the impact of Covid 19 induced restrictions on the agricultural system and food prices in India has been analyzed. The study classified the impact of lockdown on the agriculture system into four broad classifications - Farm Inputs, Farm Produce and Supply Chain, Agriculture and Allied Activities, Pandemic and Food prices. The detailed analysis across these four dimensions is discussed. Due to the shutdown of many supply routes, the availability of agricultural inputs such as fertilizer and seeds was disrupted, which jeopardized farmers' investment planning. Furthermore, the seasonal migrants who would work in urban areas enter off-season and return to their native villages for farming could not carry it on. Such a rapid chain of events created massive short-run income shortages for small and marginalized farmers across the country. The special economic package for agriculture empowerment announced by the Government of India in the tune of two lakh crore rupees, equivalent to ten per cent of India's GDP, has been the government's first response to deal with this agricultural crisis. Finally, the chapter puts forward policy suggestions to strengthen resource-poor farmers' capabilities plagued with a low-income-low-yield vicious cycle.

Keywords: COVID 19, Lockdown, Agriculture Supply Chain, Farmers Income, Food Security, Risk Assessment, Healthcare

1. Introduction

The impact of the Covid-19 on the global economy is highly devastating. The increased restriction among the nations has disrupted the economic activities causing a significant decline in economic growth [1]. The previous pandemic outbreaks were limited to certain regions (Spanish flu and Ebola). However, the spread of the Covid-19 virus was evidenced in more than 215 countries worldwide [2]. Given its deepening threat to human lives and economies, there is a need to understand the pandemic's impact on different sectors. Agriculture is one such sector that is certain to face the brunt of the crisis [2, 3]. The global trade came to be suspended, causing a threat for most of the agriculture exporting countries. With government interventions in place, the agriculture trade continued to be

IntechOpen

flat during the lockdown. The scenarios of both export and import restrictions on Agri-commodity were evidenced among major economies [4]. Few economies restricted imports to control the spread of the virus. Subsequently, these restrictions were eased for the movement of goods, while prices of staple food crops increased and a fall in prices was noted in high-value agricultural produce. Supply chain disruptions caused an immense impact on the agriculture sector of all the countries [5, 6]. This disruption leads to a decline in the income source of rural livelihood. A shortfall in the movement of agricultural produce increased the food insecurity threat among most of the developing nations.

In India, more than 80% of rural livelihood directly or indirectly depends on the agriculture sector. Food security and self-sufficiency are the main goals of

Time line (2020)	Cases	Deaths	Events	Lock down
January – February	1		Kerala Govt. declared state calamity	
1st - 16th March	2	1	Odisha declared Disaster and Delhi Govt declares closure of Educational Institutes	
March 22nd	360		14-hour 'Janata curfew'	
March 25th	606	10	A nationwide lockdown was imposed till April 14th	Lockdown 1.0
March 31st	1397	37		
April 14th	10, 000		Lockdown extended till May 3rd	Lockdown 2.0
April 29th	31,787	1008		
May 1st			Lockdown extended till May 17th	Lockdown 3.0
May 17th			Lockdown extended till May 31st	Lockdown 4.0
May 31st	1,82,143	5164		
June 8th				Unlock 1.0
June 30th	5,66,840	16,893		
July 1st				Unlock 2.0
July 31st	16,38,870	33,747		
August 1st				Unlock 3.0
August 31st	36,21,245	64,469		
September 7th				Unlock 4.0
September 30th	62,25,763	97,497		Unlock 5.0
October 31st	8,137,119	1,21,641		
November 30th	9,431,691	1,37,139		
December 31st	10,266,674	1,48,738		

Table 1.
Presents the timeline of events in India due to Covid–19 outbreak.

the Indian agriculture. The major problem in India's agriculture sector is the inefficient market system and complex supply chain issues. The movement of crops from production centers to the markets is challenging with increased players in the supply chain [7, 8]. It has been highlighted by researchers repeatedly the need for adequate storage facilities (cold storage and warehouse) and facilitating the movement of food crops without any considerable wastes [5]. The recent COVID 19 pandemics is certain to expose this bottleneck and adds additional stress to the existing crisis in the agriculture sector. The early assessment of the pandemic impact on agriculture looks profound [2, 3, 5–13]. However, disaggregated studies will provide insights for a better policy response. Boosting agricultural productivity and maximizing farm income is the critical pathway policymakers should focus on in the aftermath of the current pandemic. Against this backdrop, the present study evaluates the challenges faced by the agriculture sector for an appropriate policy response. This leads to some important questions- what was the impact of Covid-19 induced lockdowns on agriculture operations? How did it impact in terms of the income from both agriculture and its allied activities? how did the agriculture markets and food prices behave during the pandemic outbreak? The study explores the following questions using a qualitative framework, where farmer respondents are the primary source of information. Globally, restrictions were imposed to avoid the spread of the Covid-19 pandemic. **Table 1** presents the timeline of events in India due to Covid–19 outbreak. In India, a complete lockdown was first initiated from 24 March 2020 to 14 April 2020 and extended till 31 May 2020. By the end of the lockdown, the total reported cases in India were 1,82,143, with casualties of 5164. Due to fewer reported cases and low causalities, the government re-opened the economic activities with guidelines to prevent further outbreaks.

2. Materials and methods

The Covid-19 induced lockdown has a differential impact on the agriculture system in India. With restricted economic activity, the aggregate demand and supply shrank, causing a ripple effect on employment and income. This prolonged lockdown could become a larger economic crisis, especially in the primary sector of the economy. The agro-based economies found difficult in all the stages, where the availability of inputs (fertilizers, pesticides, labor, and seeds), logistics and supply chain challenges, farm operations, and allied agricultural activities are impacted in various ways. To understand these effects, the study collected information from different regions in the country. The authors focused on the follow-up interviews from the previously available baseline dataset of farmers [14, 15]. Due to the severity of the pandemic and the restriction to travel imposed by the government, field visits were not feasible. Thus, we conducted telephonic interviews with nearly 494 farmers from different states of India. The discussion with the farmers was for the period between April and May 2020. The study administered a pre-structured questionnaire (attached in appendix) involving farmers perception of the Covid-19 pandemic and its impact on farm operations, accessibility to markets, credit availability, other income sources, and support from the government. descriptive statistics Table have been included in the appendix to show the summary of the surveyed household. The study also reviewed major literature focused on the pandemic's impact on agriculture, which includes scientific articles (both quantitative and qualitative), reports from state and national level government agencies, media articles, and reports from various international agencies (World Bank, IMF). In this current situation, there is a need to ameliorate the agriculture sector, which has been lacking for many years; apparently, the direction towards sustainable development is slow in the Indian context. Against this backdrop, we outline several prima facie challenges and urge to formulate appropriate policy responses for sustainable development in the agriculture sector.

3. Results and discussion

3.1 The impact of COVID 19 on agricultural operations

The exposure to digital and social media has created awareness about the Covid-19 pandemic among the rural community. The farmers indicated their knowledge of the pandemic and its likely consequences. They expressed that precautionary measures have been instructed to them by various organizations. However, they noted their limited ability to follow these measures among the rural community. Though the respondents were aware of the precautionary measures such as washing hands using sanitiser, wearing a mask, and social distancing, they did not follow these measures thinking that Covid-19 is only an urban problem. Few farmers reported that hardly 10 to 20% in their villages followed the precautionary measures.

The agriculture sector in India faced an unprecedented challenge during the Covid-19 pandemic outbreak; the study classified four broad concerns highly experienced by the majority of the farmers. Each of these challenges is discussed in the following sections.

3.1.1 Farm inputs

The agricultural system in India varies due to its large and diversified topographic characteristics, climate, and soil. The onset of monsoon begins at the end of May in southern India. By the end of April, farmers start preparing the land and build inventory for the upcoming Kharif season. The imposed restriction created a shortage of fertilizers, pesticides, herbicides, and seeds in several regions of the country. For instance, districts in the northern interior region of Karnataka faced a huge shortfall in fertilizer, especially urea in May [16]. A similar shortage of inputs was noted in the districts of Maharashtra and Odisha [17, 18]. Several reports also cited that traders stocked up the fertilizers for higher price realization due to the lockdown. The major reason for the unavailability of the fertilizer was the restrictions imposed by the government. More than 50% of the respondents complained that disruption in the supply chain caused unavailability of at least one kind of input (For example Urea, DAP, NPK, Seeds, Sprayers, and others). This shortage also led to delay in cultivation in some regions. Further, farmers reported that even government outlets were shut down due to a shortage of fertilizer availability. Nearly 35% of the respondents expressed that they paid additional money (50 to 80% higher prices) to purchase fertilizer. However, after the initial 21 days of the first phase of lockdown, government announced the relaxation to the farm operation. This helps in building up the inventory related to farm inputs among the farming community. Though the relaxation was provided, the confusion in the implementation process caused jittery among farmers several other inputs.

The credit crunch faced by the farmers was observed from the survey due to a steep decline in agriculture prices and restriction to market access. The burden of cash flow and high labour costs caused additional stress among the farming community. Farmers hold agriculture produce for a shorter period for better price realization, while lockdown, procurement in the wholesale market was limited. This caused a glut of agricultural produces among farmers leading to a liquidity crunch to purchase the inputs for the next growing season. In the past, small farmers used to migrate to nearby towns after rabi season to form capital for the upcoming Kharif season. However, with the closure of economic activities, most of the part-time migrant laborers had to return to the villages without enough capital for the next farming season. The return of the full-time migrant workers from the urban locality caused an additional burden among the families without any source of income. Though the availability of the labourers increased in the rural community with the addition of the migrant workers, the employment creation or the farm activities involving labours decreased due to the financial constraint among the large and medium-scale farmers. The mismatch in the wages was also evident, where the migrant workers demanded higher wages. Few of the large-scale farmers reported that they used tractors and machinery due to increased labour wages. Few of the respondents owning large farmland reported that some of the lands were left barren due to increased input cost.

3.1.2 Farm produce and supply chain

The cropping pattern in India varies among the states. During March and April, rabi crop harvesting will be at its peak among major states. The pandemic outbreak coincided during this time causing a significant effect on farm production. Due to lockdown, farmers could not complete land preparation and provide irrigation on time, which caused a negative impact on crop productivity. The farmers from Uttar Pradesh and Bihar reported that wheat harvesting was in the process and they were worried about the increased restrictions due to the pandemic. Additionally, hailstorms and unseasonal rain destroyed the standing crops like green gram and black gram, where harvesting was delayed due to restriction. The primary survey on farmers in India reported that 24% of the respondents did not harvest due to lockdown-related reasons (price instability and transport cost) [19]. A similar discussion was evident from the present survey, as farmers from northern India reported that harvesting was delayed due to lower prices in the market. Farmers in southern India faced a similar problem in terms of vegetables and fruits. A significant setback was evident in the case of Mango, where harvesting and the pandemic-induced lockdown coincided during the same timeline. Additionally, mango cultivators in southern Indian states were hit drastically due to restricted travel bans, shut down in developed markets (delayed exports), and a shortage of labourers. A significant reduction in the tune of 26% was noted in the arrival of mangoes in the market during 2020–2021 compared to the previous calendar year [20]. Perishable agricultural products were more affected compared to non-perishable goods. Crops such as wheat can be stored, while perishable goods such as vegetables and fruits significantly impacted the pandemic outbreak. Farmers during the interview from all the regions said a significant loss in the cultivation of vegetables. The farmers who cultivate vegetables reported that they were left unharvested in the field due to lower demand, significant fall in the farmgate prices, and lack of market access. The lockdown restricted both interstate and intrastate movement of the vehicles resulting in disruptions in the supply chain of the vegetables and fruits. Further, increased transport charges also played a significant role in the stoppage of vegetables to reach the urban market. Though the government announced few relaxations for the movement for the vegetables in the later stage, ineffective operations in the vegetable warehouses and the limited procurement from the government caused a significant decline in the arrival of vegetables in the market. Due to low prices and no procurement in the market, farmers dumped their vegetables and fruits on the road [21]. Farmers during our discussion reported that disruption in the supply chain had led to selling the vegetables in the nearby villages, where the market prices were so low that the revenue did not cover the input cost. Furthermore, the export of vegetables and fruits was reduced by 70% in India during March 2020 and May 2021 with increased freight charges by the airline cargo companies [22].

3.1.3 Agriculture and allied activities

Agricultural allied activities such as horticulture, fishery, forestry, dairy, and floriculture generate additional income for the farming community. As discussed earlier, India is the largest producer and exporter of mango and mango pulp. The food processing industries which process mango were shut down and import was banned by major economies. This created a significant effect on the mango food chain. Similarly, India's milk supply chain, which follows a complex structure with many verticals, was disrupted due to the pandemic outbreak. The procurement by the co-operatives fell due to weak demand for dairy-related products. Moreover, the closure of the restaurants and other businesses (bakery, sweet shops, and tea par-lour) had a significant impact on the dairy industry. Farmers reported that milk was distributed among the neighbors due to weak demand in the village collection center. Farmers indicated their concern about the payment of the loans availed for the dairy business. In most regions of India, farmers avail themselves of financial support from the Self-help groups to initiate dairy farms. This is highly fragmented, where farmers own a minimum of 2–3 cows. This led to a decline in non-farm income from the dairy business and created additional stress for the repayment of the financial support.

Farm laborers who work in construction or small business enterprise in agricultural off-seasons became unemployed due to the lockdown that created an

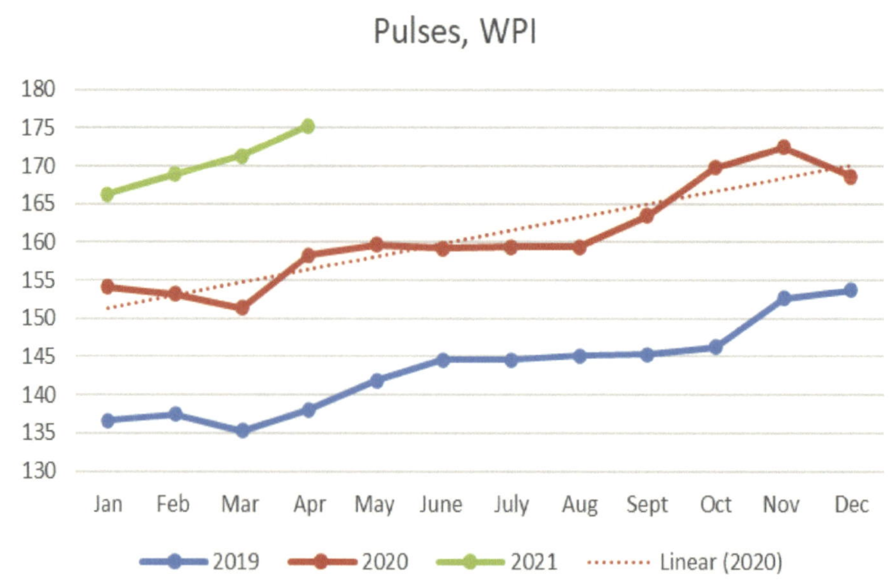

Figure 1.
Pulses WPI.

additional burden on the rural economy. Most of the daily wage laborers reported that the Government financial support was helpful, while few others complained of not getting benefits from the direct benefit transfer scheme initiated by the Government of India. The poultry sector experienced the biggest impact due to the pandemic. The projected estimate shows a loss of INR 22500 crore in the poultry sector [23]. The huge disruption in the farm inputs of poultry was also evidenced and a sharp increase in the prices can be noted due to disruption in the supply chain. Farmers in the telephonic interview stated that rumors about poultry being a source of the spread of coronavirus has declined the prices of the poultry to the

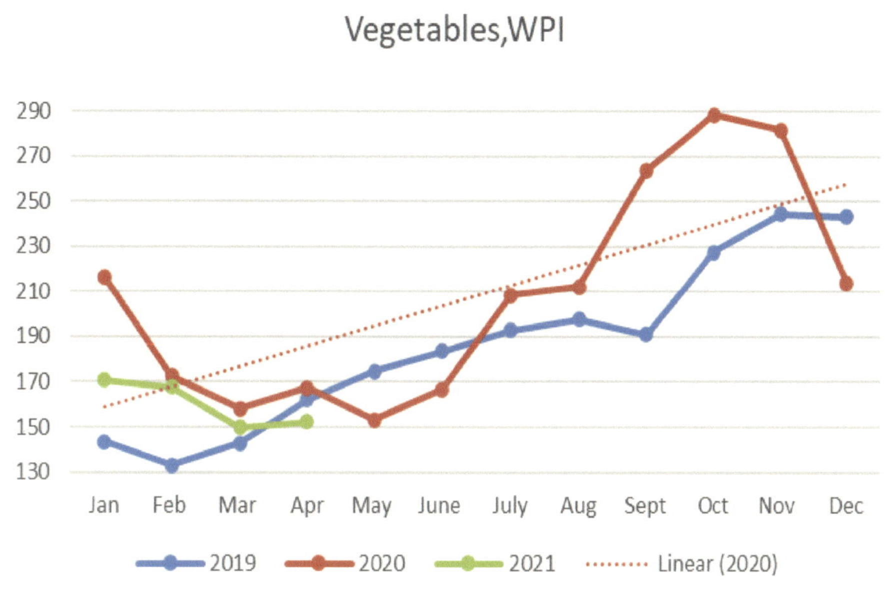

Figure 2.
Vegetables WPI.

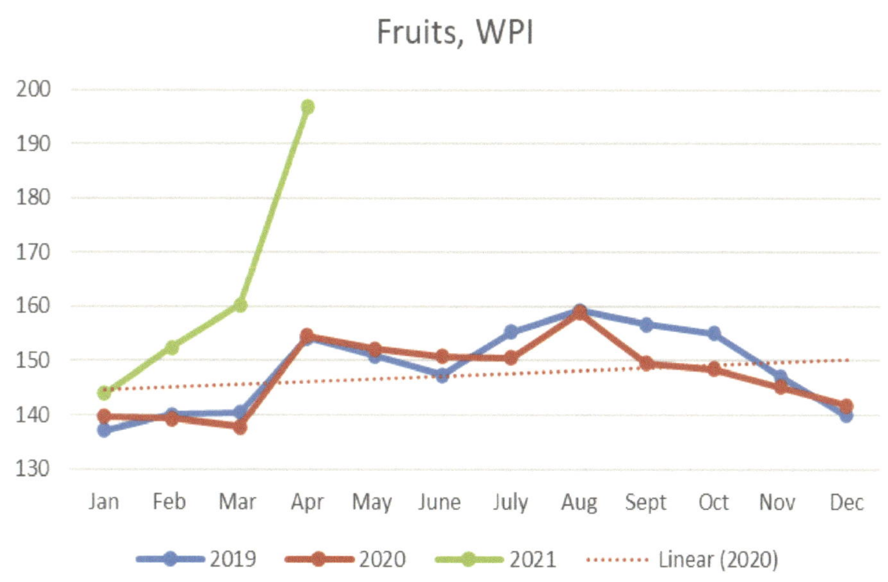

Figure 3.
Fruits WPI.

bare minimum in the rural localities. The farmers reported that the whole chicken bird was sold at Rs. 10 (0.14 USD) in the villages. It was observed from the respondents that the small and marginal farmers lost a monthly average income of INR 10000 to 30000.

3.1.4 Pandemic and food prices

The global food prices of agriculture fell drastically with weak demand [20]. Prices of corn decreased considerably due to a decline in the demand for gasoline [24].

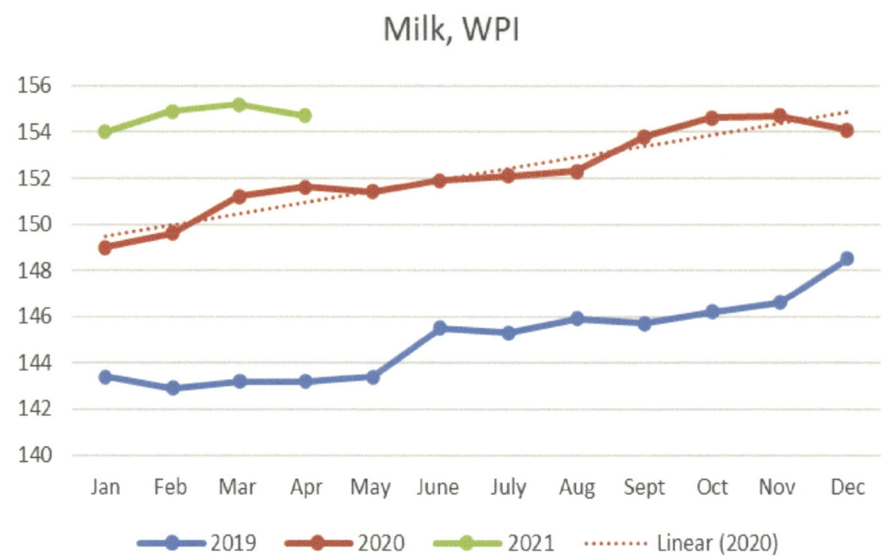

Figure 4.
Milk WPI.

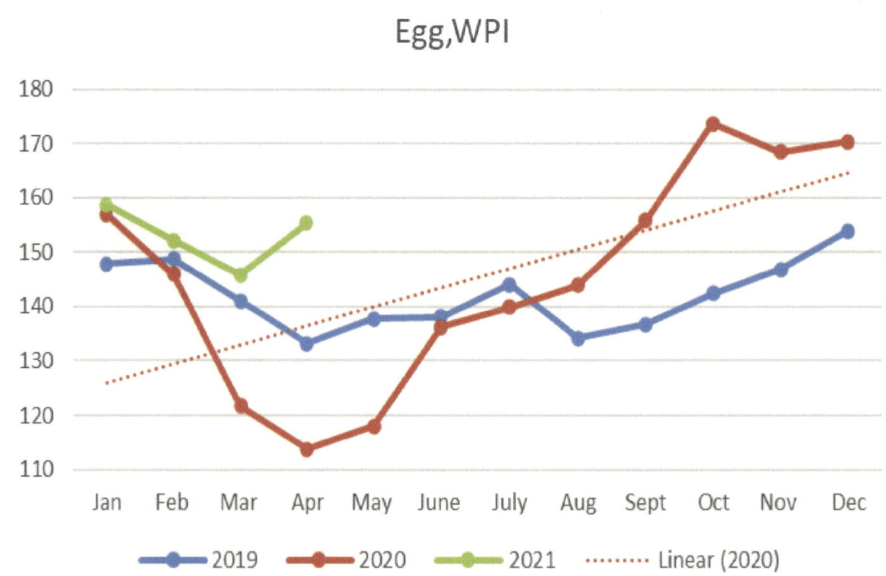

Figure 5.
Egg WPI.

Similarly, demand and supply fell drastically in the Indian context which led to a fall in the prices of agri-commodities. A decline in mandi prices was evident for most of the products. In most cases, wholesale prices have declined, and retail prices were on an upward trend. This phenomenon of the increased retail price was associated with the imposed restriction and increased transaction cost for the retailers. The daily prices analysis by the Reserve Bank of India (RBI), for 22 essential food items indicated that retail food prices rose by 2.3% from March to

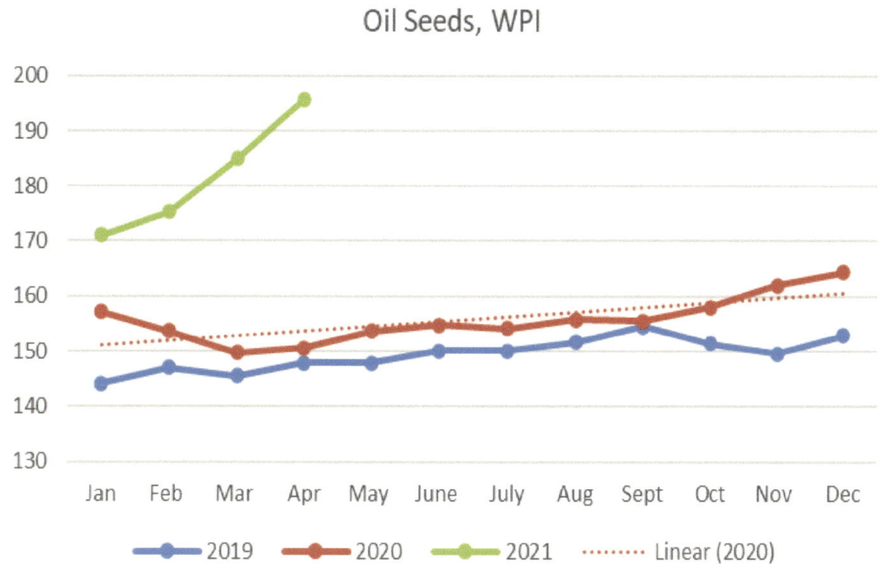

Figure 6.
Oilseeds WPI.

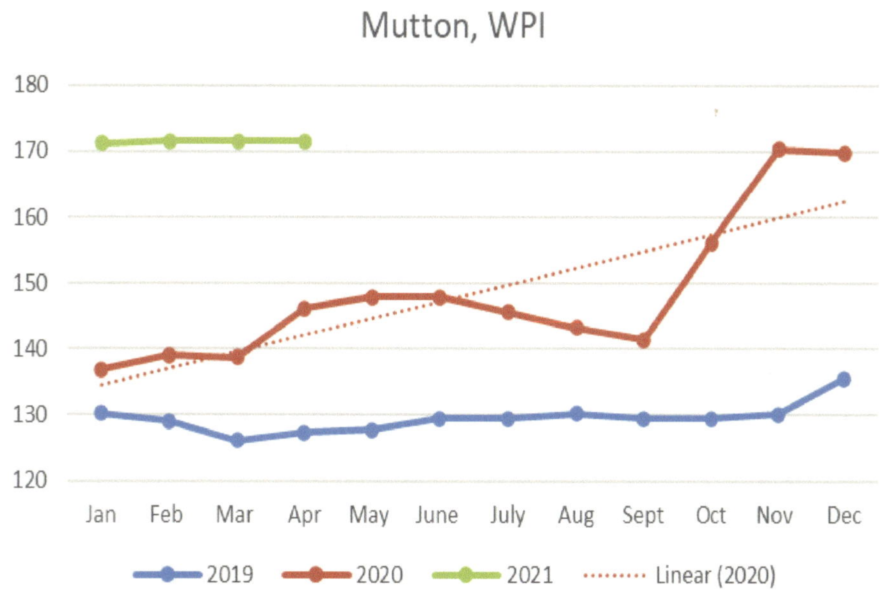

Figure 7.
Mutton WPI.

April 13, 2020 [25]. However, on a large-scale price were risen at the end consumer side, farmers saw a steep decline in the farmgate prices. Especially, in the case of vegetables and fruits, which are perishable, the farmgate price declined due to the unavailability of the transport. Farmers from the survey indicated that prices of the vegetables fell more than 50%, where they could not recover the cost of production. Due to the restriction and fewer transport vehicles, the transaction cost increased, which decreased the significant margin for the farmers in

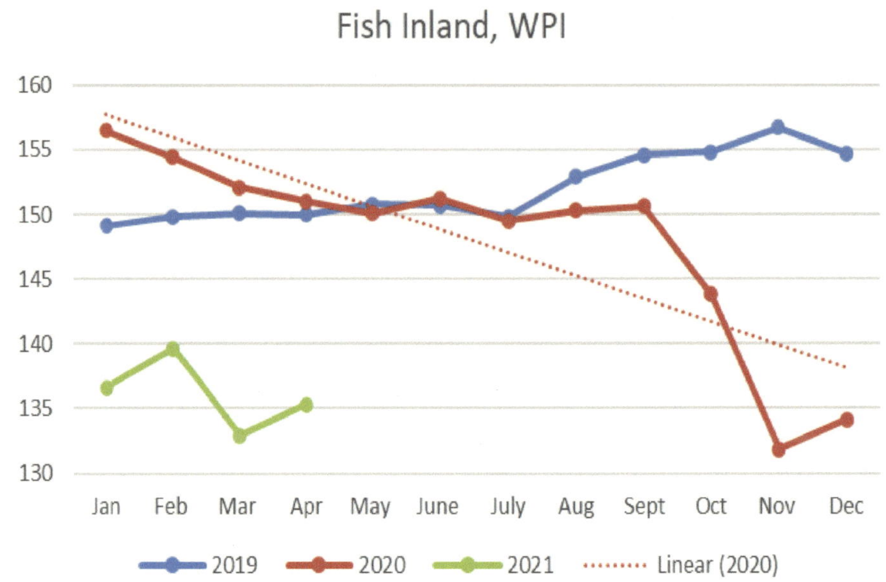

Figure 8.
Fish inland WPI.

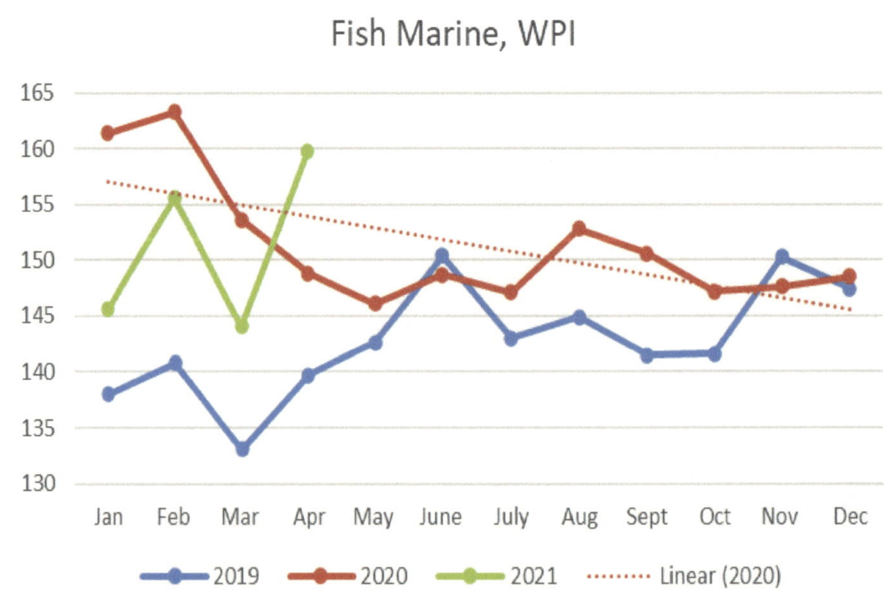

Figure 9.
Fish marine WPI.

vegetables and fruits. The wholesale price index (WPI) showed a rising trend in March and April only for pulses, fruits, milk, and beef due to the procurement by the agriculture marketing board, while in the case of cereals, a decline in WPI and increase in consumer price index (CPI) is noted [20]. This variation in the WPI and CPI was due to disruption in the supply chain and supply-side shocks. The government initiated the necessary movement of the crops from the procurement states and distributed them effectively. The prices of the fruits increased due to

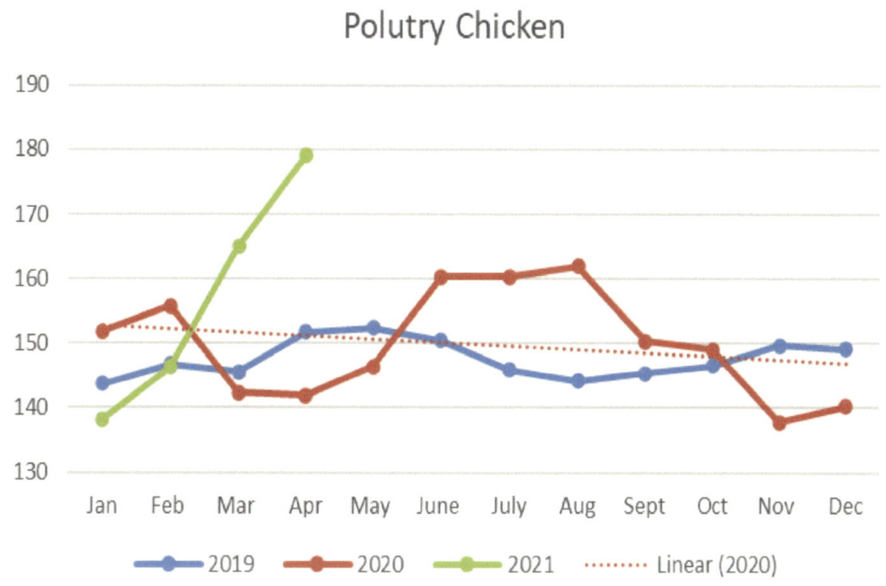

Figure 10.
Poultry Chicken.

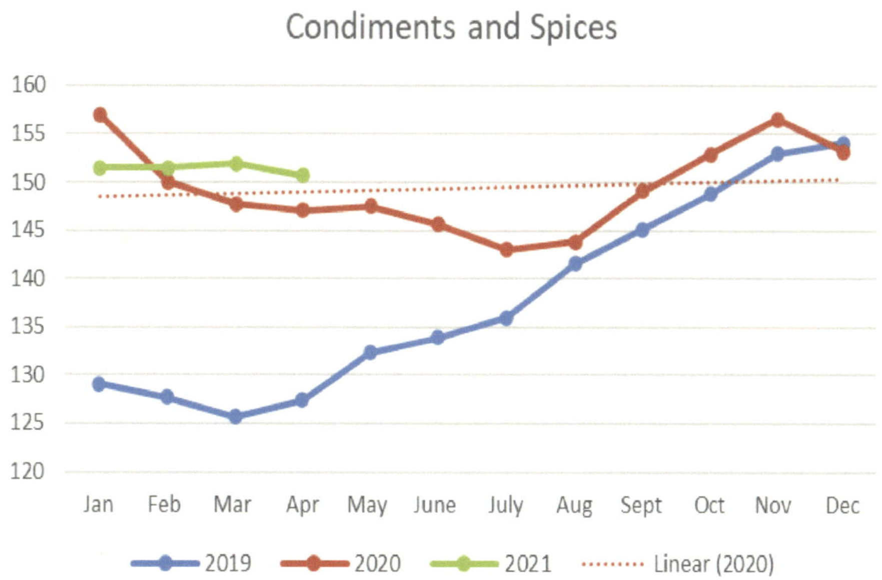

Figure 11.
Condiments and spices WPI.

supply chain disruptions, especially, apple and mango. Milk prices were hiked by Rs. 2 to 3 per liter by private dairy organizations [20]. **Figures 1–14** presents the Wholesale Price Index (WPI) of thirteen products – Cereals, Pulses, Vegetables, Fruit, Milk, Egg, Oil seeds, Mutton, Condiments and Species, Fish inland, Poultry Chicken, Wheat, and Paddy from January 2019 to April 2021. The WPI of vegetables and eggs fell drastically, where the revival of demand was evidenced post unlocking the lockdown from July 2020. The WPI of the pulses has steadily increased from the time of the pandemic outbreak, i.e., March 2020.

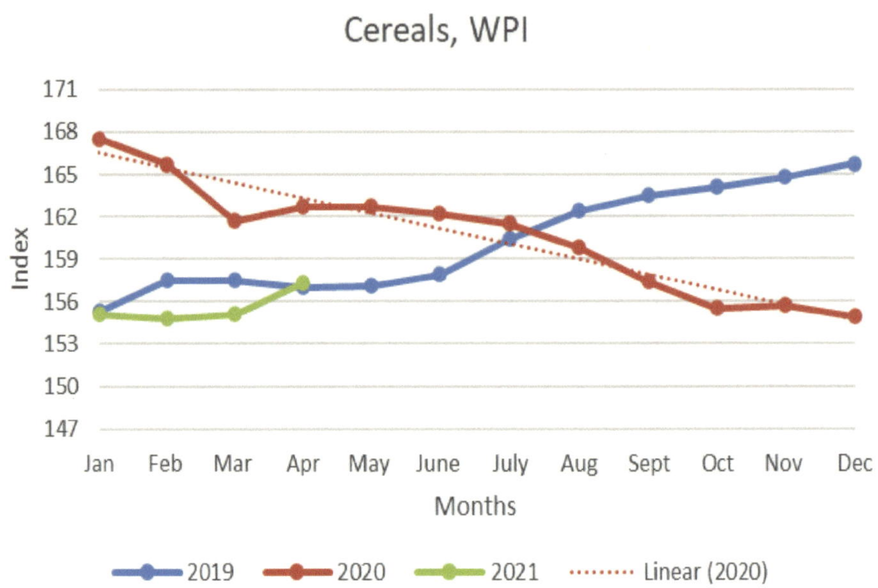

Figure 12.
Cereals WPI.

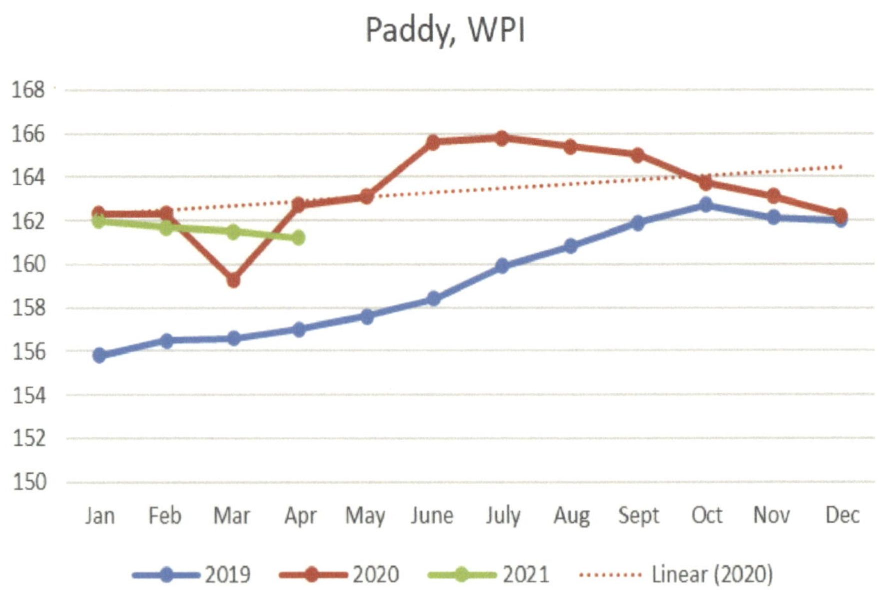

Figure 13.
Paddy WPI.

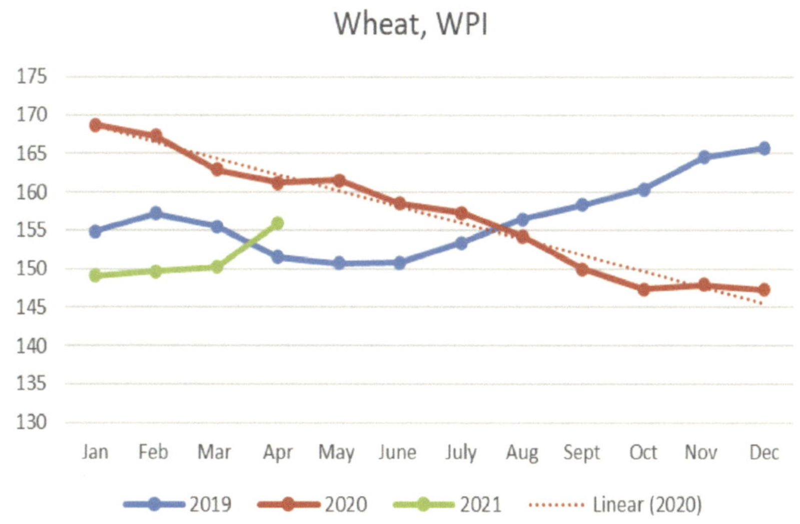

Figure 14.
Wheat WPI.

4. Review of government assistance during COVID 19 for farmers

The government relaxed the restrictions imposed due to the pandemic outbreak from April 14, 2020, for the agriculture sector after the first phase of lockdown. Though farming activities were restored in all the states, farmers were unsure about investment decisions due to the unavailability of inputs, price shocks in agro commodities, and liquidity crunch. ICAR (Indian Council of Agriculture Research) issued guidelines for farming activities with physical distance and hygiene standards. The government took several resilient measures to cope up with the current pandemic. Under the public distribution scheme, food grain was freely provided to the families below the poverty line. The scheme was successfully implemented among the states and demonstrated a strong response from the government during the crisis. Nearly 90% of the respondents from the survey indicated that they received food grains free of cost and helped them. Further, the government disbursed nearly Rs. 18253 crores under Pradhan Mantri Kisan Samman Nidhi, each farmer received Rs 6000 per year as minimum income support. Pradhan Mantri Kisan Samman Nidhi was highly recognized among the respondents from the survey. They also indicated that schemes involving Direct Benefit Transfer are beneficial, as they receive money directly to their account. Further, the government announced several measures for the farming community – Rs. 16.3 Lakh-Million package for Agriculture and Allied Sectors as stimulus packages. The fund was allocated to agriculture infrastructure projects at farm-gate and aggregation points. The main aim was to restructure the post-harvesting management infrastructures and maintain an effective value chain. The government also reported that nearly three crore farmers with agricultural loans totalling Rs. 4,22,113 crore availed the benefit of the three-month loan moratorium announced by the Reserve Bank of India.

To reduce the disruption in the supply chain, the government announced special assistance for the transportation of crops from a surplus area to a deficit area to maintain the availability of food items. The "Kisan Rath" app was launched to connect traders and farmers. The application was developed to facilitate transportation by connecting farmers to traders to sell food grains, especially perishable goods, during the lockdown. The government initiated a special financial package for agri-processing units to strengthen them during the crisis. Kisan Credit Cards (KCC) was issued to provide financial support to farmers at low interest rates. Approximately 25 lakh new KCC beneficiaries were sanctioned with a loan of Rs 2.5 lakh-Million. Other central agencies also launched rescue measures; for example, the Reserve Bank of India has directed banks to provide crop loans at 2% interest concession for the repayment from the borrowers for the extended period of 31 May 2020. NABARD also extended financial support of Rs. 29500 crores to cooperative banks and RRBs to support the agriculture sector. The government allocated Rs. 40000 crores under Mahatma Gandhi National Rural Employment Guarantee Act (MGNREGA) scheme. MGNREGA is the world's biggest livelihood scheme ensuring the "Right to work" for the rural people. The northern states such as Uttar Pradesh and Bihar saw huge inward migrants due to the suspension of the economic activities among the urban locality. To employ these migrant labourers, the central government announced to allocate a higher proportion of the budgeted money from the MGNREGA to the states with the higher recipient of migrant workers. This would act as additional income for the migrant workers until the economy stabilizes.

5. Conclusion and policy implications

COVID-19 has plunged the agricultural sector in India into certain vulnerabilities. The findings from the study show that farmers faced operational difficulties in the agriculture system. The disruption in the supply chain induced a significant fall in farmgate prices. Perishable food items, in particular, had a significant negative impact as the restrictions became longer over the months in the second quarter of 2020. Lack of accessibility to selling points of the crops and increased transport rates were the major concern among the farmers. This delay in the sale of agricultural products caused a capital crunch among the farmers to purchase inputs for the upcoming season. The non-availability of the farm inputs compounded this distress among the farming community. The migrant labor increased the burden on the rural livelihoods. In the past, migrant workers supported their families in the rural economy, which was lost due to the subsequent unemployment of these workers in urban areas. The addition of labor in the rural areas has increased in the wages among a few communities and dropped in the wages among a few others.

The lessons from the pandemic can help solve the issues in the agriculture system in India. Market access and better price realization are the long-standing issues in the Indian agriculture sector. Strengthening market access is an immediate policy concern for the governments. Reliable transport and logistics solutions need to be the primary goal to reduce further vulnerabilities in the sector. The government focused on several measures to support the farmers during the crisis. The poor infrastructure in the farm sector needs to be addressed. Being an agriculture-based economy, the cold storage chain and warehouses need to be upgraded, where an efficient cold storage chain network can enhance the market of fresh vegetables and fruits in the international market encouraging exports. Handling the Public Distribution Scheme (PDS) by reducing wastage and proper storage would be highly beneficial. At the same time, extending the financial support that emphasizes agribusiness (cold chain, warehouse, grading and standardization, food processing industries) could make agriculture self resilient. Ensuring employment in the rural areas is an utmost priority, while the MGNREGA needs to be efficiently administered and implemented in the districts with high migrant inflow.

Acknowledgements

This work is funded by the Indian Council of Social Science Research, Ministry of Education, Government of India, Grant Number (F.No.-02/25/GEN/2017-18/RP/Major).

Appendix 1

Questionnaire

Farmers during COVID19 Pandemic Lockdown: Fears and perception about their situation in the coming days?

---

1. Basic Details.

Name of the Farmer:
Social Category: Gen/SC/ST/OBC.
Gender: Male/Female.
Age:
Education.
Village:
Block:
District:
Mobile Number:
Number of Members in a Family:
Primary Income Source: Agriculture/Agriculture Labour/Business/Service/Self Employed.
Secondary Income Source: Agriculture/Agriculture Labour/Business/Service/ Self Employed.
Annual Family Income: <1 Lakh.
Between 1 lakh to 5 lakh
>5 Lakh

---

2. Cropping Details:

Crop Pattern: Mono/Multiple.

Crop Names:	Area	Starting Month	Harvesting Month	Current Status of Crop in April Month

3. Knowledge and Perception on COVID 19.

Q: Do you know about the Corona Virus Spread in Our Country? (Yes/No/Does not Know).

Q: Are you worried about the Current Pandemic? (Yes/No/Does not Know).
If yes, give three reasons for your worry –.
1.
2.
3.

Q: Whether the current Lockdown has an adverse impact on your farming activity? (Yes/No/Does not Know).

Q: If yes, how has it affected? Give three reasons –.
1.
2.
3.

Q. What is the intensity of the effect of the lockdown on your Farming Activity? (Greatly/Moderately/Neutral/No Impact).

Q: Do you feel the decision of lockdown is correct for farmers? (Yes/No).

Q: Are precautionary measures issued by the regulations are followed in your village? (Yes/No).

4. Effect of Lockdown on Agricultural Activities.

Q: Whether market opening time is overlapping with your farming time? (Yes/No).

Q: Are you in fear to go to the market due to infectious diseases? (Yes/No).

Q: Whether input dealer is charging high price during lock down?

Q: Is there access to agricultural mechanization? (Yes/No).

Q: Are you getting sufficient labour for Farming activities? (yes/No).

Q: Whether labour cost is high during Lockdown? (Yes/No).

Q: Have you started harvesting pulses/cereal (Yes/No).

If No, why not?

Q: Do hail storms and Kala Baisakhi adversely effecting your final crop due to lock down? (Yes/No).

Q: Is there excess harvesting of vegetables but no demand due to Lockdown? (Yes/No).

If yes, what will be your plan to sell them? Please explain.

Q: Whether your crops damaged due to lack of transportation to home? (Yes/No).

Q: Are you facing difficulties with cash in hand for production or labour payment? (Yes/No).

Q: Whether money lenders are charging high interest during Lockdown? (Yes/No).

Q: Whether the harvesting period is getting delayed?

Please explain.

Q: Is there any problem to prepare input seeds for next season?

Please explain.

5. Effect on Agribusiness during Lock down.

Q: where you used to sell your product before lock down? (Local market/ nearest town/ Govt Mandi/Middle man/...).

Q: Where are you selling now your product after lockdown? (Local market/ nearest town/ Govt Mandi/Middle man/........................).

Q: Is there any changes in the selling price due to lock down? (yes/No).

Q: If yes than what is the price changes? (Increased price/decreased price/ Constant) and by what percentage roughly?

Q: What is the basic problem of selling your product in the market?

a. Not selling at a desirable price

b. not more buyers/ short period of selling time

c. no cold storage to keep the excess product

d. No transport facility to export outside village

e. No government mandi to purchase at desirable rate

Q: What are the Fears of Famers during Lockdown for COVID19?

a. Expecting Increase in Input Price

b. Damage of the perishable product

c. Low price and loss

d. Fail to repay the current loan

e. Labour shortage during Harvesting

f. Fail to prepare field for next season

g. Going to loss agricultural labour works

6. Government Aid and support.

Q: What is the monetary and non-monetary support from Government so far after lockdown?

1.
2.
3.

Q. Are you aware of any schemes that the Government has announced for you after lockdown?

If yes, what are they?

1.
2.
3.

Q: What are the Government Aids provided during Lock down?

DTI (Direct Transfer of Income in Rs)
Additional PDS (Public Distribution System)
Loan waiver
Assured Market Place
Govt Sabji Mandi
Transport facility
Others

Appendix 2

Descriptive Statistics.

Variable	Mean	Std. Dev.	Min	Max
Total Area Owned	3.073	2.964	0	22
Farming experience	26.137	12.468	1	65
Age	50.863	11.688	18	82
Member in SHG	0.711	0.454	0	1
Member in NGO	0.079	0.27	0	1
Member in Govt Extension	0.70	0.459	0	1
Migration	0.261	0.44	0	1
Education	8.349	5.477	0	17
Member in Cooperative Society	0.281	0.45	0	1
Household Size	4.902	1.654	1	11
Total Sample 494				

Authors Own Creation.

Author details

Pradyot Ranjan Jena[1*], Rajesh Kalli[2] and Purna Chandra Tanti[1]

1 School of Management, National Institute of Technology Karnataka, Mangalore, Karnataka, India

2 Department of Management Studies, Madanpalle Institute of Technology and Science, Madanpalle, India

*Address all correspondence to: pradyotjena@nitk.edu.in

References

[1] Jena Pradyot Ranjan, Majhi R, Kalli R, Managi S, Majhi B. Impact of COVID-19 on GDP of major economies: Application of the artificial neural network forecaster. Economic Analysis and Policy. 2021:69: 324-339.

[2] Deaton BJ, Deaton BJ. Food security and Canada's agricultural system challenged by COVID-19. Canadian Journal of Agricultural Economics. 2020:1-7. DOI: https://doi.org/10.1111/cjag.12227.

[3] Troskie D. Impact of covid-19 on agriculture and food in the western cape. Working document. 2020.

[4] WTO. Export Prohibitions and Restrictions. World Trade Organisation. [Internet]. 2020. Available from: https://www.wto.org/english/tratop_e/covid19_e/export_prohibitions_report_e.pdf. [Accessed: 2021-06-01]

[5] Hobbs JE. Food supply chains during the COVID-19 pandemic. Canadian Journal of Agricultural Economics.2020:1-6. DOI: https://doi.org/10.1111/cjag.12237.

[6] Richards TJ, Rickard B. COVID-19 impact on fruit and vegetable markets. Canadian Journal of Agricultural Economics. 2020:1-6. DOI: https://doi.org/10.1111/cjag.12231.

[7] Gray RS. Agriculture, transportation, and the COVID-19 crisis. Canadian Journal of Agricultural Economics. 2020:1-5. DOI: https://doi.org/10.1111/cjag.12235.

[8] Mahendra Dev S, Sengupta R. Covid-19: Impact on the Indian Economy. Working Paper 2020-013.

[9] Barichello R. The COVID-19 Pandemic: Anticipating its Effects on Canada's Agricultural Trade. Canadian Journal of Agricultural Economics. 2020:219-224. DOI: https://doi.org/10.1111/cjag.12244

[10] Brewin, D. The impact of COVID-19 on the grains and oilseeds sector. Canadian Journal of Agricultural Economics. 2020:2:185:188. DOI: https://doi.org/10.1111/cjag.12239

[11] Hailu, G. Economic thoughts on COVID-19 for Canadian food processors. Canadian Journal of Agricultural Economics 2020:1-7. DOI: https://doi.org/10.1111/cjag.12241

[12] Ker AP. Risk management in Canada's agricultural sector in light of COVID-19. Canadian Journal of Agricultural Economics. 2020:1-8. DOI: https://doi.org/10.1111/cjag.12232

[13] Richards A, Martin PL. editors Migration, mechanization, and agricultural labor markets in Egypt. In Migration, Mechanization, and Agricultural Labor Markets in Egypt. 2019. DOI: https://doi.org/10.4324/9780429047107.

[14] Khosla S, Jena PR. Can Rural Livelihood Programs Dent Vulnerability to Poverty? Empirical Evidence from an Eastern Indian State, In: Proceedings of the International Seminar on Rural Development in Asia-Pacific Region, NIRDPR, Guwahati, India; August 24-28, 2020; Guwahati

[15] Tanti PC Jena, PR. Adoption of Climate-Smart Technologies in Agriculture: Evidence from an Eastern Indian State. In:31st International Conference of Agricultural Economists (ICAE), 17- 31 August 2021; New Delhi *(forthcoming)*

[16] The Times of India. Shortage of urea troubles farmers hoping to reap a bumper harvest. The Times of India. [Internet]. 2020. Available from: https://timesofindia.indiatimes.com/city/

bengaluru/shortage-of-urea-troubles-farmers-hoping-to-reap-a-bumper-harvest/articleshow/77561858.cms. [Accessed: 2021-06-01].

[17] The Indian Express. Farmers complain of urea shortage, state govt says problems in supply. The Indian Express. [Internet]. 2020. Available from: https://indianexpress.com/article/cities/mumbai/farmers-complain-of-urea-shortage-state-govt-says-problems-in-supply-6506564. [Accessed: 2021-06-01]

[18] The New Indian Express. Farmers struggle with fertilizer shortage; Odisha government remains oblivious. The New Indian Express. [Internet]. 2020. Available from: https://www.newindianexpress.com/states/odisha/2020/aug/17/farmers-struggle-with-fertiliser-shortage-odisha-government-remains-oblivious-2184364.html. [Accessed: 2021-06-01]

[19] Jaacks Lindsay M, Veluguri D, Serupally R, Roy A, Prabhakaran P, Ramanjaneyulu GV, Impact of the COVID-19 pandemic on agricultural production, livelihoods, and food security in India: baseline results of a phone survey. Food security. 2021:1-17.

[20] Ramkumar R. Agriculture and the Covid-19 Pandemic: An Analysis with special reference to India. Review of Agrarian Studies. 2020:10: 2369-2020-1856.

[21] The Hindu. Why do farmers resort to dumping produce? The Hindu. [Internet]. 2020. Available from: https://www.thehindubusinessline.com/opinion/why-do-farmers-resort-to-dumping-produce/article31365453.ece. [Accessed: 2021-06-01].

[22] The Economics Times. Fruit, veggie exports fall 70% during lockdown. The Economic Times. [Internet]. 2020. Available from: https://economictimes.indiatimes.com/news/economy/foreigntrade/fruitveggieexportsfall70during lockdown/articleshow/75880957.cms?utm_source=contentofinterest&utm_medium=text&utm_campaign=cppst. [Accessed: 2021-06-01].

[23] India Today. Covid-19: With projected losses of Rs 22,500 crore, Indian poultry sector seeks Centre's intervention. India Today. [Internet]. 2020. Available from: https://www.indiatoday.in/business/story/covid-19-with-projected-losses-of-rs-22-500-crore-indian-poultry-sector-seeks-centre-s-intervent ion-1662872-2020-04-03. [Accessed: 2021-06-01].

[24] Barrons. Corn Prices Could Drop to Their Lowest Levels in More Than a Decade, Hurting Producers. [Internet] Barrons. 2020 Available at: https://www.barrons.com/articles/corn-prices-could-drop-to-lowest-levels-in-more-than-a-decade-51585908001. [Accessed: 2021-06-01]

[25] RBI. Governor's Statement," Reserve Bank of India. [Internet]. 2020. Available from: https://www.rbi.org.in/Scripts/bs_viewcontent.aspx?Id=3853. [Accessed: 2021-06-01]

Section 10

Risk Factors for Opisthorchis Felineus Infection

Chapter 14

The World Largest Focus of the Opisthorchiasis in the Ob-Irtysh Basin, Russia, Caused by *Opisthorchis felineus*

Anastasia V. Simakova, Natalya V. Poltoratskaya, Irina B. Babkina, Tatyana N. Poltoratskaya, Alexander V. Shikhin and Tatyana M. Pankina

Abstract

The world's largest focus of opisthorchiasis caused by cat fluke *Opisthorchis felineus* Rivolta, 1884, is associated with the Ob-Irtysh basin (Russia). The chapter provides data on the history of discovery and the study of opisthorchiasis. Features of the morphology and life cycle of *O. felineus* are described. Data on the infection of intermediate hosts (mollusks and cyprinids fish) are provided. Species of fish that have important epizootological significance are indicated. The incidence of opisthorchiasis in the people of different age and social groups, clinical manifestations, pathogenesis, and complications is discussed. The climatic and social factors that contribute to maintaining the focus of opisthorchiasis are described. The measures of personal and social prevention of the people are given.

Keywords: *Opisthorchis felineus*, history and study, intermediate hosts, important epizootological significance, epizootology and epidemiology, personal and social prevention

1. Introduction

The goal of this work was to assess the current epidemiological and epizootological situations in the world largest focus of opisthorchiasis; to clarify the specific features in its clinical course, pathogenesis, and complications; to determine the natural, climatic, and social factors that enhance preservation of this focus; and to propose an algorithm for preventive activities.

The tasks of this research are to study the epizootological situation and features of the circulation of *Opisthorchis felineus* in the Ob-Irtysh basin, assess the epidemiological situation of opisthorchiasis in Russia, and give recommendations on measures to prevent the disease.

The concept of sustainable development [1] sets the control of unattended diseases as one of the global goals in the area of public health care; these diseases include the helminthic invasions in hyperendemic foci. The ongoing changes in

 IntechOpen

all spheres of production and sale of raw materials and goods have led to serious violations of sanitary rules and norms, which deteriorate the epizootic situation for parasitic invasions in the world.

Opisthorchiasis, the trematodiasis caused by *O. felineus* Rivolta, 1884, is one of the relevant problems in both Russia (with its world largest Ob-Irtysh natural focus) and worldwide despite the implemented prevention measures. The relevance of this problem is determined by both its high incidence among adults and children, severity of the resulting pathology, and its chronic course.

The socioeconomic factors, such as active migration of population, unawareness of opisthorchiasis among the newcomers to the region, poor knowledge about the rules for disinfection of local population, all-year-round consumption of fish, and homemade fish products, increase in the number of amateur fishermen and poachers, and vending of fish and fish products on unauthorized markets creates the conditions for the stable preservation of opisthorchiasis.

One of the major factors that influence the level of *O. felineus* liver fluke invasion is a high rate of fish invasion by its metacercariae. The natural and climatic conditions that have established in the Ob-Irtysh basin support the active opisthorchiasis focus there.

A vast floodplain of the Ob-Irtysh basin, rich in lakes and meadows, and a developed network of first- and second-order tributaries enhance the maintenance of the Bithyniidae mollusks at a high level.

Close coexistence and cohabitation of the first intermediate host and cyprinid fish (second intermediate host) in the same habitats provide the implementation of liver fluke life cycle. In their abundance and species diversity, the cyprinid fish are the leader group in the Ob-Irtysh basin. A high infection rate of the prevalent fish species, which are of important commercial value, with *O. felineus* metacercariae is a major risk factor, influencing the incidence of this disease among local population.

2. Brief history of opisthorchiasis discovery and research

The liver fluke was for the first time described in 1884 by Sebastiano Rivolta, an Italian scientist. He isolated the parasite from the liver of a cat and a dog and named it the liver fluke, *O. felineus*, and the corresponding disease, opisthorchiasis. K.N. Vinogradov, a professor at the Tomsk University, discovered the liver fluke in the human liver in 1891. After the discovery by Vinogradov, human cases of opisthorchiasis were repeatedly recorded in 1892–1929 in Tomsk, Biysk, Novosibirsk, Tyumen oblast, Kuznetsk raion, and other localities. During WWII, a Russian soldier from Siberia died in one of the fascist concentration camps; his autopsy demonstrated 42,000 liver flukes in his liver and pancreas.

As has been observed, the liver fluke is not met far and wide but rather near freshwater bodies. Brown in 1893 assumed that fish consumption is the source of liver fluke infection, which was later (1904) experimentally confirmed by M. Askanazy (Germany). In 1891, Vinogradov postulated the first intermediate host of liver fluke, which was experimentally confirmed by H. Vogel (Germany): he demonstrated that the first intermediate host was the mollusk *Bithynia leachii* (Sheppard, 1823).

The study of opisthorchiasis commences in 1929 after publication of the information that 100 opisthorchiasis patients were admitted to the Tobolsk hospital over 6 months. This initiated organization of specialized helminthological expeditions to the Ob-Irtysh basin, headed by K.I. Skryabin. Numerous experiments have demonstrated that this region houses the largest opisthorchiasis focus. Russian helminthologists under the guidance of Skryabin paid significant attention to the study of *O. felineus* (1927–1929). The liver fluke larvae were for the first time discovered in the muscle of fish individuals inhabiting Siberian water bodies by N.N. Plotnikov and L.K. Zerchaninov in 1932.

All these efforts allowed for discovery of a considerable incidence of opisthorchiasis among people, cats, and dogs along the Irtysh and Ob rivers up to the polar circle. In 1973, a cat was autopsied by an expedition organized by Skryabin in the north of the Tomsk oblast; eight cysts containing liver flukes were found in its liver; one of the cysts, medium in its size (similar to a walnut), contained 654 parasites.

The following scientists contributed to the studies of the epidemic situation of opisthorchiasis: S.D. Titova (publications of 1946–1980), V.S. Myasoedov (publications of 1953, 1959, and 1960), M.P. Miroshnichenko (1954, 1955, and 1956), T.A. Bocharova (1971–2005), G.I. Golovko (1981–1986), and so on. The population migration to the oil and gas areas in the north of the Tomsk oblast increased the attention to this disease [3, 18–22, 24, 43].

3. Life cycle of *O. felineus*

The liver fluke *O. felineus* has an intricate life cycle, which involves three hosts: the definitive host and two intermediate hosts; the life cycle comprises two free-living stages, the egg and cercaria (**Figure 1**).

Infected domestic and wild animals that fed on fish and infected people, which are the definitive host of the liver fluke, are the sources of invasion. One trematode lays approximately 2000 eggs per day. The eggs are not viable when dry and are rapidly killed by sunlight but retain their viability for 15 months in a water body at a temperature of 4–7°C; all eggs die after 29 months [2].

When entering water with human and animal feces, the liver fluke eggs can be ingested with detritus by the first intermediate host, a Bithyniidae (genera *Codiella* and *Opisthorchophorus*) mollusk [2].

In the Ob-Irtysh basin, the mollusks susceptible to the invasion inhabit only standing perennial silt water bodies. The mollusks are unable to migrate for a long distance and form local clusters. Presumably, the infection rate of mollusks depends on the population density and the distance from human dwellings [3].

The infection rate of Bithyniidae mollusks in the upper reaches of Ob and Irtysh rivers within the Altai Krai is 2%, amounts to 6.1% within the Novosibirsk oblast, and varies in the range of 0.3–20.2% in the Irtysh basin in the Omsk oblast [4, 5]. The density of the mollusk population in the floodplain water bodies in the Tomsk oblast is 8100 individuals/m^3; however, the prevalence of invasion is extremely low (3.7%), and the intensity is very high (on the average, 8130 ± 470 cercariae/mollusk). Coinvasions are extremely rare [6]. The infection rate of mollusks in the Tura and Pyshma river floodplains varies from 4 to 9%; the infection characteristics in the Khanty-Mansiysk Autonomous Okrug are also low, to 6.7% [7].

In the mollusk gut, miracidia, free-swimming larvae, hatch from the eggs (**Figure 1**). A miracidium hatched from the egg enters the mollusk body cavity by passing through the gut wall to undergo a regressive metamorphosis there. It loses its larval organs (glands, epidermal plates, cilia, etc.) preserving only the germline cells and protonephridia to change into a mother sporocyst with a length up to 2 mm [2].

Young sporocysts are transversely constricted to give smaller sporocysts, which propagate and form rediae. Rediae are sack-like structures with a large mouth and gut. When leaving the mother sporocyst, rediae migrate to the liver of mollusk to parthenogenetically reproduce.

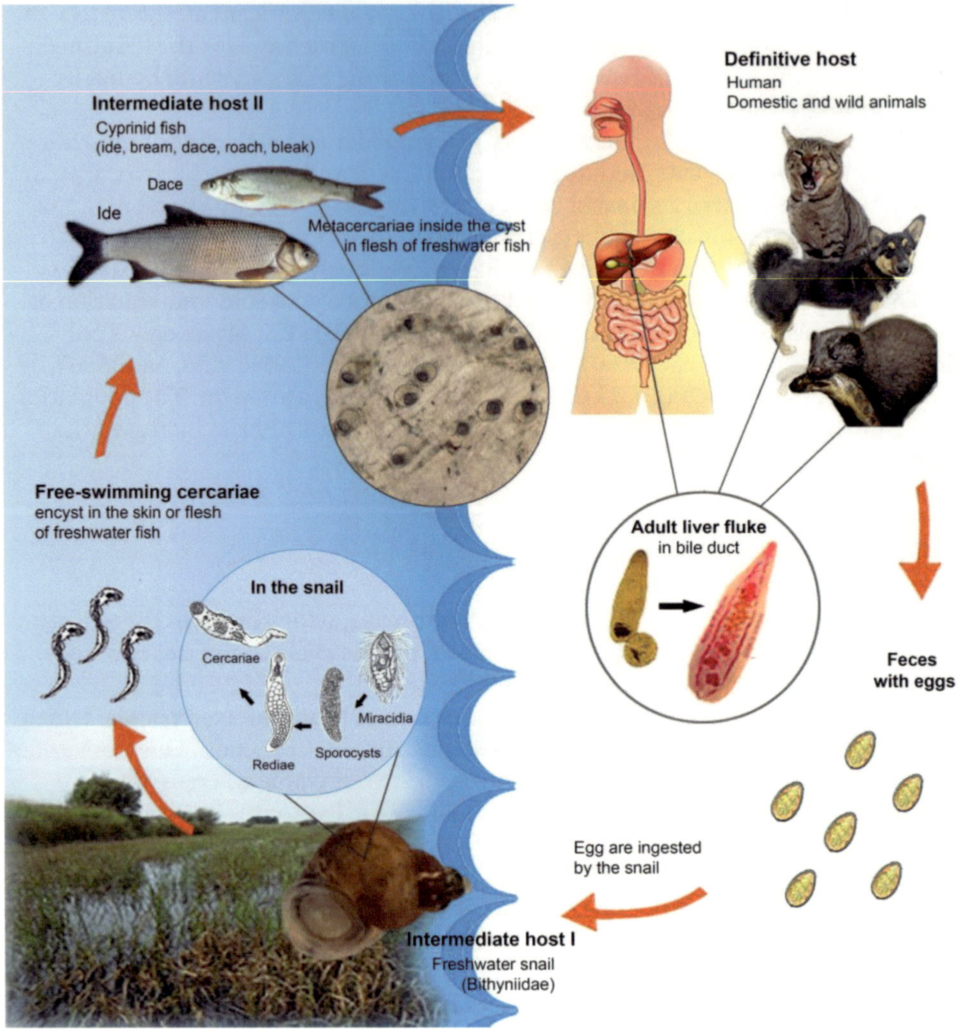

Figure 1.
Life cycle of O. felineus.

In the redia, tailed motile larvae—cercariae—are formed of the germ balls. The developmental stage in the mollusk takes 2–2.5 months (**Figure 1**) [2].

With the maturation, cercariae leave the redia through the pore to migrate in the mollusk body leaving it for water, where they swim for 30–50 h. Up to 3500 cercariae can leave the mollusk during 24 h. The release of cercariae has two peaks, namely a pronounced midsummer peak and a flat spring one [2].

When encountering a cyprinid fish (ide, dace, roach, bream, Siberian roach, Caspian roach, tench, common rudd, common carp, asp, common bleak, etc.), the cercaria attaches to it; detaches its tail; loses its eyes and sensory organs; and penetrates into the muscles to form the inner and outer (a capsule of connective tissue) membranes and to transform into the next phase, metacercaria (**Figure 1**).

The metacercariae have a size of 0.23–0.38 × 0.18–0.28 mm and are very survivable. The metacercariae become invasive 3–6 weeks after entering the fish and now are able to infect the definitive hosts—domestic and wild carnivores and omnivorous animals and humans. Metacercariae retain their viability in the fish body for 1–3 years and even to 9 years according to some data [8].

As is known, only cyprinid species are suitable intermediate hosts for the metacercariae. Approximately 20 species of both aboriginal and alien cyprinid species of commercial or noncommercial value inhabit the rivers and lakes of the Ob-Irtysh basin, the most important fish species of commercial significance are the ide, bream, crucian carp, roach, and, to a lesser degree, dace [2].

The rate of the fish infection by liver fluke metacercariae has been studied with different intensities in different periods. A large volume of data on the prevalence of fish infection in the Ob-Irtysh basin was accumulated in the 1990s to 2000s. Our data and the earlier results suggest high rates of infection of the ide, dace, and roach. The prevalence of ide and dace infection amounted to 20–100% and of roach, 2–80% with the intensity of infection of 1–1780 metacercariae per individual. These fish species are among the major carriers of *O. felineus* metacercariae and significantly contribute to the preservation of the opisthorchiasis focus. In addition, the bream and common bleak, alien species for this region, also appeared to be susceptible to the infection by liver fluke metacercariae and, correspondingly, have been involved in the maintenance and spreading of opisthorchiasis in Western Siberia [8–25].

The definitive hosts are infected orally by consuming the cyprinid fish muscles infected by liver fluke. The metacercarial membrane is finally destroyed in the host stomach, and the young helminth migrates along bile ducts to the liver and gall bladder to reach the sexual maturity in 20–25 days (**Figure 1**) [2].

The intensity of invasion of definitive hosts and their role in maintaining the strength of opisthorchiasis focus are different. As is assumed, in addition to humans who account for 56.6% of the invasion, cats (15.8%), dogs (3.6%), and pigs (to 0.9%) are also significant contributors to opisthorchiasis [26]. The total prevalence of cat invasion in the opisthorchiasis focus of the Khanty-Mansiysk Autonomous Okrug in the 2000s amounted to 48.2% (males were more frequently affected than females). The prevalence of dog invasion was lower, amounting to 17.14% [27]. An analogous study in Novosibirsk demonstrated the total prevalence of cat invasion of 7.9% with the intensity of 69.9 flukes and of dog invasion of 3.4% with the intensity of 23.8 flukes. Males appeared more affected among cats and females among dogs. The invasion parameters increase with animal age [28].

In addition to domestic carnivores, wild carnivores (common fox, wolf, brown bear, lynx, polecat, sable, mink, muskrat, bank vole, and others) also contribute to the liver fluke circulation in natural foci. These animals play different roles in the epizootic process in opisthorchiasis: the animals living in the floodplain and constantly "supplying" the infectious material to the biotopes of the first intermediate host are actual players of the opisthorchiasis circulation in the Ob-Irtysh basin, whereas the remaining animals are potential sources of invasion. In general, foxes and muskrats account for the largest number of invaded wild animals. The rate of invasion in the floodplain of Ob river and its tributaries reaches 77% on the background of a growth in the prevalence characteristics from the upper to lower reaches. The intensity of invasion amounts to 10–500 liver flukes per individual. The invasion of the muskrat in Western Siberia reaches 33% [29]; however, this issue requires further studies.

Thus, a complex multihost life cycle of this parasite enhances its long-term retention in wildlife and preservation of the natural opisthorchiasis focus in the Ob-Irtysh basin.

4. Epidemiology of opisthorchiasis in Russia

Opisthorchiasis is an important social problem in Russia. Two-thirds of the world distribution range of this pathogen concentrates in this country [30]. Opisthorchiasis accounts for approximately 80% of all helminthic diseases. According to the official statistical data, up to 26,000 cases are annually recorded. The actual number of opisthorchiasis patients taking into account the correction factor is 15-fold higher [31].

In total, 106,362 cases of invasion were detected in 2014–2018. The maximum number of cases was recorded in 2014 (25,545 cases) and minimum, in 2017 (18,755 cases). The incidence rate of opisthorchiasis among population in 2018 decreased by 25.3% as compared with 2014, varying from 12.79 to 17.51 per 100,000 population (**Table 1**).

The natural foci of opisthorchiasis are adjacent to the Ob, Irtysh, Ural, Volga, Kama, Don, Dnepr, Severnaya Dvina, and Biryusa rivers [32–42].

Approximately 80% of the opisthorchiasis cases are recorded in the territories adjacent to the Ob, Irtysh, and Tom river basins and their tributaries [43], housing the administrative centers of the Omsk, Novosibirsk, Tyumen, Tomsk, and Kemerovo oblasts and Khanty-Mansiysk and Yamalo-Nenets Autonomous Okrugs. Most part of the local population is affected (80–95%) [44–46]. The total incidence rate over 2014–2018 was 84,331 opisthorchiasis cases, accounting for 79.3% of the total cases in the Russian Federation.

The Khanty-Mansiysk Autonomous Okrug heads the list of percentage of opisthorchiasis incidence (2.6–4.6) followed by Yamalo-Nenets Autonomous Okrug (1.2–2.3%), Novosibirsk oblast (1.1–1.5%), Tomsk oblast (1.0–1.6%), Tyumen oblast (0.9–1.3%), Omsk oblast (0.7–1.0%), Kemerovo oblast (0.5–0.7%), and Altai Krai (0.3–0.5%) [47–51].

The incidence rate of opisthorchiasis in the analyzed regions varies, with the maximum exceeding 1.3–1.8-fold the minimal value. The highest incidence rates are recorded in the hyperendemic regions of Yamalo-Nenets (124.2–226.7) and Khanty-Mansiysk (259.2–461.5) Autonomous Okrugs, Tyumen oblast (90.7–132.2), Tomsk oblast (104.7–158.4), Novosibirsk oblast (112.2–148.8), and Omsk oblast (72.8–103.3). The Kemerovo oblast (49.8–66.23) and Altai Krai (33.09–45.48) are the regions with a high level of invasion. The incidence of opisthorchiasis in these regions severalfold exceeds the mean level for the Russian Federation with the Khanty-Mansiysk Autonomous Okrug heading the list (19–26-fold) followed by Yamalo-Nenets Autonomous Okrug (9–13-fold), Tomsk and Novosibirsk oblasts (7–10-fold), Omsk and Tyumen oblasts (5–8-fold), Kemerovo oblast (3–5-fold), and Altai Krai (2–3-fold).

According to the statistical data for 2014–2018, a decrease in the absolute characteristics and incidence rate was in general observed in all hyperendemic regions, which is explainable by inadequate diagnosing, registration, and recording of the cases as a result of decreased attention to the problem of opisthorchiasis.

Opisthorchiasis is mainly diagnosed among the adult population (over 90% cases in people aged 39–59); however, the level of child morbidity is rather high. Opisthorchiasis has been recorded in all age cohorts of children up to 17 years, with the age cohort of 7–14 years accounting for 60–80% of all cases recorded in children. In the Tomsk oblast, the children to 17 years old are the most affected as compared with other regions (29.7% in 2014–40.8% in 2018). In the mid-Ob river region, opisthorchiasis is detectable in children starting from 3 years (25–30%) with an increase at the age of 12–14 years (50–60%) to 100% in the adults [52]. In the child population of the city of Urai (Khanty-Mansiysk Autonomous Okrug), the most affected cohort is 7–14 (38%) and 14–17 (34%) years old versus 23 and 5% for the cohorts of 3–6 and 2–2 years [53]. An increase in the prevalence of infection among the children of 1–2 years (from 3.8 to 6.1%) is observed in the Tomsk oblast. Cases of opisthorchiasis in the children under 1 year have been recorded in Khanty-Mansiysk Autonomous Okrug (six cases in 2017).

Region of Russian Federation	2018		2017		2016		2015		2014	
	Total*	IR**	Total*	IR**	Total*	IR**	Total*	IR**	Total*	IR**
Russian Federation	19,077	12.99	18,755	12.79	20,846	14.24	22,139	15.15	25,545	17.51
Yamalo-Nenets Autonomous Okrug	838	155.6	666	124.2	766	143.4	875	162.0	1228	226.7
Khanty-Mansiysk Autonomous Okrug	5046	299.6	4309	259.2	4454	272.5	6024	374.0	7370	461.5
Tyumen oblast	1483	98.9	1341	90.7	1384	95.1	1518	106.2	1831	132.2
Tomsk oblast	1129	104.7	1251	116.0	1336	124.1	1557	145.5	1686	158.4
Novosibirsk oblast	3252	116.6	3118	112.2	4109	148.8	3930	143.1	3505	128.3
Kemerovo oblast	1386	51.43	1704	62.91	1800	66.23	1357	49.8	1547	56.58
Omsk oblast	1427	72.8	1450	73.27	1469	74.24	1622	81.99	2035	103.1
Altai Krai	869	36.7	818	34.3	959	40.2	791	33.09	1091	45.48

**Morbidity data according to Form 2 "Data on infectious and parasitic diseases" approved by Order 52 of the Russian Federal State Statistics Service of January 28, 2014.*
***IR is the incidence rate of disease per 100,000 population.*

Table 1.
Absolute values and incidence rate of opisthorchiasis in the Russian Federation and Western Siberian region in 2014–2018.

In 2008–2017, 43 cases of acute opisthorchiasis were recorded in the middle Ob basin. Among those infected, the proportion of women and men was 48.8 and 51.2%, respectively. In terms of age, the maximum number of cases of acute opisthorchiasis was recorded among people aged 20–39 years (74.4%), followed by those aged 40–49 and 50–59 years (9.3% each group), and people aged 15–19 years (7.0%).

The largest number of cases of opisthorchiasis was recorded in May (20.9%) and June (32.6%), and less often opisthorchiasis was recorded in September and November (11.6% each). In other months, the infection was observed sporadically (1–2 cases). In 2008–2017, from 52.8% (2011) to 80.9% (2017) of people with recorded opisthorchiasis underwent dehelmintization (original data).

Since most rural population, including children, are involved in fishing, regular consumption of frozen and slightly salted freshwater fish is widespread; correspondingly, the incidence rate increases with age, and the cases of superinvasion are observable [54, 55].

The morbidity patterns in the municipal entities of autonomous okrugs and oblasts are considerably different. However, the corresponding levels observed in the municipal entities of the north are higher by an order of magnitude. The significant differences in morbidity in different municipal entities of oblasts and autonomous okrugs are associated with different quality of clinical diagnostics, recording, and registration of opisthorchiasis cases rather than with the difference in diet pattern [56]. The facts that the child morbidity rate is higher than that in adults are explainable by that adult population rarer seeks medical help. Since the diet of children and adults does not significantly differ, it is likely that the adult population is highly affected with the prevalence of chronic disease courses [56].

The urban population on the average accounts for 75–78% of the opisthorchiasis cases [31, 57]. However, the incidence among the rural population is higher than the urbane population. Characteristic of the urban life style is rarer consumption of freshwater fish and better adherence to good cooking practice [54].

5. Clinical manifestations, pathogenesis, and complications of human opisthorchiasis

Opisthorchiasis is a food-borne disease, with the pathogen transmission via eating the fish infected with the liver fluke metacercariae. The susceptibility to invasion is ubiquitous. The duodenal content induces larvae to excyst there wherefrom they migrate through the ampulla of Vater to the bile excretory ducts owing to a positive chemotaxis to bile. In 3–5 h, liver flukes (100%) are detectable in the liver, pancreas, and gall bladder (20–40%) [58, 59].

After 3–4 weeks, liver flukes turn into sexually mature maritae, producing eggs [58].

Clinical manifestations of opisthorchiasis are manifold and depend on individual specific features of the host organism as well as infection intensity and duration [34, 60, 61]. Humans are unable to develop immunity to this pathogen; correspondingly, repeated consumption of the fish carrying metacercariae merely increases invasion [62, 63]. The counts of maritae in an individual can vary from solitary parasites to several tens and even hundreds [63].

The incubation period of opisthorchiasis is on the average 2–3 weeks [58, 61]. The early (acute) and late (chronic) phases of this disease are distinguished [64]. The early phase lasts from several days to 4–8 weeks and longer [60], while the chronic phase may last for 10–20 and more years [64]. The disease may have unapparent or overt manifestations [58, 61, 65, 66].

Characteristic of the subclinical case of opisthorchiasis early phase is a subfebrile temperature and insignificant eosinophilia on the background of normal leukocyte counts [58]. A subclinical course is observed in the children who have received the antigen during their embryonic development or the antibodies with mother's milk [67–69]. This is the explanation why the manifestation of opisthorchiasis in the indigenous population of the north (Khanty and Mansi) is primary chronic with poor symptomatics and aggravation under adverse conditions, such as stress, infections, or surgery [58, 60, 61, 70, 71].

An overt course of opisthorchiasis is usually observable in the patients who moved to the opisthorchiasis focus from the regions not endemic for the disease [58]. The acute phase starts abruptly and continues for 1–3 months or rarer, for 6–9 months [58, 62, 63]. A systemic allergic response determines development of inflammation in the lungs, gastrointestinal tract, musculoskeletal system, skin, and cardiovascular system [64]. The patients experience fever (from subfebrile to febrile for 1–3 weeks), eosinophilia (20–40%; sometimes, to 90%), intoxication, dyspeptic disorders (nausea, vomiting, and epigastric burning), moderate arthralgia and myalgia, and exanthems of various types [58, 60, 61, 64]; hepatocholangitic syndrome (right subcostal pain, increased liver, elevated transaminase activities, and elevated alkaline phosphatase activity) [58, 64], bronchopulmonary syndrome (hyperemic pharynx, retropharyngeal granulation, rhinitis, asthmatic bronchitis, eosinophilic infiltration in the lungs, and exudative pleurisy), and cardiovascular changes (palpitation, cardiac pain, hypotonia, and diffuse dystrophic changes in the myocardium detectable by electrocardiography) are observable [72].

A severe form of the acute opisthorchiasis can be represented by typhoid, hepatocholangitic, and gastroenteritic clinical variants [73]. Severe toxic and allergic responses appear as toxic epidemic necrolysis (Lyell's syndrome), Stevens-Johnson syndrome, acute myocarditis, Quincke's edema, or hives [60].

In the absence of treatment, the acute phase transforms into a chronic one [63], which can continue for 20 years [61] and proceed either latently or with clinical manifestations [62]. A latent course is more frequent characteristic of the aboriginal population in the opisthorchiasis foci and in young people [60]. Patients have no complaints, and laboratory tests are normal. Opisthorchiasis is diagnosed in these cases only by chance during a periodic health examination or examination for other diseases [62]. In practice, this is the situation for 8% of several thousands of patients [63].

Characteristics of a latent opisthorchiasis are periods of remission and exacerbation [62]. In an endemic focus, opisthorchiasis initially follows a chronic course without any acute manifestations. Clinical symptoms may appear 10–20 years after infection. Patients frequently develop the symptoms of cholangitis and cholecystitis (80–87% of the cases) [74, 75], including right subcostal pain, heaviness in the stomach, nausea, fat intolerance, dryness and bitter taste in the mouth [58], abdominal distention, frequent liquid stool [63], vomiting, eructation, hepatomegaly, and jaundice during exacerbation [73]. Part of the opisthorchiasis patients develops pancreatitis with a wave-like course (frequent alternation of remission and exacerbation periods); 45–50% of the patients experience gastritis, duodenitis, and gastric and duodenal ulcers [73, 76]. In case of gastric involvement, patients frequently develop intestinal dyspepsia and dysbacteriosis, with the absence of bifidobacteria or their decrease and an increased content of facultative opportunistic pathogenic microflora, such as *Staphylococcus epidermidis* and *Staphylococcus aureus* [74]. Patients complain of undue fatigability, petulance, sleep loss, headache, hyperhidrosis (frequently local, for example, sweaty hands), excessive salivation, pronounced dermographism, tremor (eyelids, tongue, and/or fingers), vasomotor vascular response, and subfebrile temperature [76, 77].

The immunological response to antigens clinically manifests itself as an allergic syndrome, with skin itching, hives, recurrent Quincke's edema, arthralgia, alimentary allergy, moderate eosinophilia, and specific IgE in the blood [61]. A constant presence of the liver fluke antigen wears off the immune system and decreases its ability to suppress infection [69, 78, 79].

Chronic opisthorchiasis is a factor that is able to induce liver cancer development [63]. The early manifestations of liver cancer are an increase in the right subcostal pain and epigastria; their constant unceasing character, especially during nighttime; sensation of discomfort and heaviness; and pronounced dyspeptic disorders (anorexia, idiopathic weight loss, early satiety, abdominal distension, alternation of constipation and diarrhea, and so on). Weakness, general uneasiness, and sleep disorders rapidly worsen. The prescribed treatment of chronic opisthorchiasis fails to bring relief [80]. Hepatomegaly is characteristic of the liver cancer (the liver is dense, nodular, and painful); typical manifestations are hypochromic anemia, eosinophilia, accelerated ESR, and, in the case, of cancer, lymphopenia [80].

In pancreatic cancer, patients more frequently experience weakness, vomiting, and progressive weight loss. In part of patients, vomiting is caused by impaired gastric emptying because of the tumor compression or its invasion to the duodenum. Patients lose 5–32 kg over 2–3 months [80].

The main sign of pancreatic cancer is jaundice; it is persistent, increasing in its intensity, and accompanied by a high body temperature and chill. The fever and itching exhaust patients so that they lose sleep and experience growing adynamia and apathy. The liver may be increased; it has smooth surface and is less dense [80]. Characteristic of jaundice is a high concentration of bilirubin in the blood as well as increased alkaline phosphatase, aspartate aminotransferase, and alanine aminotransferase activities. Amylase activity is also increased in the liver and pancreatic cancers; thymol and sublimate tests are changed, which suggest an advanced cancer process [80].

Pathogenesis is determined by the combined impact of parasites on the host body (mechanical, toxic, and neuroreflectory) and host body responses (immunopathological) [60, 61, 64].

In the early phase, the immunopathological mechanisms with development of the immediate type allergic response are more pronounced [61, 64]. The liver fluke antigens enter the blood through mucosa and sensitize the organism (gastrointestinal tract, lungs, kidneys, liver, etc.) [60, 61]. The liver fluke metabolites induce toxic and allergic syndrome [58, 64], which are accompanied by edema, proliferation, desquamation of bile duct epithelium, and metaplasia of bile ducts with formation of goblet cells and small gland-like structures [58].

In the late phase, the liver fluke metabolites induce an immune inflammation in many organs and systems [81, 82]. The immunopathological effect appears as a secondary immunodeficiency with prevalence of a delayed type allergic response; characteristics of this response are vascular involvement and regeneration of cell elements in the connective tissue with development of extensive fibroplasia [73, 83].

Mechanical and toxic factors in the late stage become the most important [61, 64]. Young liver fluke individuals damage the bile duct walls by their spinules and the sexually mature individuals and by their oral and ventral suckers. Liver flukes consume the mucosal secretions and bile duct epithelium [45]. A mechanical stimulation of the walls of bile and pancreatic ducts interferes with the motor and secretory functions of the gastrointestinal tract [60].

Inflammatory and proliferative processes are induced and developed in the mucosal lesions, as well as peroxidation is activated and antioxidant defense is damaged [60, 84].

Clusters of liver flukes, their eggs, and crusts of desquamated epithelium in the ducts create a mechanical barrier for the outflow of bile and secretion, thereby enhancing the development of proliferative cholangitis and canaliculitis accompanied by different degrees of fibrosis in these organs [60].

Frequently, the pancreas responds to the presence of liver flukes and their metabolites by certain pathological changes. Both the exocrine and endocrine functions of the pancreas are damaged during pancreatitis [67, 85, 86].

Persistent hypertension develops in the duodenum, stomach, esophagus, and biliary system on the background of chronic duodenal stasis [61], creating the favorable conditions for secondary infections (*Escherichia coli*, staphylococci, yeast-like fungi, and others) [60].

The liver fluke invasion has a negative effect in the mother-placenta-fetus system [87], increasing the probability of gestoses and miscarriage [88].

The involvement of gastrointestinal tract affects digestion and absorption, leading to dysmetabolic sensitization. As a consequence, allergic skin lesions are developed, including urticarial rash in the early phase and chronic hives with exacerbation periods and remissions in the late phase [85, 86]. The urticarial rash rather frequently transforms into papular and vesicular rash. In some cases, hives can follow a hemorrhagic pattern owing to release of erythrocytes, which fall apart and form pigment spots [61, 79, 89].

The host immunopathological response is the cause underlying the dystrophy and necrosis of the epithelium of biliary tract and pancreatic ducts [79, 89, 90].

The sclerotic processes leading to the development of chronic hepatitis are prevalent in the late phase. Superinvasion and reinvasion lead to development of an active hepatitis as a result of an immune inflammation in the liver [61, 68, 91].

Complications of opisthorchiasis most frequently develop in the chronic stage. This disease belongs to the group of carcinogenic helminthiases [55, 59, 92, 93]. Liver tumors [55, 57, 94] as well as stomach, pancreas, and breast tumors most frequently develop on the background of liver fluke superinvasion [95, 96].

The carcinogenesis on the background of opisthorchiasis involves multifactorial mechanisms comprising inflammatory, mechanical, and secretory-excretory processes [84, 97].

In case of superinvasion, maritae provide a sustainable basis of the food substrate—permanent proliferation and differentiation of liver and pancreatic stem cells as well as the stem cells in the organs beyond their ecological niche [55].

An overt inflammation determines a constant response as the regenerative cell proliferation [55, 98].

Activated macrophages and polymorphonuclear leukocytes produce reactive oxygen species, proteolytic enzymes, proinflammatory cytokines, and growth factors. Reactive oxygen and nitrogen species and oxysterol production play the decisive role in the disturbance of the function of proto-oncogenes, the DNA regions the abnormalities in which induce cancer transformation of liver cells [45, 66]. As a result, adjacent cells are altered, and an active regeneration of injured tissues is triggered [97, 99].

Maritae interfere with the bile outflow in a purely mechanical manner. The stagnant bile in the ducts interacts with free radicals to form endogenous carcinogens, which has a mutagenic effect on the DNA of cholangiocytes [100, 101]. Eggs can penetrate to the periductal tissues via the ulcerations at the sites of liver fluke sucking and cause there a granulomatous inflammation [93]. The liver fluke excretory and secretory antigens (by themselves or via the interaction with free radicals) initiate cell proliferation during a liver fluke superinvasion [57] and display direct cytotoxic and mutagenic effects [96, 98, 102–104].

Hemozoin, a liver fluke pigment, is able to induce a carbonyl (extracellular) stress [105, 106]. A long-term injury of cholangiocytes and a mitogenic effect of growth factors are the cause underlying the complications, such as epithelial hyperplasia, periductal fibrosis, and strictures, and cysts of bile ducts followed by cholestasis, as well as lead to development of cholangiocarcinoma [80, 84, 105, 107, 108].

Morphologically, up to 80% of all tumors in opisthorchiasis cases are cholangiocarcinomas [109]. The risk of cholangiocarcinoma development correlates with the duration and intensity of liver fluke invasion [109–111]. The external factors enhancing cholangiocarcinoma development in opisthorchiasis cases are alcohol (demonstrated for *Opisthorchis viverrini*) and food nitrosamines (independent risk factor), especially in the endemic regions [98, 112, 113].

In 1970–2005, 1170 patients underwent surgery because of the complications of opisthorchiasis, which accounts for 24.6% of the total opisthorchiasis cases (4756). The patients with cholangiocholecystitis (70.3%), cholecystopancreatitis (18.4%), and hepatocholecystitis (11.3%) received a conservative treatment. A repeated invasion was observable in the overwhelming majority of patients; most of the opisthorchiasis cases (75%) were of the working age with the overall age range of 21–87 years [114].

Opisthorchiasis is complicated by liver abscesses, ascending cholangitis, hepatitis, and gastric and duodenal ulcers [115]. Frequently met surgical complications of opisthorchiasis are opisthorchiasis pancreatitis, observed in 16% cases [115]. A dangerous complication of opisthorchiasis cysts in the liver is abscesses and their rupture followed by bile peritonitis [114].

6. Prevention of opisthorchiasis

The prevention measures against opisthorchiasis comprise in the following:

- detection and treatment of opisthorchiasis cases in the disease focus;
- dehelminthization of domestic carnivores; and
- protection of water bodies from feces, proper keeping of the areas of settlements, use of sewage containers in river vessels, decontamination of sewage, and prohibition of using the content of outhouse latrines for fertilization of vegetable gardens [63].

The degree of human protection is determined by the level of their knowledge about the measures ensuring the invasion prevention and their sanitary culture [64].

The personal precautions mainly reduce to good cooking practices in fish processing, which ensures fish disinfection [63]. A special attention must be paid to teaching the population to properly process fish at home [64].

The disinfection is attained by thermal treatment, freezing, smoking, and salting [58].

The fishes with a weight of up to 1 kg must be frozen at a temperature of −28°C for 41 h or at −35°C for 10 h. In a household refrigerator, metacercariae retain viability for over 1 month [64].

Fish (in the case of a large individual, cut into pieces of no more than 2 cm) should be stewed for at least 20 min from the moment of boiling or fried as small flattened pieces (or minced) for 20 min in a large volume of oil. Fish pies must be kept in the oven (200°C) for at least 60 min [63].

Fish salting requires at least 2 weeks (2 kg salt per 10 kg fish; [64]). Before cold smoking, fish is disinfected by either salting or freezing [63].

Hot smoking requires a temperature of 70–80°C for 2–2.5 h [64].

The preservation meeting the Codex Alimentarius rules also guarantees safety from the liver fluke metacercariae [58].

It is always necessary to carefully wash your hands and kitchen utensils after processing raw fish [64].

It is strongly recommended to avoid consumption of raw fish, weakly or shortly salted fish, or raw minced fish as well as the frozen fish as stroganina (cut into thin slices), and other local variants of raw frozen fish as well as freshly caught fish in any home-made slightly salted, smoked, or dried variants prepared without observing the described technologies and by unknown persons [63].

Unfortunately, insufficient attention has been recently paid to education of population, which naturally resulted in an increase in the number of opisthorchiasis cases [116].

7. Natural, climatic, and social factors enhancing preservation of the opisthorchiasis focus

The activity of epizootic process in Western Siberia depends on the parameters of water regime in this territory. The vastness of the Western Siberian floodplains increases from south northward as well as the regular pattern, volume, and duration of spring floods; duration of summer-fall floods in the floodplains; and good water heating [57, 64]. The Western Siberian rivers are rather slow, with a long freeze-up period, preventing aeration, and winter deficiency in oxygen. Poor soil draining and excessive moistening enhance an abundance of water in the region and an increased number of floodplain water bodies, favorable for the development of Bithyniidae mollusk population [57].

In addition, large-scale hydrotechnical engineering activities (construction of channels, cascade artificial water reservoirs, dead dams without byways, and littering of water bodies with household and construction waste) create favorable conditions for mollusk development [57, 64].

Water and soil contamination with the liver fluke eggs significantly contribute to sustainable circulation of the opisthorchiasis agent in natural biocenoses; the liver fluke eggs have been detected in 1.13 ± 0.1% of the soil samples, 15.4 ± 0.9% of wastewater and silt samples, and 1.34 ± 0.2% of water from water bodies. The intensity of wastewater and sediment seeding with liver fluke eggs was maximal and varied from 2000 to 4000 eggs/m^3; this value for the soil specimens was significantly lower, 0–40 eggs/kg soil. Because of poor disinvasion efficiency, the wastewater discharged into water bodies remains uncontaminated, thereby maintaining the circulation of this pathogen in nature [57, 117].

A high level of population infection with opisthorchiasis is aggravated by social factors, namely, a decrease in population living standards and an increase in the share of fish and home-made fish products in the diet of the inhabitants of the cities and villages adjacent to rivers. Population buys fish in shops or unofficial markets or harvests it by themselves. In particular, 52% of opisthorchiasis cases bought the fish in unofficial markets; 34% of them were infected as a result of amateur fishing; and 14.0% received the fish shipped from a northern part of the region [57].

The main risk factors of opisthorchiasis are a high infection rate of the cyprinid fish species and the eating behavior pattern, i.e., prevalence in insufficiently disinfected fish in the common diet; in addition, the cyprinid fish is typically accessible to population, as is demonstrated by all-year-round fishing. In particular, over half (58.36 ± 2.81%) of the questioned subjects were amateur fishermen, and 41.44 ± 3.33% of them have their own fishing gear (nets, dragnets, etc.). This explains why the cohort of fishermen, water transportation workers, amateur fishermen, and their family members form the risk group with the maximum infection rate in the epicenter of the Ob-Irtysh opisthorchiasis focus. In the Khanty-Mansiysk Autonomous Okrug, the opisthorchiasis rate in the most important risk groups—buoy keepers and motor fishing fleet workers with their families—amounts to 75.6 ± 2.7 and 67.8 ± 3.8%, respectively [57]. In the southern part of the focus, the infection rate of the Tobolsk fish processing plant workers was 78 ± 0.3%; of the amateur fishermen in the Tobolsk raion, 36.6 ± 3.2%; and of the persons constantly involved in fishing in the Tyumen raion, 30.8 ± 3.8 and 50.0 ± 8.1% [57].

A high risk of opisthorchiasis is characteristic of the socially vulnerable cohorts, which eat the fish products conditionally approved as fit for human consumption, processed and prepared without taking into account the good cooking practice [57, 118–120]. In many households, weakly salted (in particular, large batches of ungutted fish salted in barrels), undercooked, freshly frozen, and freshly harvested cyprinid fish are the common all-year-round component of their diet. Infection can take place when testing minced fish "for salt" and accidental ingestion of liver fluke larvae from hands or kitchen utensils during fish processing. Children can be infected when cooking fish broth by themselves, making a kind of barbecue, or eating fresh fish [64, 85]. A high invasion rate of the indigenous northern population in Siberia is determined by the local tradition of eating stroganina, sliced frozen raw fish [64].

Population has little knowledge about the prevention measures. Only 27.93 ± 4.25% of the adult population is aware of the thermal processing practice, and 7.74 ± 1.31% knows the proper rules for fish salting and drying [57]. As has been shown, 89.0% of the opisthorchiasis cases either neglected the good fish cooking and salting practice or do not know them at all, and 1% of the infected subjects consume raw fish (stroganina) [57].

The effect of urbanization on the epidemic process is rather ambiguous [57]. One of the factors of an autogenic impact on the function of parasitic liver fluke system is the migration of population. Migration "supplies" the cohorts with a high risk of infection and poorly or completely unaware of how to prevent the invasion (who eat the improperly cooked fish) to the territories with a high risk of opisthorchiasis. An increase in population enhances the decrease in its morbidity owing to "dilution" of the aboriginal population by a large influx of uninfected newcomers, involved in shift work or expeditions [57].

Improvement of the sanitary knowledge owing to development of the medical network and sanitary education activities at the locations of newcomer cohorts decreases the risk for opisthorchiasis [57].

Low rates of dehelminthization result in an increase in the number of infection sources. Human pollution of the habitat increases the risk of infection of the population. In particular, 90% of the opisthorchiasis subjects listed for regular medical check-up in the Khanty-Mansiysk Autonomous Okrug ignored the prescribed treatment [31]. In the city of Langepas (Khanty-Mansiysk Autonomous Okrug), the incidence of opisthorchiasis increased 1.2-fold because of the problems with providing the necessary drugs, refuse of the treatment, and ignore the therapy without any particular reason [121].

8. Discussion

Opisthorchiasis is an anthropozoonous natural focal biohelminthosis caused by trematodes of *O. felineus*. Invasion has been recorded mainly in the Ob-Irtysh basin since 1891.

The main source of opisthorchiasis caused by *O. felineus* is a person infected with opisthorchiasis, all fish-eating mammals (dogs, cats, foxes, muskrats, etc.) can also be the final hosts. In addition to human distributing up to 56.6% of invasive material, cats (15.8%), dogs (3.6%), and pigs (up to 0.9%) are assumed to be another source of infection [26]. Intermediate and additional hosts of *O. felineus* inhabit water bodies, and foci of opisthorchiasis are concentrated near rivers.

The first intermediate host in the focus is freshwater mollusks, subclass Prosobranchiata, family Bithyniidae, genera *Codiella* and *Opisthorchophorus*. The mollusk invasion prevalence is very low, whereas the invasion intensity is very high. One mollusk lays up to 8000 cercariae [4–7].

The second intermediate host is fish of the family Cyprinidae. The prevalence of invasion of fish population ranges from 20 to 100%, while the invasion intensity varies from one to several hundred metacercariae (original data).

Russia has the highest incidence of this helminth. Natural foci of opisthorchiasis are located near the rivers Ob, Irtysh, Urals, Volga, Kama, Don, Dnieper, Severnaya Dvina, and Biryusa [32–42]. The world's largest focus of opisthorchiasis is located in the Ob-Irtysh basin.

The transmission mechanism of the infection fecal-oral route, and the transmission route is food. Infection occurs when a person eats raw or insufficiently thermally processed and freshly salted cyprinid fish, containing live larvae (metacercaria).

Natural susceptibility of people to opisthorchiasis is high. The population does not show durable immunity after curing. These helminths have adverse effects on human health, mainly affecting the hepatobiliary system and pancreas. Clinical manifestations of the acute phase of opisthorchiasis last from several days to 4–8 weeks or more, and the phase of chronic opisthorchiasis lasts 15–25 years or more. The duration of the incubation period (in the early phase of the disease) is 2–4 weeks (up to 6 weeks). Allergic reactions, mechanical, and neuroreflex effects of helminths play the main role in the pathogenesis of opisthorchiasis and cause biliary dyskinesia, temporary and complete cessation of bile flow, glandular proliferation in the epithelium of the biliary, and pancreatic ducts and other glandular organs. Pathological processes affect the liver (impaired secretion of enzymes and protein, reduced cholesterol synthesis, and antioxidant function of the liver), pancreas (impaired secretion of enzymes, including insulin), stomach and intestines (erosive gastritis and colitis), and skin (itching, cracks, and psoriasis). Severe complications of opisthorchiasis include biliary peritonitis, liver abscesses, liver cirrhosis, primary liver cancer (less commonly pancreas cancer), acute destructive pancreatitis, bronchial asthma, and diabetes mellitus. Due to the character of infection and a high degree of mutual adaptation of the host and the parasite, opisthorchiasis often proceeds latently (without clinical symptoms).

Among people of various professions, fishermen, river fleet personnel, agricultural workers, and forest industry workers are primarily infected. In endemic areas, opisthorchiasis can be recorded at the age of 1–3 years. The infection rate attains its highest level by 25 years and keeps stable up to 50–60 years. The prevalence among the local population can reach 100% (original data).

The most important prerequisites for an intensive epidemic process in these territories are natural and social factors:

- abundance of rivers and lakes rich in fish and mollusks (the highest infection rate among population is recorded in territories with numerous flood meadows and former riverbeds and places where the floodplain is more developed);

- hydrotechnical transformations;

- intensive contamination of rivers and floodplain lakes by helminths' eggs from permanent and temporary settlements, cities, etc. located on their banks;
- prevalence of insufficiently disinfected fish in the diet and cyprinid fish consumed by the population;
- specific ethnic or traditional behavior associated with food and nutrition that determines the nature of distribution and the infection rate among the population in endemic foci;
- poor knowledge of preventive measures; and
- infection is possible beyond these foci when exporting fish.

Simple personal preventive measures will contribute to prevention of opisthorchiasis.

9. Conclusions

The optimal natural and climatic conditions together with social and economic factors create the favorable conditions for preservation of the world largest Ob-Irtysh focus of the opisthorchiasis caused by the trematode *O. felineus*.

Acknowledgements

The work was supported by the Ministry of Education and Science of the Russian Federation (project no. 6.7525.2017/8.9), program for elevating the competitive ability of Tomsk State University, and Russian Science Foundation.

Author details

Anastasia V. Simakova[1,2*], Natalya V. Poltoratskaya[1,3], Irina B. Babkina[1], Tatyana N. Poltoratskaya[3], Alexander V. Shikhin[3] and Tatyana M. Pankina[3]

1 Department of Biology, Tomsk State University, Tomsk, Russia

2 Tomsk Oil and Gas Research and Design Institute, Tomsk, Russia

3 Federal State Institution of Health "Center for Hygiene and Epidemiology in the Tomsk region", Tomsk, Russia

*Address all correspondence to: anastasiasimakova@yahoo.com

References

[1] Report of United Nations. Department of Economic and Social Affairs Population Division; 2015. p. 149

[2] Beer SA. The Biology of Opisthorchiasis Agent. Moscow: KMK; 2005. p. 336 [in Russian]

[3] Zavoikin VD, Beer SA, Bocharova TA. Comparative opisthorchiasis situation in the largest Ob river tributaries. In: Human Opisthorchiasis: Proceedings of the Scientific Conference, Tomsk. 1979. pp. 60-62 [in Russian]

[4] Drozdov VN. Infection of Bithynia by liver fluke cercariae in the water bodies of the Irtysh River basin. In: Proceedings of the Scientific Conference on Medical Parasitology, Tyumen. 1964. pp. 76-78 [in Russian]

[5] Fedorov VG. The infection of Bithynia leachi mollusk by liver fluke cercariae in the water bodies of the Ob River upper reaches. In: The Problems in Natural Focality of Human Helminthiases, Tyumen. 1969. p. 71 [in Russian]

[6] Zavoikin VD, Zelya OP, Sokerina OA. Current state of the issue of opisthorchiasis in Western Siberia. In: Relevant Problems in Infectology and Parasitology: Proceedings of the First International Anniversary Conference, Tomsk. 2001. p. 99 [in Russian]

[7] Potseluev AN. The effect of hydrological regime and anthropogenic factors on the ecology of the first intermediate host of opisthorchiasis agent: A case study of the Ob-Irtysh Basin. [Candidate of Sciences (Med.) thesis]. Moscow; 1991. p. 21 [in Russian]

[8] Fattakhov RG. The distribution of opisthorchiid metacercariae in cyprinid fish in Western Siberia. In: Parasites and Diseases of Hydrobionts in the Ice Sea Province. Novosibirsk: Nauka; 1990. pp. 128-131 [in Russian]

[9] Krivenko VV, Filatov VG. Cyprinid fish are intermediate hosts of trematodes in the Tura–Pyshma interfluve. In: Parasites and Diseases of Hydrobionts in the Ice Sea Province. Novosibirsk: Nauka; 1990. pp. 131-135 [in Russian]

[10] Fattakhov RG. The distribution of *Opisthorchis felineus* (Riv., 1884) and *Metorchis bilis* (Braun., 1790) larvae in populations of the roach Rutilus rutilus (L.) and sunbleak Leucaspius delineates (Heck). In: The Tasks and Problems in Fish Management in Siberian Inner Water Bodies. Tomsk: Izd. Tomsk. Univ.; 1996. pp. 109-110 [in Russian]

[11] Fattakhov RG. Invasion of fish by opisthorchiasis agent in Russia and several adjacent countries. Meditsinskaya Parazitologiya i Parazitarnye Bolezni. 2002;**1**:62

[12] Gafina TE. On the current state of the helminth fauna of the main commercial; fish species in the Ob Reservoir tail pond. In: The Tasks and Problems in Fish Management in Siberian Inner Water Bodies, Tomsk. 1996. pp. 105-106 [in Russian]

[13] Fedorov VG, Belov GF, Naumov VA. The problem of human trematodiases in Western Siberia. In: Topical Problems in Infectology and Parasitology, Proc. of the First International Conference devoted to 110th Anniversary of Prof. K.N. Vinogradov's Discovery of Liver Fluke in Humans, Tomsk. 2001. p. 34 [in Russian]

[14] Sous' SM. Analysis of the specific morphoecological features of opisthorchiasis and metorchiasis in the Novosibirsk oblast. Sibirskiy Ekologicheskiy Zhurnal. 2006;**4**:399-407

[15] Sous' SM, Bocharova TA. The dynamics of cyprinid infection by liver

fluke metacercariae in water bodies of the Tomsk and Novosibirsk oblasts. In: Current Problems in Hydrobiology of Siberia. Tomsk: Izd. Tomsk. Univ.; 2001. pp. 149-150 [in Russian]

[16] Sous' SM, Rostovtsev AA. Opisthorchiasis, metorchiasis, and fish tapeworm disease. Prevention. In: Parasites of Fish in the Novosibirsk Oblast. Tyumen: Gosrybtsentr; 2006 [in Russian]

[17] Karpenko SV, Chechulin AI, Yurlova NI, et al. Characteristics of Opisthorchosis Nidus in the South of Western Siberia. Sibirskiy Ekologicheskiy Zhurnal. 2008;**5**:675-680

[18] Bocharova TA. The role of some cyprinid species in the opisthorchiasis epidemiology in the Tomsk oblast. In: Topical Problems in Infectology and Parasitology, Proc. of the First International Conference devoted to 110th Anniversary of Prof. K.N. Vinogradov's Discovery of Liver Fluke in Humans, Tomsk. 2001. p. 141 [in Russian]

[19] Bocharova TA. The muscle parasitic fauna of the cyprinid fish in the lower Tom River basin. In: Parasitological studies in Siberia and the Far East. Proc of Interregional Conference. Novosibirsk. 2002. pp. 29-32 [in Russian]

[20] Bocharova TA. An epidemiological state of the opisthorchiasis foci in the Tomsk oblast. In: Topical Problems in Medical Biology, Tomsk. 2002. pp. 67-69 [in Russian]

[21] Bocharova TA. The dynamics of muscle infection in some cyprinid species in the lower Tom River basin. Vestnik Tomskogo Gosudarstvennogo Universiteta. 2003;**8**:22-24

[22] Bocharova TA. The role of small water flows in the opisthorchiasis focus of the lower Tom River basin. In: Topical Problems in Biology, Medicine, and Ecology, Tomsk. 2004. pp. 404-405 [in Russian]

[23] Bocharova TA. The effect of microwave beams on the survivability of trematode larvae in the muscles of the common dace in the Tom River lower reaches. In: Parasitological Studies in Siberia and the Far East. Proc. of the 11th Interregional Conference, Novosibirsk. 2005. pp. 29-31 [in Russian]

[24] Bocharova TA. Opisthorchiasis Agent and Other Muscle Parasites of the Cyprinid Fish in the Lover Tom River Basin. Tomsk: Izd. Tomsk. Univ.; 2007. 66 p [in Russian]

[25] Simakova AV, Babkina IB, Babkin AM, Interesova EA. Infestation of alien cyprinid fishes with trematode Opisthorhis felineus Rivolta, 1884 in the middle Ob River basin. Russian Journal of Biological Invasions. 2019;**10**(2):178-180. DOI: 10.1134/s2075111719020115

[26] Krivenko VV. Biological Properties of liver fluke eggs and the role of some definitive host species as sources of invasion material during opisthorchiasis in Western Siberia. [Candidate of Science (Biol.) thesis]. Moscow; 1984 [in Russian]

[27] Shibitov SK. Opisthorchiasis of carnivorous animals in Western Siberia: Prevalence, pathogenesis, diagnostics, and control measures. [Candidate of Sciences (Vet.) thesis]. Moscow; 2013 [in Russian]

[28] Zubareva IM. Main helminthiases of domestic carnivorous animals in large cities (a case study of Novosibirsk). [Candidate of Sciences (Vet.) thesis]. Novosibirsk; 2004 [in Russian]

[29] Fedorov KP, Pashkevich VY, Konyukhov EN. Helmithofauna of the muskrat in Western Siberia. Problems in Ecology. 1976;**4**:113-120

[30] Resolution no. 179 of the Federal Service for Supervision of Consumer Rights Protection and Human Well-being of December 12, 2016 "On Prevention of Distribution of the Parasitic Diseases Transmitted via Fish and Fish Products in the Russian Federation" [in Russian]

[31] Letter no. 1/12315-2018-27 of the Federal Service for Supervision of Consumer Rights Protection and Human Well-being of September 24, 2018 "On implementation of the Resolution of the Chief State Sanitary Inspector of the Russian Federation of December 12, 2016 "On Prevention of Distribution of the Parasitic Diseases Transmitted via Fish and Fish Products in the Russian Federation"" [in Russian]

[32] Beer SA. Parasitological monitoring in Russia (basics of the concept). Medical Parasitology and Parasitic Diseases. 1997;**1**:3-8

[33] Mordvinov VA, Yurlova NI, Ogorodova LM, Katokhin AV. *Opisthorchis felineus* and *Metorchis bilis* are the main agents of liver fluke infection of humans in Russia. Parasitology International. 2012;**61**: 25-31. DOI: 10.1016/j.parint.2011.07.021

[34] Fedorova OS, Kovshirina YV, Kovshirina AE, Fedotova MM, Deev IA, Petrovskii FI, et al. Analysis of the prevalence of *Opisthorchis felineus* invasion and malignant neoplasms of the hepatobiliary system in the Russian Federation. Bulletin of Siberian Medicine. 2016;**15**(5):147-158

[35] State Report "On the Sanitary and Epidemiological Well-being of the Population of the Yamalo-Nenets Autonomous Okrug in 2014-2018" [Internet]. [in Russian]. Available from: http://89.rospotrebnadzor.ru [Accessed: 25 September 2019]

[36] State Report "On the Sanitary and Epidemiological Well-being of the Population of the Khanty-Mansiisk Autonomous Okrug–Yugra in 2014-2018" [Internet] [in Russian]. Available from: http://86.rospotrebnadzor.ru [Accessed: 30 September 2019]

[37] State Report "On the Sanitary and Epidemiological Well-being of the Population of the Tyumen Oblast in 2014-2018" [Internet]. [in Russian]. Available from: http://72.rospotrebnadzor.ru [Accessed: 30 September 2019]

[38] State Report "On the Sanitary and Epidemiological Well-being of the Population of the Tomsk Oblast in 2014-2018" [Internet]. [in Russian]. Available from: http://70.rospotrebnadzor.ru [Accessed: 30 September 2019]

[39] State Report "On the Sanitary and Epidemiological Well-being of the Population of the Novosibirsk Oblast in 2014-2018" [Internet] [in Russian]. Available from: http://54.rospotrebnadzor.ru

[40] State Report "On the Sanitary and Epidemiological Well-being of the Population of the Kemerovo Oblast in 2014-2018" [in Russian]. Available from: 42.rospotrebnadzor.ru [Accessed: 30 September 2019]

[41] State Report "On the Sanitary and Epidemiological Well-being of the Population of the Altai Krai in 2014-2018" [Internet] [in Russian]. Available from: http://55.rospotrebnadzor.ru [Accessed: 30 September 2019]

[42] State Report "On the Sanitary and Epidemiological Well-being of the Population of the Tomsk Oblast in 2014-2018" [Internet] [in Russian]. Available from: http://22.rospotrebnadzor.ru [Accessed: 30 September 2019]

[43] Beer SA. Stages in the evolution of distribution ranges of some opisthorchiids and opisthorchiasis

paleo foci. In: Relevant Problems in Opisthorchiasis. Tomsk: Izd. Tomsk. Univ.; 1986. pp. 12-15 [in Russian]

[44] Bronshtein AM. Communication 3. Incidence of opisthorchiasis and diphyllobothriasis among the population of the village of Vanzetur, Khanty-Mansiisk Autonomous Okrug. Medical Parasitology. 1986;**5**:10-14

[45] Il'inskikh EN. Relevant topics in the study of opisthorchiasis in Siberia. Bulletin of Siberian Medicine. 2002;**1**:63-70

[46] Osipova LP, Ofitserov VI, Tkachenko TN, Zhadanov SI, Rugin VP. Enzyme immunoassay of liver fluke invasions among the population of the Shuryshkarskii raion of Yamalo-Nenets Autonomous Okrug. Medical Parasitology and Parasitic Diseases. 2004;**1**:14-17

[47] On the Sanitary and Epidemiological Well-being of Population of the Russian Federation in 2014: State Report. Moscow: Federal Service for Surveillance on Consumer Rights Protection and Human Wellbeing (Rospotrebnadzor); 2015 [in Russian]

[48] On the Sanitary and Epidemiological Well-being of Population of the Russian Federation in 2015: State Report. Moscow: Federal Service for Surveillance on Consumer Rights Protection and Human Wellbeing (Rospotrebnadzor); 2016 [in Russian]

[49] On the Sanitary and Epidemiological Well-being of Population of the Russian Federation in 2016: State Report. Moscow: Federal Service for Surveillance on Consumer Rights Protection and Human Wellbeing (Rospotrebnadzor); 2017 [in Russian]

[50] On the Sanitary and Epidemiological Well-being of Population of the Russian Federation in 2017: State Report. Moscow: Federal Service for Surveillance on Consumer Rights Protection and Human Wellbeing (Rospotrebnadzor); 2018 [in Russian]

[51] On the Sanitary and Epidemiological Well-being of Population of the Russian Federation in 2018: State Report. Moscow: Federal Service for Surveillance on Consumer Rights Protection and Human Wellbeing (Rospotrebnadzor); 2019 [in Russian]

[52] Khodzhayan AB, Kozlova SS, Golubeva MV. Medical Parasitology and Parasitic Diseases: Textbook. GEOTAR-Media: Moscow; 2014. p. 448 [in Russian]

[53] Abdelgantsev RF. Specific epidemiological features of opisthorchiasis in the city of Urai. In: Proceedings of the Regional Workshop on the Relevant Problems in Epidemiological Surveillance of Parasitic Diseases in Siberian and Ural Federal Regions, Surgut. 2018. pp. 67-69 [in Russian]

[54] Fedotova MM. The role of *Opisthorchis felineus* invasion in the development of food sensitization in children. [Candidate of Sciences (Med.) thesis]. Tomsk; 2014 [in Russian]

[55] Bychkov VG, Molokova OA, Kalenova LF, Kulikova SV, Kurchatova AN, Bazhin AS, et al. The results of antihelminthic effect of cynaropicrin on opisthorchiasis (preclinical studies). Health and Education Millennium. 2016;**18**(1):260-266 [in Russian]

[56] Uskov PA, Nikitin AA, Letyushev AN. Opisthorchiasis in the Omsk oblast: Epidemiological aspects. Relevant problems in epidemiology and microbiology. National Priorities of Russia. 2013;**9**(2):136-138 [in Russian]

[57] Belyaeva MI. Specific ecological and biological features in formation of

opisthorchiasis endemic foci in Western Siberia. [Doctor of Sciences (Biol.) thesis]. Moscow; 2017 [in Russian]

[58] Bronshtein AM, Tokmalaev AK. Human Parasitic Diseases: Protozoiases and Helminthiases. Textbook. Izd. RUDN: Moscow; 2002 [in Russian]

[59] Grigor'eva IN. Opisthorchiasis: Traditions and innovations. Experimental and Clinical Gastroenterology. 2012;**4**:54-59

[60] Kuznetsova VG, Krasnova EI, Paturina NG. Opisthorchiasis in clinical practice of an infectious disease physician. In: Attending Physician. Moscow: Otkrytye sistemy; 2013. p. 74 [in Russian]

[61] Filimonova LA, Borisenko NA. Opisthorchiasis: Clinical manifestations. Siberian Medical Review. 2006;**2**(39):812 [in Russian]

[62] Diunov AG, Zharikov GP, Tikhomirova SV. Medical Parasitology for the First Year Students. Yaroslavl: Avers Plus; 2011 [in Russian]

[63] Mamonov YP, Mamonova EY, Kalinina MY. Opisthorchiasis Is a Natural Danger in the Khanty-Mansiisk Autonomous Okrug–Yugra. Nizhnevartovsk: NGGU; 2008 [in Russian]

[64] Moiseenko AV. Opisthorchiasis (Textbook for Students). Izd. TGMA: Tyumen; 1999 [in Russian]

[65] Sergiev VP. Human Parasitic Diseases (Protozoiases and Helminthiases): Manual for Physicians. Foliant: St. Petersburg; 2006 [in Russian]

[66] Bogdanov AO, Prokudina DV, Baikov AN, Saltykova IV. Molecular mechanisms that mediate cholangiocarcinoma development during chronic liver fluke invasion. Siberian Oncological Journal. 2015;**6**:83-90

[67] Pal'tsev AI. The pathology of digestive organs in chronic opisthorchiasis: Pathomorphosis, diagnostics, therapy, and prevention. [Doctor of Sciences (Med.) thesis]. Novosibirsk; 1995 [in Russian]

[68] Trukhmanov AS. Gastroesophageal reflux disease: Clinic, diagnosis, treatment. Diseases of Digestive Organs. Russian Medical Journal. 2001;**3**(1):19-25

[69] Khardinova SA, Beloborodova EI, Pesterev PI. Morphofunctional changes in the gastrointestinal tract in combined therapy of psoriasis and chronic opisthorchiasis. Medical Parasitology and Parasitic Diseases. 2005;**4**:48-51

[70] Parfenov SB, Ozeretskovskaya NN, Shuikina EE. Comparative characterization of clinical and immunological parameters in different cohorts of opisthorchiasis patients in its focus. Communication 2. Indigenous population. Medical Parasitology and Parasitic Diseases. 1989;**2**:42-45

[71] Parfenov SB, Ozeretskovskaya NN, Shuikina EE. Comparative characterization of clinical and immunological parameters in different cohorts of opisthorchiasis patients in its hyperendemic focus. Communication 4. Transplacental transmission of *Opisthorchis felineus* antigens. Medical Parasitology and Parasitic Diseases. 1991;**3**:42-44

[72] Nikolaeva NI, Nikolaeva VP, Gigileva AV. Opisthorchiasis: Etiology, clinics, diagnostics, and therapy. Russian Journal of Parasitology. 2005;**5**:23-26

[73] Kalyuzhina MI. The state of digestive organs in the patients during residual period of chronic opisthorchiasis. [Doctor of Sciences (Med.) thesis]. Tomsk; 2000 [in Russian]

[74] Kuznetsova VG. Pathogenetic mechanisms and the specific clinical

features of the opisthorchiasis consequences. [Doctor of Sciences (Med.) thesis]. Novosibirsk; 2000 [in Russian]

[75] Pal'tsev AI. Chronic opisthorchiasis from the standpoint of a systemic approach: Clinics, diagnostics, Pathomorphosis, and therapy. Russian Journal of Medicine. 2005;**2**:96-101 [in Russian]

[76] Svyatenko IA, Beloborodova EI. Specific features of the clinical and endoscopic pattern in gastroesophageal reflux disease during chronic opisthorchiasis. Siberian Medical Journal. 2010;**1**:41-44

[77] Yablokov DD. Human Opisthorchiasis. Tomsk: Izd. Tomsk. Univ.; 1979 [in Russian]

[78] Leutskaya ZK. Some Aspects of Immunity in Helminthiases. Moscow: Nauka; 1990 [in Russian]

[79] Kulaga VV, Romanenko IM. Allergic Skin Diseases. Zdorov'e: Kiev; 1997 [in Russian]

[80] Brazhnikova NA, Tolkaeva MV. Cancer of liver, biliary tract, and pancreas in chronic opisthorchiasis. Bulletin of Siberian Medicine. 2002;**2**:71-77

[81] Migdalovich MG. The clinical significance of immunoregulatory function of the blood neutrophils in opisthorchiasis patients before and in dynamics after biltricide therapy. [Candidate of Sciences (Med.) thesis]. Chelyabinsk; 1995 [in Russian]

[82] Sutarung S, Haswell-Elkins MR, et al. Relationships between the synthesis of N-nitrosodimethylamine and immune responses to chronic infection with carcinogenic parasite, *Opisthorchis viverrini*, in men. Carcinogenesis. 1998;**19**(3):485-491

[83] Zubov NA. To pathomorphosis in opisthorchiasis. Medical Parasitology and Parasitic Diseases. 1996;**2**:23-26

[84] Baikova OA, Nikolaeva NN, Grishchenko EG, Nikolaeva LV. The cholangiocarcinoma associated with chronic opisthorchiasis and clonorchiasis. Health and Education Millennium. 2018;**20**(4):27-32 [in Russian]

[85] Lepekhin AV, Mefodiev VV, Filatov VG, Buzhak NS. Epidemiology, Clinics, and Prevention of Opisthorchiasis. Tomsk: Izd. Tomsk. Univ.; 1992 [in Russian]

[86] Suvorov AI, Krylov GG, Bychkov VG. Duodenogastroesophageal reflux disease as a complication of opisthorchiasis superinvasion. Medical Parasitology and Parasitic Diseases. 2004;**4**:17-19

[87] Bekarova AM, Binbasova TA, Buslaeva GN. Pediatrics. Selected Lections. GEOTAR-Media: Moscow; 2009 [in Russian]

[88] Solov'eva AV. Chronic Opisthorchiasis and Pregnancy: Manual for Physicians. GEOTAR-Media: Moscow; 2007 [in Russian]

[89] Pytskii VI, Andrianova NV, Artomasova AV. Allergic Diseases. Meditsinskaya nauka i obrazovanie: Moscow; 1991 [in Russian]

[90] Parfenov SB. Specific features in the course of opisthorchiasis and immune status of the patients of different population cohorts as the basis for development of differential approach to its therapy. [Candidate of Sciences (Med.) thesis]. Moscow; 1990 [in Russian]

[91] Glumov VY. Morphology, morphogenesis, and pathogenesis of chronic hepatitis and liver cirrhosis during opisthorchiasis. [Doctor of Sciences (Med.) thesis]. Moscow; 1981 [in Russian]

[92] Watanapa P, Watanapa WB. Liver fluke-associated cholangiocarcinoma.

British Journal of Surgery. 2002;**89**(8):962-970

[93] Kaewpitoon N, Kaewpitoon SJ, Pengsaa P, Sripa B. *Opisthorchis viverrini*: The carcinogenic human liver fluke. World Journal of Gastroenterology. 2008;**14**(5):666-674

[94] Khadieva ED, Lukmanov IR, Sabirov AK, Bychkov VG. Gastrointestinal stromal tumors (GISTs). Medical Science and Education in the Ural. 2010;**3**:165-167 [in Russian]

[95] Sabirov AK. Histological, immunohistological, and molecular genetic markers in breast cancer on the background of liver fluke invasion. Medical Science and Education in the Ural. 2010;**1**:82-83 [in Russian]

[96] Zuevskii VP, Bychkov VG, Tselishcheva PV, Khadieva ED. Opisthorchiasis as a promoter of gastro-carcinogenesis. Medical Parasitology and Parasitic Diseases. 2015;**4**:7-10

[97] Sripa B, Brindley PJ, Mulvenna J, Laha T, Smout MJ, Mairiang E, et al. The tumorigenic liver fluke *Opisthorchis viverrini* - multiple pathways to cancer. Trends Parasitol. 2012;**28**(10):395-407. DOI: 10.1016/j.pt.2012.07.006

[98] Smout JM, Sripa B, Laha T, et al. Infection with the carcinogenic human liver fluke, *Opisthorchis viverrini*. Molecular bioSystems. 2011;**7**(5):1367-1375

[99] Pal S, Bhattacharjee A, Ali A, Mandal NC, Mandal SC, Pal M. Chronic inflammation and cancer: potential chemoprevention through nuclear factor kappa B and p53 mutual antagonism. Journal of Inflammation (Lond). 2014;**11**:1-28. DOI: 10.1186/1476-9255-11-23 [eCollection 2014]

[100] Wonkchalee O, Boonmars T, Kaewkes S, Chamgramol Y, Pairojkul C, Wu Z, et al. *Opisthorchis viverrini* infection causes liver and biliary cirrhosis in gerbils. Parasitology Research. 2011;**109**(3):545-551. DOI: 10.1007/s00436-011-2282-y

[101] Jusakul A, Loilome W, Namwat N, Haigh WG, Kuver R, Dechakhamphu S, et al. Liver fluke-induced hepatic oxysterols stimulate DNA damage and apoptosis in cultured human cholangiocytes. Mutation Research. 2012;**731**(1-2):48-57. DOI: 10.1016/j.mrfmmm.2011.10.009

[102] Tielens AG, van den Heuvel JM, van den Bergh SG. The energy metabolism of *Fasciola hepatica* during its development in the final host. Molecular and Biochemical Parasitology. 1984;**13**(3):301-307

[103] Ninlawan K, O'Hara SP, Splinter PL, Yongvanit P, Kaewkes S, Surapaitoon A, et al. *Opisthorchis viverrini* excretory/secretory products induce toll-like receptor 4 upregulation and production of interleukin 6 and 8 in cholangiocyte. Parasitology International. 2010;**59**(4):616-621. DOI: 10.1016/j.parint.2010.09.008

[104] Daya M, Loilome W, Techasen A, et al. Progranulin modulates cholangiocarcinoma cell proliferation, apoptosis, and motility via the PI3K/pAkt pathway. Onco Targets and Therapy. 2018;**11**:395-408

[105] Maksimova GA, Zhukova NA, Kashina EV, Lvova MN, Katokhin AV, Tolstikova TG, et al. Role of *Opisthorchis felineus* on induction of bile duct cancer. Parazitologiia. 2015;**49**(1):3-11

[106] Saltykova IV, Ogorodova LM, Ivanov VV, et al. Carbonyl stress phenomena during chronic infection with *Opisthorchis felineus*. Parasitology International. 2017;**66**(4):453-457

[107] Sripa B, Kaewkes S, Sithithaworn P, Mairiang E, Laha T,

Smout M, et al. Liver fluke induces cholangiocarcinoma. PLoS Medicine. 2007;**4**(7):1148-1155. DOI: 10.1371/journal.pmed.0040201

[108] Onishchenko SV, Darvin VV, Lysak MM. Acute cholangitis in the patients residing in an endemic opisthorchiasis focus. Annals of Surgical Hepatology. 2009;**2**:38-43

[109] Glumov VY, Kotrikov VV, Tret'yakova NA. Pathogenesis and morphology of the primary liver cancer developing of the background of opisthorchiasis. Problems in Oncology. 1974;**9**:46-49

[110] Sriamporn S. Epidemiologic study of liver cancer using a population-based cancer registry as a guide in Khon Kaen, Thailand. Health Reports. 1993;**5**(1):51-58

[111] Bouvard V, Baan R, Straif K, et al. A review of human carcinogens—Part B: Biological agents. Lancet Oncology. 2009;**10**(4):321-322

[112] Sriraj P, Aukkanimart R, Boonmars T, et al. Does a combination of opisthorchiasis and ethyl alcohol consumption enhance early cholangiofibrosis, the risk of cholangiocarcinoma? Parasitology Research. 2013;**112**(8):2971-2981

[113] Buisson Y. Control of *Opisthorchis viverrini* infection for cholangiocarcinoma prevention. Bulletin de la Société de pathologie exotique. 2017;**110**(1):61-67. DOI: 10.1007/s13149-017-0544-8

[114] Merzlikin NV, Brazhnikova NA, Al'perovich BI, Tskhaiyu VB. Surgical Diseases. GEOTAR-Media: Moscow; 2015 [in Russian]

[115] Aftaeva LN, Mel'nikov VL, Nikol'skaya MV. Opisthorchiasis in the perspective of severe complications. Proceedings of higher education institutions. Volga region. Medical Science. 2018;**4**(48):27-32 [in Russian]

[116] Arinzhanov AE, Lyadova AY. Opisthorchiasis: Epidemiology, prevention, treatment. Territory of Science. 2016;**6**:7-13 [in Russian]

[117] NachevaLV,BibikOI,StarchenkovaTE, Dodonov MV. Helminthiases among Kuzbass population. Medicine in Kuzbass. 2007;**1**:22-29 [in Russian]

[118] Onishchenko GG. Incidence of parasitic diseases in the Russian Federation and the main directions in the activities on its stabilization. Medical Parasitology. 2002;**4**:3-10

[119] Onishchenko GG. On the measures for strengthening prevention of parasitic diseases in the Russian Federation. Medical Parasitology and Parasitic Diseases. 2003;**3**:35

[120] Guzeeva TM. The state of incidence of parasitic diseases in the Russian Federation and the goals for reorganization of the service. Medical Parasitology and Parasitic Diseases. 2008;**1**:3-11

[121] Tsareva TP, Grebneva VN. Epidemiological surveillance of acute and chronic opisthorchiasis in the City of Langepas. Analysis of the causes of infection and the conditions and factors of infection in the periods of increased incidence. In: Relevant Issues of Epidemiological Surveillance of Parasitic Diseases in the Siberian and Ural Federal Regions. Proceedings of Regional Conference, Surgut. 2018. pp. 69-72 [in Russian]